Dedicated to my wife, Teresa, and to all those who strive to be caring, compassionate physicians.

Carlos Ayala, MD

I dedicate this book to my parents, Dr. Richard and Carole, to my brother, Jason, and to my mentors, Drs. Edwards, Filler, Schiller, and Wirshing.

Brad Spellberg, MD

Preface

The transition from the basic science to the clinical years of medical school is perhaps the most dramatic step students take toward becoming a physician. The USMLE Step 1 is the first barrier one must overcome during this transition, and this is quickly followed by the nerve-racking switch from the classroom to the wards. This book is intended to smooth the transition from 2nd to 3rd year by helping you prepare for USMLE Step 1 and by easing your assimilation into the culture of clinical medicine that is prevalent on the wards.

We wrote this book as medical students, during our own preparation for the USMLE Step 1 examination, and subsequently as we rotated through our 3rd year clerkships. We compiled information from numerous sources to develop an organ-based clinical pathophysiological approach to patient treatment. Our intent was to provide a necessary and concise review of the major pathological conditions most commonly tested on the boards and commonly "pimped" on the wards. **This versatile book will prove useful not just for USMLE Step 1, but also for your rotations as you begin the 3rd year and look forward to USMLE Step 2**. *Pathophysiology for the Boards and Wards* is not an all-encompassing textbook of pathophysiology, but instead will provide you with the main concepts and pathognomonic findings of testable and "pimpable" diseases. In addition, we provided a list of highly detailed pearls of wisdom that will separate you from the competition during your clerkships.

We welcome any feedback you may have about *Pathophysiology for the Boards and Wards.* Please feel free to contact the authors with your comments or suggestions.

Boards and Wards
c/o Lippincott Williams & Wilkins
351 W. Camden Street
Baltimore, MD 21201

We are confident that you will find this book useful in your preparation for the boards and wards. Good luck to all of you!!!

Acknowledgments

The authors extend their most sincere gratitude to Gary Schiller, MD, Associate Professor of Medicine at UCLA, and Richard Spellberg, MD, Clinical Professor of Medicine at UCLA, for their critical review of the original manuscript.

Contributors

Jennifer W. Jung
Class of 2003
Thomas Jefferson University: Jefferson Medical College
Philadelphia, Pennsylvania

John Nguyen
Class of 2002
University of Texas Medical Branch
Galveston, Texas

Victor R. Rodriquez
Class of 2003
Tufts University School of Medicine
New England Medical Center
Boston, Massachusetts

Contents

Tables

Algorithms

Abbreviations

↑ (↑↑)	Increases/High (Markedly Increases/Very High)
↓ (↓↓)	Decreases/Low (Markedly Decreases/Very Low)
→	Causes/Leads to/Analysis shows
1°/2°	primary/secondary
Ag/Ab	Antigen/Antibody
BP	Blood Pressure
Bx	Biopsy
CA	Carcinoma
CN	Cranial Nerve
CNS	Central Nervous System
CXR	Chest X-Ray
DDx	Differential Diagnosis
Dx	Diagnosis
dz	Disease
HTN	Hypertension
Hx/FHx	History/Family History
ICP	Intracranial Pressure
infxn	Infection
Nml	Normal
PE	Physical Exam or Pulmonary Embolus
PMN	Polymorphonuclear Leukocyte (neutrophil)
pt(s)	Patient(s)
Px	Prognosis
Rx	Prescription/Indicated Drug
Si/Sx/aSx	Sign/Symptom/asymptomatic
Tx	Treatment/Therapy
Utz	Ultrasound

1. NEUROLOGY

I. Cellular Neurobiology

A. Cell types and responses to injury
   1. Neurons undergo a variety of responses to cellular injury
      a. Manifestations of axonal damage
         (1) Distal wallerian degeneration of axon & myelin
         (2) Proximal central chromatolysis → cell body swelling, nucleus & Nissl body (rough endoplasmic reticulum) pushed to periphery
         (3) Prolonged axon injury → retrograde cell body decay
      b. If synaptic input is lost, get transsynaptic degeneration
      c. Cell bodies injured directly by anoxia, glutamate excitotoxicity, apoptosis, metabolic storage diseases (Tay-Sachs, etc.)
   2. Astrocytes regulate fluid/ion balance in brain parenchyma
      a. Foot processes help comprise blood-brain barrier (BBB)
      b. Respond to injury like fibroblasts: proliferate & hypertrophy = gliosis
      c. **Gliosis is an acute response**, depicted by staining with glial fibrillary acidic protein (GFAP)
      d. Reactive astrocyte is also called a "gemistocyte," looks glassy, hypertrophic, with pink cytoplasm
   3. **Microglia respond subacutely to injury**
      a. They are derived from reticuloendothelial scavenger cells
      b. They become gitter cells (foamy macrophages), glial fibrillary acidic protein
      c. BOTH gitter cells & reactive astrocytes persist for months to years following injury
   4. Oligodendrocytes myelinate central nervous system (CNS) neuronal axons
      a. One oligodendrocyte myelinates multiple axons
      b. Oligodendrocyte damage causes primary (1°) demyelinating diseases, axon remains undamaged
      c. 1° demyelination may be autoimmune or viral induced
      d. Secondary (2°) demyelination occurs following damage to the axon

II. Infarct & Hemorrhage

A. Introduction

1. Stroke ≡ a sudden, nonconvulsive focal neurologic deficit (see Table 1.1)
2. Infarcts are more common than hemorrhages
3. Liquefactive necrosis 2° to infarct → gliosis, shrinkage of affected tissue, cyst formation, and compensatory dilation of lateral ventricles

B. Transient ischemic attack

1. Transient ischemic attack (TIA) ≡ neurologic event that lasts less than 24 hours (usually less than 1 hour), resolves completely
2. Is recurrent, can herald stroke
3. Due to emboli from carotid or vertebral arteries, rarely cardiac emboli
4. **Classic carotid emboli symptom (Sx) = ipsilateral blindness (amaurosis fugax)** with contralateral hemiparesis & paresthesias
   a. Amaurosis fugax is a classic visual sign of TIA
   b. Described as if a shade was pulled down over the eye, blinding it
   c. Resolves in a matter of minutes
5. **Classic vertebrobasilar emboli Sx = drop attacks, bilateral blindness & confusion, vertigo**

Table 1.1 Vascular Distribution of Strokes

Cerebral Artery		Lobe Symptom
Middle	Parietal	Contralateral hemiplegia
	Temporal	Homonymous hemianopsia
	Temporal	Dominant hemisphere → aphasia
	Temporal	Nondominant → sensory neglect and apraxia (inability to follow commands even if comprehended and patient is physically capable)
Anterior	Parietal	Contralateral hemiplegia
	Frontal	Urinary incontinence
	Frontal	Grasp reflex
Posterior	Occipital	Homonymous hemianopsia

6. Aphasia seen when dominant hemisphere damaged—left hemisphere dominant in 99% of right-handed people & in >50% of left-handed people
7. Differential diagnosis (Dx) = seizures, neoplasms, migraine, vertigo
8. Treatment (Tx) is multimodal
   a. Correct underlying disorder; e.g., hyperlipidemia, hypertension, diabetes, valve abnormality
   b. Administer aspirin or warfarin for thrombus prophylaxis
   c. If carotid is 70% occluded & patient has symptoms, perform surgical endarterectomy

C. Infarcts
1. Most common CNS vascular disease is atherosclerosis, usually occurs in carotid or vertebral arteries
2. Bland infarcts are due to thrombotic occlusion, which is more common than embolic
3. Hemorrhagic infarcts are due to embolization, frequently lodged at bifurcation of major arteries
   a. Middle cerebral artery (MCA) bifurcation is particularly common (see Figure 1.1)
   b. Hemorrhage due to infarct followed by reperfusion
   c. **Most common emboli come from carotid atheroma**
      (1) Others come from cardiac mural thrombi, septic heart valve vegetations, or fat emboli after long bone fracture
      (2) More rarely can be from infectious or marantic endocarditis (metastasizing cancer cells)
4. Watershed infarcts occur at border of areas supplied by different arteries (e.g., MCA–anterior cerebral artery (ACA)
   a. Usually occur following prolonged hypotension (e.g., surgery), when area is reperfused
   b. Due to reperfusion, they are often hemorrhagic & bilateral
5. Lacunar infarct = small infarct in deep gray matter, strongly associated with hypertension & atherosclerosis
6. Edema occurs 2–4 days after infarct, watch for this clinically (e.g., ↓ consciousness, projectile vomiting, pupillary changes)
7. Precise clinical presentation depends on affected vessel
8. Posturing
   a. Decorticate (cortical lesion) causes flexion of arms
   b. Decerebrate (midbrain/corticospinal tract lesion) causes extension

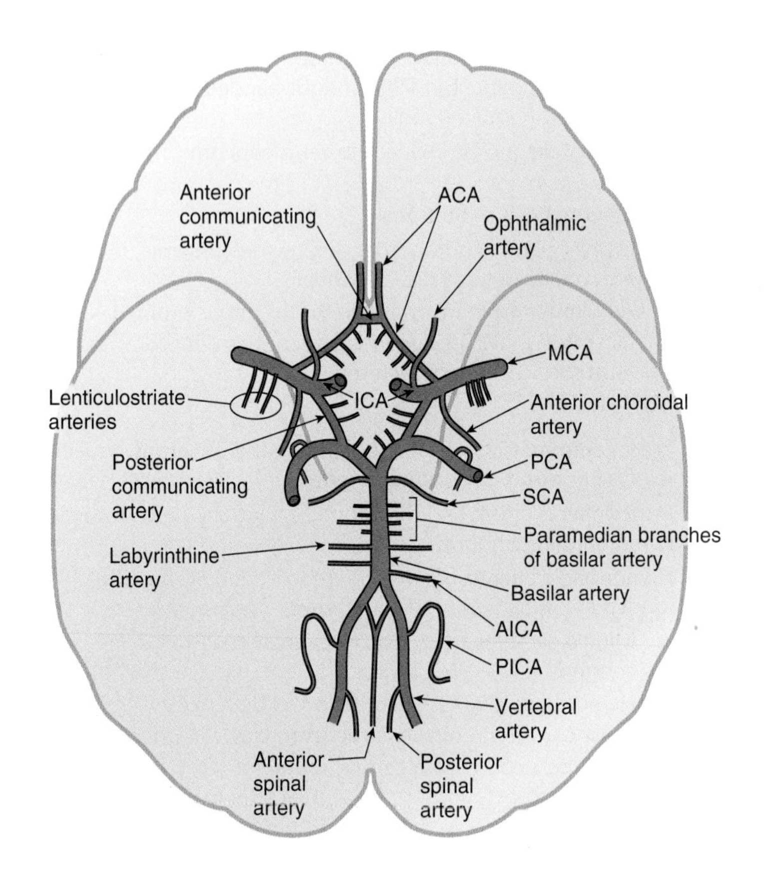

Figure 1.1 Circle of Willis
ACA = anterior cerebral artery; AICA = anterior inferior cerebellar artery; ICA = internal carotid artery; MCA = middle cerebral artery; PCA = posterior cerebral artery; PICA = posterior inferior cerebellar artery; SCA = superior cerebellar artery. (Reproduced with permission from Pritchard TC, Alloway KD. Medical Neuroscience. Madison, Connecticut: Fence Creek Publishing, 1999:78. © Fence Creek Publishing, LLC.)

D. Intracranial hemorrhage
  1. Four classes = epidural, subdural, subarachnoid, intracerebral
  2. Epidural hemorrhage
    a. Caused by traumatic rupture of middle meningeal **artery** (rarely rupture of superior longitudinal sinus)
    b. **This is a medical emergency!!!!!**

c. **Computed tomography (CT) shows biconcave disk-shaped hemorrhage that does not extend across suture lines** (see Figure 1.2A)

3. Subdural hemorrhage
   a. Caused by **trauma (can be trivial in elderly)** or blood dyscrasias, coagulopathy, alcoholism, birth injury
   b. Occurs in the cortical bridging **veins**
   c. Contrast to epidural, Sx may start 1–2 weeks after trauma
   d. If presents acutely, subdural prognosis (Px) worse than epidural due to ↑ incidence of coexisting brain injury
   e. **CT shows crescent-shaped hemorrhage that extends across cranial suture lines** (see Figure 1.2B)
4. Subarachnoid hemorrhage
   a. Due to berry aneurysm rupture, trauma, parenchymal hemorrhage, or congenital arteriovenous malformation (see Figure 1.3)
   b. Usually occurs in anterior circle of Willis (often at MCA branch point)
   c. Berry aneurysms → **severe headache, isolated cranial nerve (CN) III palsy**
   d. Dx = CT, can also check cerebrospinal fluid (CSF) for blood from sentinel bleeds
   e. **Classic CSF finding = xanthochromia = yellow discoloration due to degraded red blood cells from old bleed** (also see if CSF protein >150 mg/dL or serum bilirubin >6 mg/dL)
   f. Rupture of berry aneurysms → ↑ intracranial pressure (ICP) and chemical meningitis from blood in CSF
   g. Tx = surgical excision of aneurysm or fill sac with metal coil
   h. Mycotic aneurysms can also bleed
      (1) These occur at site of bacterial/fungal vessel wall infection, often 2° to septicemia due to endocarditis
      (2) *Salmonella* has a predilection to go for vessel walls
5. Intracerebral hemorrhages
   a. Most often due to hypertension, but can be due to trauma, arteriovenous (AV) malformations, blood dyscrasias & thrombocytopenia
   b. Occurs at small arteries of deep gray/white matter & the pons
   c. Most often occurs in the lenticulostriate distribution = basal ganglia, thalamus, & external & internal capsules

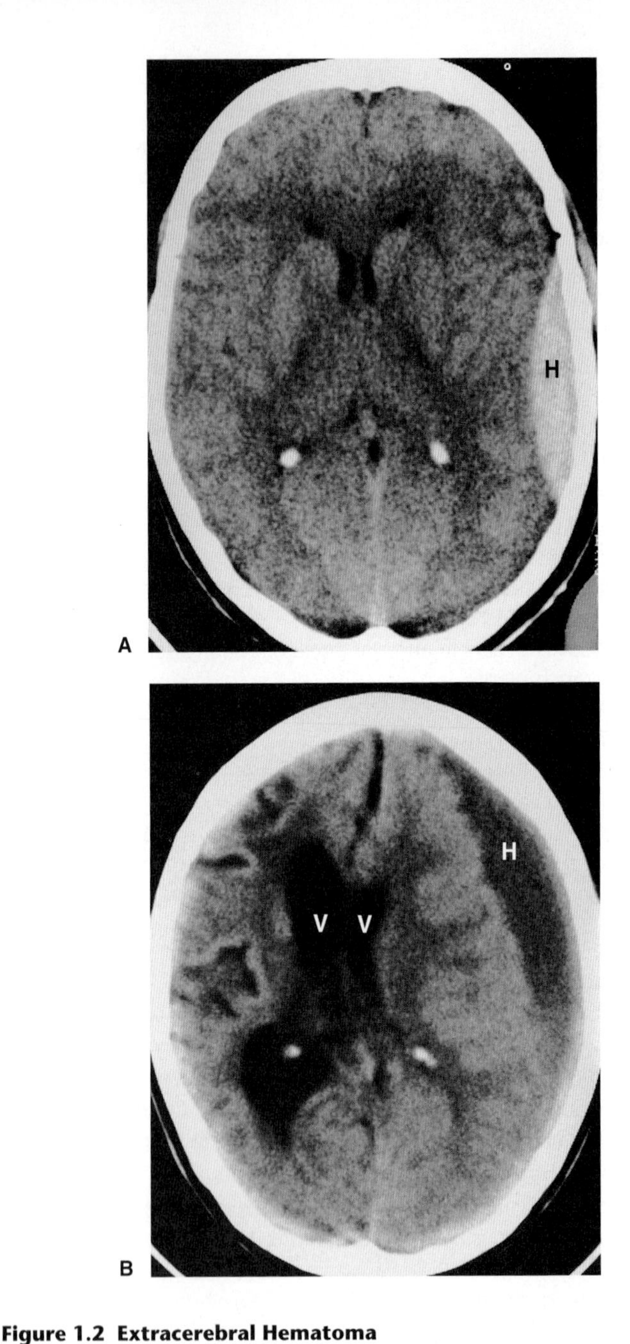

Figure 1.2 Extracerebral Hematoma
A. CT scan showing a high-density lentiform area typical of an acute epidural hematoma (H). **B.** CT scan in another patient taken 1 month after injury showing a subdural hematoma (H) as a low-density area. Note the substantial ventricular displacement. V = ventricles. (From Armstrong P, Wastie M. Diagnostic Imaging. 4th ed. Oxford: Blackwell Science, 1998.)

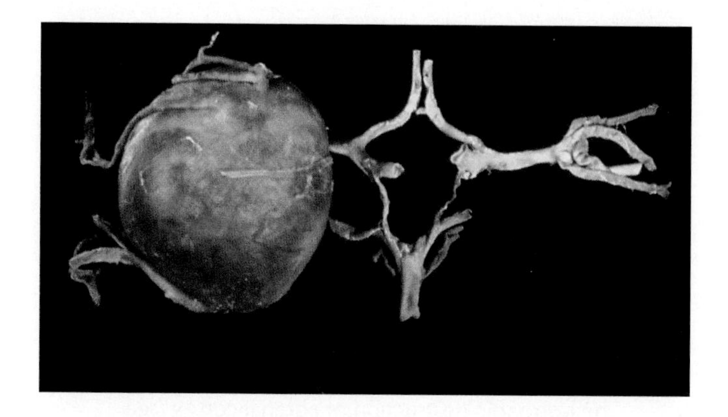

Figure 1.3 Giant Saccular Aneurysm
A large aneurysm of the middle cerebral artery created a mass lesion (on the left), which produces symptoms that may be mistaken clinically for those of a tumor. (From Rubin E, Gorstein F, Rubin R, et al. Rubin's Pathology: Clinicopathologic Foundations of Medicine. 4th ed. Baltimore: Lippincott Williams & Wilkins, 2005.)

   d. If hypertension present, will see vessel wall thickening (lipohyalinosis) and small aneurysms (Charcot-Bouchard aneurysms)
6. Hemorrhage complication → herniation, can be rapid & fatal
   a. Subfalcine herniation of the cingulate gyrus
   b. Transtentorial herniation of the uncus
   c. Cerebellar tonsillar herniation through the foramen magnum

III. Infection & Inflammation

A. Bacterial meningitis
1. 50% due to *Streptococcus pneumonia*, 25% due to *Neisseria meningitidis, Haemophilus influenzae* is rare now due to vaccination, *Listeria* seen in neonates, elderly and immunocompromised patients (pts), and group B streptococcus (*S. agalactiae*) and *Escherichia coli* are the #1 and #2 causes of neonatal meningitis
2. Sx = fever, headache, nuchal rigidity
3. Signs = **meningismus** (patient cannot touch chin to chest), ⊕ **Kernig's sign** (pt is supine with hip and knees flexed to 90°, examiner cannot extend knee), ⊕ **Brudzinski's sign** (pt is supine, when examiner flexes neck, pt involuntarily flexes hip and knees)

4. CSF → ↑ polymorphonuclear neutrophils, ↑ protein, ↓ glucose (≤1/2 serum glucose)
5. *Neisseria meningitidis*
   a. Gram-negative diplococci, ⊕ capsule, oxidase ⊕, culture on chocolate agar
   b. 5% of population carries in nasopharynx, airborne transmission
   c. Occurs most often in first year of life, or in epidemics in close populations (military barracks)
   d. Classic presentation = petechial rash on trunk, lower extremities & conjunctivae
   e. Beware of **Waterhouse-Friderichsen syndrome** = hemorrhagic destruction of adrenal cortex (see Endocrinology, Section III.C.3.a.1)
   f. Tx: if CSF → gram-negative cocci, start empiric Pen G
   g. All close contacts with patient (family members, etc.) get rifampin or quinolone prophylaxis, because these antibiotics penetrate into nasopharyngeal secretions better than Pen G
6. *Streptococcus pneumonia*
   a. Gram-positive diplococci, ⊕ capsule, catalase -, α-hemolytic
   b. Most common cause of meningitis in adults, can progress from otitis media, sinusitis, or bacteremia
   c. Splenectomy, impaired humoral immunity, cerebral trauma & advanced age are predispositions
   d. Tx: if CSF → gram-positive cocci, start empiric ceftriaxone (cefotaxime) + vancomycin (needed due to alarming increase in β-lactam resistance)
7. *Haemophilus influenzae type B*
   a. Gram-negative rod, ⊕ capsule, culture on **chocolate agar + heme (factor X) & NAD (factor V)**
   b. Formerly #1 cause of meningitis in children 6 months to 2 years
   c. Vaccine has dramatically ↓ incidence recently, consists of polysaccharide linked to carrier protein
   d. **Beware of epiglottitis, a medical emergency**
   e. Tx: if CSF → gram-negative cocco-bacillus, start empiric ceftriaxone (or cefotaxime)
8. *Streptococcus agalactiae* (group B Strep, GBS)
   a. Gram-positive cocci, ⊕ carbohydrate capsule
   b. **Most common cause of neonatal meningitis**

c. Causes sepsis within 1 week of birth, meningitis in 1 week to 3 months old
d. Acquired during delivery: **preterm delivery, premature rupture of membranes, prolonged labor, chorioamnionitis are major risk factors for transmission of this disease!**
e. 50% of babies suffer postmeningitic neurologic sequelae
f. Tx = ampicillin

9. *Escherichia coli*
   a. Gram-negative rod, ⊕ capsule, motile, ferments lactose (pink colony on MacConkey's agar)
   b. Common cause of neonatal meningitis, transmitted during delivery
   c. Tx: if CSF → gram-negative rods, start empiric ceftazidime + gentamicin
10. *Listeria monocytogenes*
    a. Can cause an aseptic picture due to difficulty gram staining & difficulty culturing out of CSF, usually Dx made by culturing blood
    b. Seen in immunosuppressed (diabetes, glucocorticoid treatment, acquired immunodeficiency syndrome [AIDS]), elderly, neonates
    c. Tx: if CSF → gram-positive rods, start ampicillin
11. **Start empiric antibiotics immediately, do not wait for CSF results before giving the first dose of antibiotics**
    a. Empiric treatment of all patients with community acquired suspected bacterial meningitis is ceftriaxone (or cefotaxime)
    b. If the patient is a neonate, elderly, or immunocompromised, add ampicillin for *Listeria* and *S. agalactiae* coverage
    c. If CSF cell count, glucose, or protein are concerning for bacterial meningitis and gram stain is negative, add vancomycin due to concern for β-lactam–resistant *S. pneumonia*
    d. If gram stain is positive, change antibiotics as previously described under each specific organism

B. Aseptic meningitis
   1. Viral meningitis
      a. Echovirus most common cause, others include Coxsackie virus, adenovirus, herpes simplex virus (HSV), human immunodeficiency virus (HIV), Ebstein-Barr virus, cytomegalovirus (CMV)

b. CSF → 1) lymphocytosis, 2) normal glucose, 3) +/−↑ protein
c. Tx = supportive

2. Subacute/chronic meningitis
   a. Differential diagnosis (DDx) = tuberculosis (TB), fungal, spirochetal, noninfectious (e.g., sarcoid, vasculitis, malignancy, drugs)
   b. TB meningitis
      (1) Second only to lung disease in TB organ frequency
      (2) Usually occurs in the elderly due to reactivation
      (3) CSF → (1) lymphocytosis; (2) glucose ≤ 1/2 of serum glucose; (3) ↑ protein; (4) almost always acid-fast bacillus stain negative but culture may be positive; 5) PPD often negative in the face of active tuberculosis
      (4) Dx: culture positive or polymerase chain reaction +
      (5) Magnetic resonance imaging for TB and all granulomatous meningitis shows "basilar meningitis"
      (6) Tx = isoniazid, rifampin, pyrazinamide, ethambutol
   c. Fungal meningitis
      (1) Typically due to *Cryptococcus*, *Coccidioides immitis*, less commonly *Histoplasma*
      (2) HIV patients frequently get *Cryptococcus*
      (3) *Coccidioides* occurs in people in the southwestern United States, *Histoplasma* in the Mississippi River Valley
      (4) Dx
         (a) *Cryptococcus* (see Figure 1.4): 1) serum or CSF cryptococcal antigen (CRAG) very sensitive and specific; 2) India Ink test moderately sensitive but very specific, shows large halo around the organism which is the capsule, that doesn't take up the ink; 3) culture very sensitive and specific but takes longer than antigen
         (b) *Coccidioides*: diagnosed by antibody test, rarely culture positive
         (c) *Histoplasma*: diagnosed by urine antigen test, rarely culture positive
   d. Spirochetal disease due to syphilis, leptospirosis, or Lyme disease
      (1) Syphilis diagnosed by serum RPR/FTA and CSF VDRL, treatment with intravenous penicillin

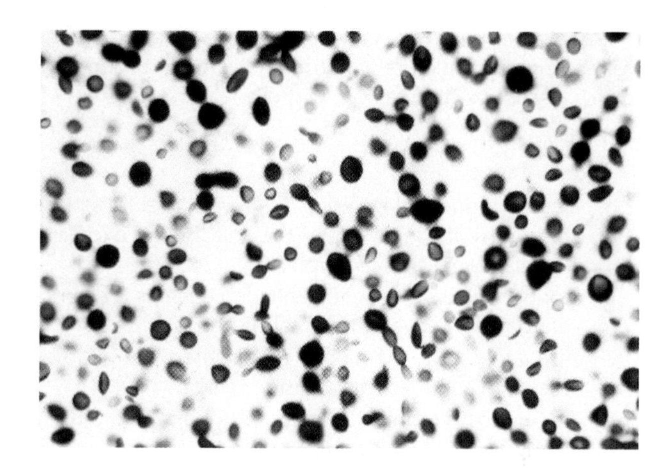

Figure 1.4 Cryptococcal Meningitis
The cryptococcal organisms vary in size (between 5 and 15 μm in diameter). They reproduce by budding. (From Rubin E, Gorstein F, Rubin R, et al. Rubin's Pathology: Clinicopathologic Foundations of Medicine. 4th ed. Baltimore: Lippincott Williams & Wilkins, 2005.)

- (2) Leptospirosis causes aseptic meningitis + renal failure + transaminitis + myalgias, Dx by antibody test, treatment with intravenous penicillin
- (3) Lyme disease caused by *Borrelia burgdorferi*, causes meningitis in late stage, along with bilateral facial nerve paralysis, myocarditis, treatment is with ceftriaxone

e. Noninfectious
- (1) Sarcoid diagnosed by biopsy, treatment is steroids
- (2) Vasculitis diagnosed by biopsy or serologies, treatment is steroids
- (3) Malignancy diagnosed by CSF cytology, commonly seen with leukemia, lymphoma, breast cancer
- (4) Drug-induced meningitis typically due to nonsteroidal anti-inflammatory drugs or sulfa antibiotics, others more rare

3. Amebic meningitis due to *Naegleria fowleri*
   - a. Infects swimmers (often children) in warm lakes
   - b. Often in California & southern states
   - c. Typical outcome is death within 24 hours
   - d. No effective Tx, amphotericin B can be attempted

4. Complications of meningitis = cerebral edema, syndrome of inappropriate antidiuretic hormone secretion, seizures, deafness, vestibular dysfunction, hydrocephalus & ↓ IQ

C. Encephalitis

1. Toxoplasmosis
    a. Causes congenital encephalitis, transmitted transplacentally (transplacental infections = the ToRCHS = **To**xoplasmosis, **R**ubella, **C**MV, **H**erpes, **S**yphilis)
    b. Congenital Si/Sx = neonatal hydrocephalus & mental retardation, periventricular calcifications
    c. Also adults exposed via cat feces, subsequently causes disease in acquired immunosuppression
    d. **Is the most common cerebral lesion in AIDS patients**
    e. **Presents as ring-enhancing mass lesions, usually multiple, causing focal neurologic changes**
    f. Toxoplasmosis antibody test is very sensitive for disease
    g. Tx = sulfadiazine + pyrimethamine or trimethoprim/sulfamethoxazole (Bactrim)
    h. **AIDS pts with CD4 < 200/μL get trimethoprim/sulfamethoxazole prophylaxis**
2. Lymphocytic meningoencephalitis due to viral, TB, or syphilis
    a. If it is viral, look for perivascular inflammation on biopsy
    b. Will also see lymphocytic infiltrate in CNS leukemia, lymphoma, systemic lupus erythematosus, lymphocytic choriomeningitis
3. Viral encephalitis
    a. HSV
        (1) Affects **temporal lobe**, inferior frontal lobe
        (2) Causes acute **hemorrhagic encephalitis**
        (3) Histology → **Cowdry intranuclear** inclusion bodies
        (4) **HSV is the most common cause of viral encephalitis,** especially in younger ages
        (5) **Classic Sx = olfactory hallucinations & personality changes**
        (6) Look for RBCs in CSF, temporal spikes on electroencephalography
        (7) Tx = acyclovir
    b. Rabies
        (1) Affects midbrain & floor of fourth ventricle, causes hippocampal degeneration

(2) Histology → **Negri body inclusions** (eosinophilic **cytoplasmic** inclusions in cerebellum & hippocampus) (see Figure 1.5)

(3) **Classic Sx = hydrophobia**, literally fear of drinking despite great thirst, due to painful laryngeal & pharyngeal spasms stimulated by attempts to drink

(4) Tx = coadministration of passive & active vaccines aborts rabies if given prior to symptom onset

c. CMV

(1) Occurs in immunosuppressed

(2) Infection during pregnancy → fetal microcephaly, retardation, hepatosplenomegaly, chorioretinitis

(3) Histology → giant cells with eosinophilic inclusions in **both cytoplasm & nucleus** (see Figure 1.6)

(4) Tx = ganciclovir

d. Arthropod encephalitis viruses (equine, California, St. Louis, Japanese, West Nile)

(1) All are mosquito-borne arboviruses (RNA)

(2) Tx is symptomatic, high mortality rates

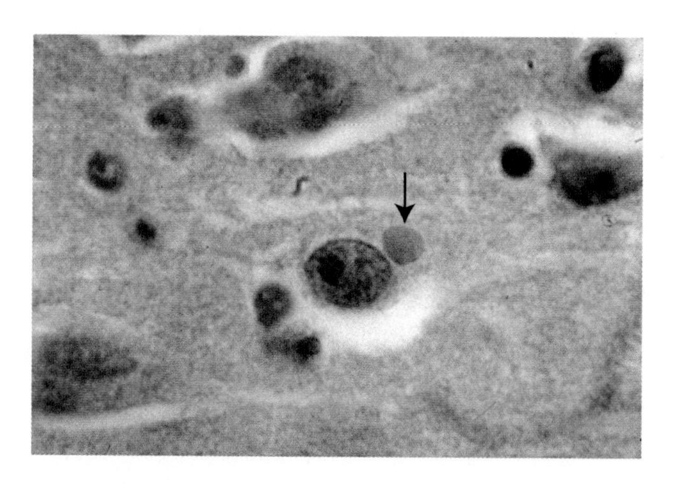

Figure 1.5 Negri Bodies
Rabies encephalitis is characterized by round, eosinophilic cytoplasmic inclusions that resemble an erythrocyte (arrow). (From Rubin E, Gorstein F, Rubin R, et al. Rubin's Pathology: Clinicopathologic Foundations of Medicine. 4th ed. Baltimore: Lippincott Williams & Wilkins, 2005.)

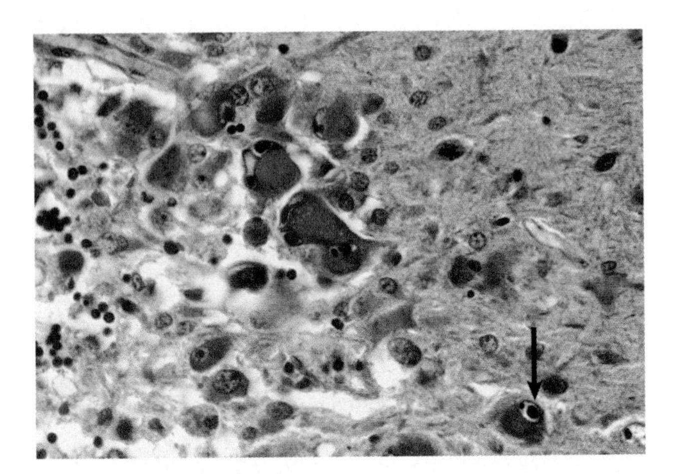

Figure 1.6 Intranuclear Inclusions
Cytomegalovirus induces intranuclear inclusions with prominent clear halos (arrow). These inclusions are demonstrated in the Purkinje cells of a patient with acquired immunodeficiency syndrome (AIDS). (From Rubin E, Gorstein F, Rubin R, et al. Rubin's Pathology: Clinicopathologic Foundations of Medicine. 4th ed. Baltimore: Lippincott Williams & Wilkins, 2005.)

e. HIV
   (1) Penetrates blood brain barrier by living in monocytes, causing progressive dementia = AIDS-related dementia
   (2) No Tx to reverse dementia once it starts
f. Progressive multifocal leukoencephalopathy (PML)
   (1) Usually seen in AIDS, but not caused by HIV
   (2) Diffuse white matter demyelination due to JC virus (a papovavirus)
   (3) Histology → **nuclear inclusions in oligodendrocytes**
   (4) No effective Tx
g. Subacute sclerosing panencephalitis
   (1) Due to measles, occurs in children
   (2) Both gray & white matter are involved, slowly progressive, & usually fatal
   (3) Sx = multiple neurologic deficits & grand mal seizures
   (4) Histology → **Damson's inclusion bodies**
   (5) No effective Tx

4. Creutzfeldt-Jakob ("kuru" or "spongiform encephalopathy")
   a. Caused by prion = infectious protein molecule that cannot be destroyed by normal sterilization techniques
   b. Si/Sx → personality change, dementia, myoclonus, spongiosis, ataxia, tremor, cerebellar degeneration, intracytoplasmic vacuoles
   c. No effective Tx
5. Neurosyphilis can be due to 2° or tertiary (3°) disease
   a. 2° syphilis causes lymphocytic meningitis
   b. 3° syphilis is of 2 types: meningovascular & parenchymal
      (1) Meningovascular syphilis
         (a) Causes meningeal adhesions, CN palsies
         (b) **Pathognomonic finding is Argyll Robertson pupil (miotic, irregular, unequal, ⊕ accommodation but nonreactive)**
         (c) Also causes Heubner's arteritis (small vessel intimal thickening & lymphocyte infiltration)
      (2) Parenchymal syphilis presents in 2 forms
         (a) Tabes dorsalis
            (i) Bilateral demyelination of posterior spinal cord, usually lumbar involvement is heaviest
            (ii) Si/Sx = ↓ proprioception/reflexes/vibration sense, pain, hypotonia, paresthesias, neurogenic bladder
         (b) Dementia paralytica
            (i) Cortical atrophy, neuron loss, gliosis & granular change of the ventricles
            (ii) Sx = psychosis, dementia, personality change

D. Abscess
   1. Brain abscess: location points to etiology
      a. Hematogenous spread causes multiple abscesses at gray-white matter junction
      b. Temporal lobe involvement suggests middle ear extension
   2. Risk factors for abscess development include congenital right-to-left shunt (lung filtration bypassed), otitis media, paranasal sinusitis, metastases, trauma, & immunosuppression
   3. Abscess comprised of 1) necrotic core, 2) granulation ring, 3) outer fibrosis/gliosis with edema
   4. Major complications = ↑ ICP & rupture into ventricle

5. **Brain abscesses are invariably fatal if untreated**
6. Abscesses must be surgically drained
7. Causes include *Streptococcus* (#1), *S. aureus* (trauma, endocarditis, Tx = oxacillin), *Bacteroides fragilis* or *Peptostreptococcus* (Tx = metronidazole), & Enterobacteriaceae (extension from otitis media, Tx = cefotaxime)
8. Helminthic infections
   a. Cysticercosis (*Taenia solium*)
      (1) Eggs transmitted by fecal-oral route
      (2) **Seizures in a Latin American immigrant is due to neurocysticercosis until proven otherwise**
      (3) Tx = steroids for edema, anti-helminthic therapy controversial
   b. Schistosomiasis
      (1) Waterborne larval forms directly penetrate skin, acutely → itching & dermatitis at site of infection
      (2) Causes eosinophilic granulomas in the brain
      (3) Tx = praziquantel
   c. Hydatid cysts (*Echinococcus*)
      (1) Acquired by dog feces
      (2) Can cause focal neurologic symptoms & seizures
      (3) If cysts rupture they can cause fatal anaphylaxis
      (4) Tx = careful surgical excystation, mebendazole

IV. Tumors

A. General characteristics
   1. In adults majority of intracranial tumors are supratentorial, while in children they are infratentorial
   2. Most common intracranial tumors overall are metastatic, most common 1° intracranial tumors are glioblastoma multiforme, meningioma, acoustic neuroma
   3. Most common cerebral tumor in AIDS is B-cell lymphoma
   4. Embryology (see Table 1.2 and Figure 1.7)
   5. General symptoms
      a. ↑ ICP → headache (worse in morning after waking), nausea/vomiting, **bradycardia with hypertension & Cheyne-Stokes respirations (Cushing's triad),** papilledema
      b. Local compression → focal neural deficits, frequently compression of CN III → fixed, dilated pupil

Table 1.2 Embryologic Derivatives of Neurologic Cancers

Tissue Derivative	Neoplasms
Neural tube	Gliomas: astrocytoma, glioblastoma, ependymoma, pineal tumors, medulloblastoma, ganglioneuroma, oligodendroglioma
Neural crest	Meningioma, schwannoma, neurofibroma
Mesoderm	CNS lymphoma, hemangioblastoma, lipoma, chordoma
Ectoderm	Craniopharyngioma, pituitary adenoma
Germ cell	Teratoma, germinoma

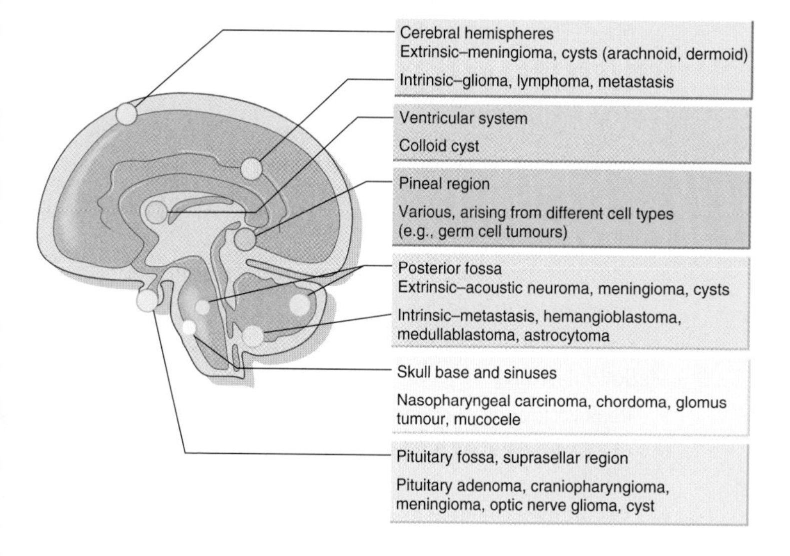

Figure 1.7
Most probable histological type of primary tumor at different sites in the brain (metastases can occur at any site). (Adapted from Axford JS. Medicine. Oxford: Blackwell Science, 1998.)

B. Intracranial neoplasms
   1. Glioblastoma multiforme (grade IV astrocytoma)
      a. Most common 1° intracranial neoplasm, peaks in late middle age
      b. Almost invariably lethal, usually within 1–2 years (without resection of mass, death in weeks)
      c. Impossible to completely resect due to microinfiltrates beyond the margins of the tumor mass
      d. **CT → central necrosis of the mass surrounded by bright ring of enhancement**—main differential = abscess
      e. Histology → pseudopalisading
      f. Associated with intestinal polyps in Turcot's syndrome
   2. Oligodendroglioma
      a. More common in cerebral hemispheres & grows slowly so associated with many calcifications visible on x-ray
      b. Most frequent in middle-aged people
      c. Histology → large, round nuclei with a clear halo of cytoplasm (**fried egg morphology**)
   3. Ependymoma
      a. Most frequently in the fourth ventricle
      b. Causes hydrocephalus if CSF flow obstructed at fourth ventricle
      c. Histology → **microscopic rosettes around lumen**
   4. Papilloma of choroid plexus
      a. Most often in children, similar to ependymoma
      b. Arises in ventricular system
      c. Usually ↑ ICP & hydrocephalus present
   5. Medulloblastoma
      a. Peak incidence in children
      b. Occurs in cerebellar vermis in children, hemispheres in adults
      c. Histology → rosettes
   6. Meningiomas
      a. Second most common primary intracranial neoplasm
      b. Benign, slow growing tumor, usually easily resectable
      c. Arise in arachnoid granulations, found adjacent to venous sinuses
      d. Histology → **whorls of fibrous tissue** & calcified **psammoma bodies** (other psammoma body diseases

(dzs) = ovarian serous papillary cystadenocarcinoma, papillary adenocarcinoma of thyroid, mesothelioma)

7. Neuroblastoma
   a. Related to neuroblastomas of adrenal gland
   b. *N-myc* amplification seen
8. Retinoblastoma
   a. Occurs in children, 60% sporadic, 40% familial
   b. Familial cases are due to inheritance of *rb* deletion, so bilateral tumors common
9. Hemangioblastoma
   a. Often seen in von Hippel-Lindau syndrome, an inherited disorder with hemangioblastomas in many organs (see Dermatology, Section IV.D.4)
   b. Can ectopically produce erythropoietin → erythrocytosis
10. Craniopharyngioma
    a. Most common supratentorial tumor in children
    b. Compresses optic chiasm & hypothalamus
11. Prolactinoma
    a. Most common pituitary tumor
    b. Classic Sx = **bilateral gynecomastia in males, amenorrhea in females, galactorrhea (either sex), impotence, bitemporal hemianopsia** due to CN III effacement & daily headaches
    c. Tx: first line = bromocriptine (D_2 agonist inhibits prolactin secretion), second line = surgery (for lack of medical response)
12. Lymphoma
    a. Most common brain neoplasms in AIDS patients
    b. **AIDS patients have 100x ↑ incidence of lymphoma**
    c. Causes subacute focal neurologic changes, can ↑ ICP
    d. **MRI → ring-enhancing mass lesion difficult to distinguish from a single toxoplasmosis lesion** (multiple lesions more likely to be toxo, although both diseases can be present simultaneously)
    e. Tx = radiation therapy, poor Px
13. Metastatic neoplasm
    a. 20% of intracranial neoplasms are metastases
    b. Most common 1° = lung, breast, melanoma, renal cell, colon, thyroid
    c. Form discrete, spherical nodules, often localized at junction of grey & white matter

C. Peripheral nerve tumors
   1. Schwannoma (neurilemoma)
      a. Benign tumors, most commonly intracranially localized to CN VIII (acoustic neuroma)
      b. Third most common primary intracranial tumor
      c. Seen at cerebellar pontine angle
      d. Can cause tinnitus, deafness, vertigo, hydrocephalus, & ↑ ICP
   2. Neurofibroma
      a. Can be part of von Recklinghausen's neurofibromatosis (type 1 neurofibromatosis = NF1)
      b. Malformation of nerve fibers due to diffuse, generalized proliferation of Schwann cells in a loose fibrillar pattern
      c. Antoni A type is tightly woven, Antoni B is more loose
      d. NF1 has variable expressivity, can clinically range from asymptomatic to "elephant man"
         (1) Classic NF1 lesions = café au lait spots (brown macules), axillary/inguinal freckling, subcutaneous nodules (neurofibromas) plexiform neuromas, Lisch nodules of iris
         (2) More severe disease presents with gliomas, optic tumors, scoliosis, & bone defects
      e. NF2 lesions = bilateral acoustic neuromas

V. Hydrocephalus

A. General characteristics
   1. Definition = ↑ CSF, leading to increased intracranial pressure
   2. **Classic CT/MRI finding is dilated ventricles**
   3. In children separation of cranial bones leads to grossly enlarged calvarium
   4. Causes: (1) ↑ CSF production (rare, choroid plexus tumors), (2) ↓ CSF resorption

B. Classification
   1. Communicating (free flow from ventricles & subarachnoid space)
      a. Hydrocephalus ex vacuo = ventricular dilatation after significant neuronal loss (e.g., Alzheimer's, strokes)
      b. Normal pressure hydrocephalus
         (1) **Classic triad: bladder incontinence, dementia, ataxia ("wet, wacky, wobbly")**
         (2) Causes: 50% idiopathic, also meningitis, cerebral hemorrhage, trauma, atherosclerosis

(3) Due to ↓ CSF resorption across arachnoid villi
(4) Incontinence due to pressure on subcortical fibers in frontal lobe

c. Pseudotumor cerebri
(1) Spontaneous ↑ ICP without ventricular obstruction or intracranial mass
(2) **Commonly seen in obese, young females**, idiopathic (massive quantities of vitamin A can cause it)
(3) Sx = headache, papilledema, with or without monocular blindness
(4) **CT → no ventricular dilation (may even be shrunken)**
(5) Tx = symptomatic (acetazolamide or surgical lumboperitoneal shunt), dz is typically self-limiting

2. Noncommunicating (block between ventricles & subarachnoid space → CSF outflow obstruction at one of several points)
   a. Foramina of Luschka/Magendie, due to chronic meningitis or subarachnoid hemorrhage
   b. Tumor effacing fourth ventricle, can be ependymoma or medulloblastomas in cerebellar vermis
   c. Congenital narrowing of aqueduct of Sylvius
   d. Foramen of Munro, rare, due to glioma or colloid cyst, causing ipsilateral lateral ventricle hydrocephalus
   e. Foramen magnum, frequently in the Arnold-Chiari syndrome, due to brainstem herniation
3. Congenital hydrocephalus
   a. Arnold-Chiari malformation (see below)
   b. Stenosis of aqueduct of Sylvius → third & lateral ventricle dilation
   c. Atresia of foramina of Luschka/Magendie, causing third & fourth ventricle dilation
4. Acquired hydrocephalus usually due to tumor or meningeal scarring following meningitis or subarachnoid hemorrhage

VI. Congenital/Perinatal Disorders

A. Chromosomal disorders (see Table 1.3)

B. Malformations

1. Arnold-Chiari malformation (see Figure 1.8)
   a. Caudally displaced cerebellum, elongated medulla passing into foramen magnum with the fourth ventricle, flat skull base, hydrocephalus, meningomyelocele, & aqueductal stenosis
   b. Bilateral vocal cord paralysis (hoarseness and stridor)

Table 1.3 Congenital Neurologic Disorders

Karyotype	Disease	Deformations
Trisomy 13	Patau's	Arrhinencephaly,* holoprosencephaly
Trisomy 18	Edward's	Arrhinencephaly,* corpus callosum agenesis, microcephaly
Trisomy 21	Down's syndrome	Malformed temporal gyri, premature Alzheimer's changes, frequent cardiac involvement including atrial septal but more commonly ventricular septal defects, psychomotor retardation

*Arrhinencephaly = congenital lack of olfactory cortex.

2. Neural tube defects
   a. Associated with ↑ α-fetoprotein levels in maternal serum
   b. Preventable by folic acid supplements during pregnancy
   c. Spina bifida = failure of posterior vertebral arches to close
   d. Meningocele = failure of neural canal closure so lumbar cord covered only by sac of meninges & skin
   e. Meningomyelocele = herniation of cord tissue into the sac causing paraplegia & risk of meningitis
   f. Syringomyelia
      (1) Spinal cord cavitation (= syringobulbia in medulla)
      (2) Sx = weakness, thenar atrophy, spastic lower limbs, ↓ pain/temperature sensation, normal position/vibration sense
      (3) Wall of cavitation → gliosis, cavity not connected with central canal (contrast to hydromyelia)

C. Fetal alcohol syndrome
   1. Characterized by facial abnormalities & developmental defects
   2. Classic physical finding is **smooth filtrum of lip**
   3. Also → microcephaly, atrial septal defect, mental/growth retardation

D. Tuberous sclerosis
   1. Autosomal dominant multinodular proliferation of multinucleated astrocytes
   2. Form small tubers = white nodules in cortex & periventricular areas
   3. Characterized by seizures & mental retardation in infancy
   4. Can be associated with rhabdomyosarcoma in children

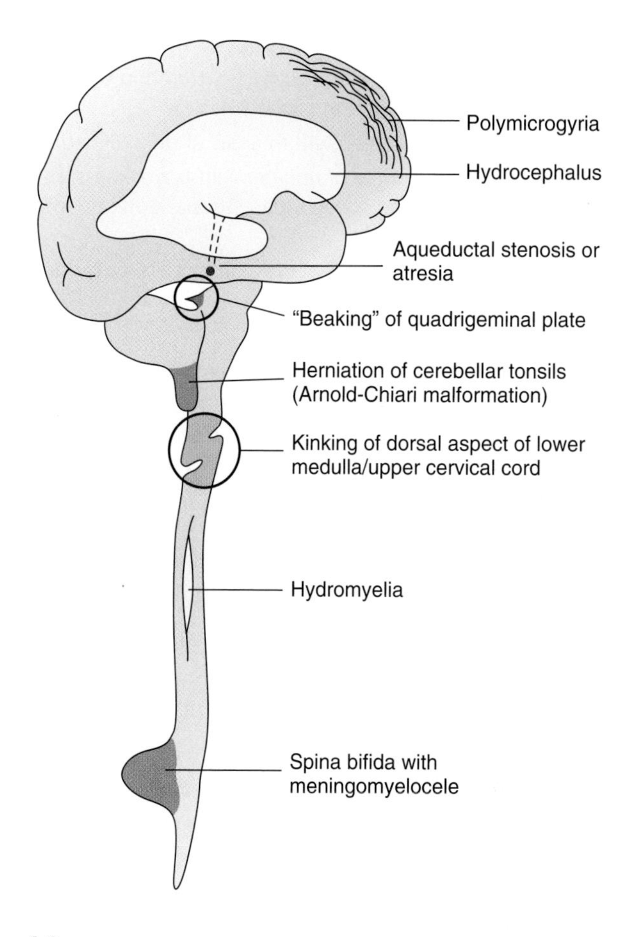

Figure 1.8
Arnold-Chiari malformation and associated lesions. (From Rubin E, Gorstein F, Rubin R, et al. Rubin's Pathology: Clinicopathologic Foundations of Medicine. 4th ed. Baltimore: Lippincott Williams & Wilkins, 2005.)

VII. Demyelinating Diseases

A. Multiple sclerosis (MS)
   1. Unknown etiology, but has some genetic predisposition
   2. Also environmental predisposition, more common in people who live the first decade of life in northern, temperate latitudes
   3. **↑ CSF immunoglobulins often manifest as multiple oligoclonal bands on electrophoresis**

4. Periventricular areas of demyelination, with multiple focal plaques of demyelination irregularly scattered in the brain & spinal cord (disseminated in space & time)
5. Preservation of axons seen within areas of demyelination
6. Relapsing chronic course of unilateral limb weakness, nystagmus, tremor, scanning speech, paresthesia, optic neuritis, urinary incontinence
7. Acute lesions contain lymphocytes, gitter cells, & products of lipids
8. Chronic lesions demonstrate gliosis
9. Not necessarily a relentlessly progressive degenerative disease, long periods of remission sometimes seen

B. Devic's syndrome (variant of multiple sclerosis)
   1. Acute spinal cord & optic nerve demyelination → blindness & paraplegia
   2. More common in Asians

C. Schilder's diffuse cerebral sclerosis
   1. Begins in early childhood, associated with adrenoleukodystrophy (see Appendix B) or adrenal atrophy in males
   2. Most commonly found in occipital lobes & corpus callosum
   3. Sx = visual, motor, auditory & psychiatric disorders

D. Hemorrhagic encephalomyelitis
   1. Hyperacute allergic reaction following measles or smallpox
   2. Brain shows edema, petechiae, capillary congestion, demyelination, & hemorrhage

E. Postvaccine encephalomyelitis
   1. Resembles hemorrhagic encephalomyelitis but occurs after immunization
   2. Predominant perivascular dz within white matter
   3. Absence of necrosis with preservation of axons

F. Guillain-Barré syndrome
   1. Acute inflammatory demyelinating dz involving peripheral nerves
   2. Highest incidence in young adults
   3. **Most often preceded by viral infection**, immunization, gastroenteritis, or allergic reactions, considered to be autoimmune
   4. **Symptoms = Muscle weakness and paralysis beginning in lower part of lower extremities & ascending upward, loss of reflexes**

5. Respiratory failure & death can occur, but most pts recover
6. **CSF protein markedly elevated without an increase in cells seen (albumin-cytologic dissociation)**

G. Central pontine myelinolysis
1. Diamond-shaped region of demyelination in basis pontis
2. **Seen after rapid correction of hyponatremia & in liver transplant pts**

VIII. Metabolic & Nutritional Disorders

A. Anoxia/hypoglycemia
1. Anoxia & hypoglycemia have similar effects on brain
2. Widespread cortical neuron loss & cortical laminar necrosis
3. Purkinje cells are lost in cerebellum

B. Carbon monoxide poisoning
1. Presents in pts enclosed in burned areas, or during the start of a cold winter (people using their new gas heaters)
2. Causes bilateral pallidal necrosis
3. Sx = headache, nausea, vomiting, mental disturbances, cherry-red lips
4. Dx = carboxyhemoglobin levels must be obtained
5. Tx = 100% oxygen

C. Thiamine deficiency
1. Usually 2° to alcoholism
2. Beriberi peripheral neuropathy due to Wallerian degeneration
3. Wernicke's encephalopathy: **Wernicke's triad = confusion (confabulation), ophthalmoplegia, ataxia**
4. Wernicke's is related to lesions of mamillary bodies

D. Vitamin B_{12} deficiency
1. Subacute degeneration of posterior columns & lateral corticospinal tract
2. Si/Sx = bilateral paresthesias, numbness, weakness, ↓ vibration sense, ataxia, all worse in lower extremities

E. Wilson's disease (hepatolenticular degeneration)
1. Underlying defect in copper metabolism → accumulation
2. Dx = ↓ serum ceruloplasmin

3. Causes lesions in basal ganglia, presents with extrapyramidal symptoms (tremors, rigidity), psychosis, & manic-depression
4. **Pathognomonic finding → Kayser-Fleischer ring circumscribing cornea**
5. Treatment = Penicillamine

F. Hepatic encephalopathy (see Gastroenterology and Liver, Section VI.B.8.d. (5))
   1. Seen in cirrhosis, may be due to brain toxicity 2° to excess ammonia & other toxins not degraded by malfunctioning liver
   2. Sx = limb rigidity, hyperreflexia, **asterixis** (flapping of extended wrists)

G. Sphingolipidosis
   1. Tay-Sachs
      a. Hexosaminidase A defect → ↑ ganglioside GM2
      b. Sx = blindness, **cherry-red spot on macula**, mental & motor deterioration, paralysis
      c. Histology → Periodic acid-Schiff (PAS) ⊕ lipid-laden neurons, multilamellar cytoplasmic bodies in CNS, & myenteric plexus ganglia
      d. Dx by biopsy of rectum, or enzymatic assay
   2. Batten's disease (neuronal ceroid lipofuscinosis)
      a. Progressive neurodegeneration disorder
      b. Neurons distended by lipofuscin-like material thought to be abnormal complex of adenosine triphosphate synthase
      c. Cerebral cortical astrocytosis, PAS⊕ neurons & macrophages
   3. Niemann-Pick disease = deficiency in sphingomyelinase
      a. See foamy histiocytes containing sphingomyelin, hepatosplenomegaly
      b. **50% have cherry-red spot on macula similar to Tay-Sachs**

H. Leukodystrophy
   1. Krabbe leukodystrophy
      a. Autosomal recessive deficiency in β-galactocerebrosidase
      b. Si/Sx = peripheral demyelination, myoclonus, paralysis, blindness, retardation → pts invariably die as infants
      c. No evidence of storage of materials
      d. Loss of myelin with gliosis & presence of PAS⊕ globoid cells (curved tubular inclusions within macrophages)

2. Metachromatic leukodystrophy
   a. Autosomal recessive deficiency in arylsulfatase A → accumulation of galactocerebroside sulfate
   b. Loss of myelin → progressive paralysis & death by age 10
   c. **PAS⊕ macrophages demonstrating metachromasia**
   d. Metachromatic granules present in kidney tubular epithelium & peripheral nerves
   e. **Urine stains positive with toluidine blue**

IX. Degenerative Diseases

A. General characteristics
   1. Glutamate excitotoxicity causes neuron injury in some models
   2. Trinucleotide repeats seen in Huntington's (CAG), Friedreich's ataxia (GAA), & spinocerebellar degeneration (CAG)
   3. Clinically present with dementia (Table 1.4)
      a. Dementia ≡ global decline in cognition, involving memory, personality, motor, or sensory functions
      b. Delirium is the only other cause of global decline in cognition, can be difficult to differentiate from dementia

Table 1.4 Dementia versus Delirium

	Dementia	Delirium
Course	Constant, progressive	Sudden onset, waxing/waning daily
Reversible?	Usually not	Almost always
Circadian?	Constant, no daily pattern	Usually worse at night (sun-downing)
Consciousness	Normal	Altered (obtunded)
Hallucination/ Delusion	Usually not	Often, classically visual
Tremor	Often not	Often present (i.e., asterixis)
Causes	Alzheimer's, multi-infarct, Pick's disease, alcohol, brain infection/tumors, malnutrition (thiamine/B_{12} deficiency)	Systemic infection/neoplasm, drugs (often nosocomial), CVA, heart dz, alcoholism, uremia, electrolyte imbalance, hyper/hypoglycemia

CVA, cerebrovascular accident; dz, disease.

B. Alzheimer's disease (senile dementia of alzheimer type)
   1. Most common cause of both presenile (<65 years) & senile dementia
   2. Genetics involved may include amyloid gene on chromosome 21, amyloid β-protein, A4/β protein
   3. Starts in temporal lobe & hippocampus, spreads to entire cortex
   4. Cellular changes = neurofibrillary tangles (neocortical & hippocampal), granulovacuolar degeneration (primarily in hippocampus), plaques & amyloid angiopathy (the only extraneuronal sign)
   5. All of these signs occur in normal aging but to a lesser degree
   6. Occurs in Down's syndrome pts at younger ages (age 30–40 years)

C. Pick's disease
   1. Clinically similar to Alzheimer's, more in women, younger age onset (50s)
   2. Swollen neurons have Pick body inclusions seen with silver stain
   3. Predominates in frontal (more personality changes seen) & temporal lobes

D. Parkinson's disease
   1. Loss of dopaminergic neurons in substantia nigra
   2. Dz is idiopathic, but Parkinson-like disease (parkinsonism) can result from intoxication (e.g., manganese, synthetic heroin, phenothiazine)
   3. Pathologically see depigmentation of substantia nigra & **Lewy bodies →27cytoplasmic inclusions seen with antiubiquitin antibodies** (see Figure 1.9)
   4. Si/Sx = **bradykinesia** (slow movement), **cog-wheel rigidity, classic "mask-like" facial expression** (flat affect), **shuffling gait, "pill-roll" resting tremor**, can lead to dementia
   5. Tx = levodopa/carbidopa, benztropine, selegiline
   6. Px = poor, typically chronically progressive, Tx palliates Sx

E. Huntington's chorea
   1. Gene on chromosome 4 is the cause
   2. Atrophy of striatum (especially caudate nucleus), neuronal loss, & gliosis
   3. Movement disorder & dementia
   4. ↑ CAG triplet repeats seen; the more repeats, the more severe the Sx

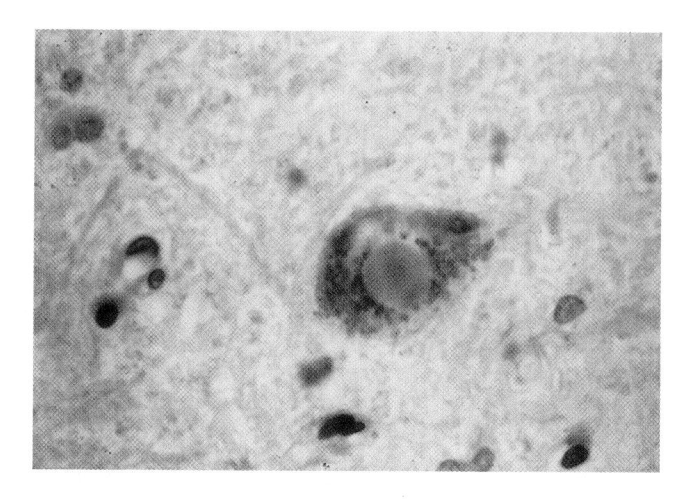

Figure 1.9 Parkinson's Disease
A microscopic section of the substantia nigra from a patient with PD shows a Lewy body (a spherical eosinophilic inclusion surrounded by a halo within the cytoplasm of a pigmented dopaminergic neuron). (From Rubin E, Gorstein F, Rubin R, et al. Rubin's Pathology: Clinicopathologic Foundations of Medicine. 4th ed. Baltimore: Lippincott Williams & Wilkins, 2005.)

5. Huntington's disease gene encodes a protein widely expressed in CNS, function unknown
6. **Not a demyelinating disorder**

F. Amyotrophic lateral sclerosis (Lou Gehrig's disease, motor neuron disease)
1. Most common motor neuron disease
2. Degeneration of upper & lower motor neurons
3. Muscle weakness with fasciculations (anterior motor neurons) eventually progresses to denervation atrophy of muscle
4. Lateral cortical spinal tract degeneration (lateral sclerosis) causes hyperreflexia, spasticity
5. Bulbar (lower brain stem) dz → difficulty speaking & swallowing
6. Superoxide dismutase gene mutation seen in some patients
7. Congenital variant, Werdnig-Hoffmann disease, shows only lower motor neuron Sx due to anterior horn cell loss, no upper motor signs/cortical spinal tract degeneration

G. Spinocerebellar degeneration (Friedreich's ataxia)
  1. Cerebellar & spinal cord dorsal column atrophy
  2. An example of this class of disorders is Friedreich's ataxia
     a. Friedreich's ataxia onsets between ages 5 & 25 years
     b. Multiorgan disease → pes cavus (hollowing of instep), diabetes, kyphoscoliosis, dim proprioception, tremors, ↓ tendon reflexes, ⊕ Babinski sign & cardiomyopathy

2. HEAD AND NECK

I. Embryology (see Table 2.1)

Table 2.1 Branchial Derivatives

Level	Groove (Ectoderm)	Arch (Mesoderm)	Pouch (Endoderm)	Artery
1	Pinna External auditory meatus	Meckel's cartilage Mandible, malleus, incus Masticator muscles, mylohyoid, anterior belly of digastric CN V_3	Eustachian tube Middle ear cavity	Maxillary
2		Reichert's cartilage Styloid process, stapes Stapedius, anterior tongue muscles, muscles of facial expression, stylohyoid, posterior belly of digastric CN VII	Palatine tonsil	Stapedial & hyoid
3		Posterior tongue muscles, stylopharyngeus CN IX	Vallecular recess Thymus Inferior parathyroids	Common carotid Proximal internal carotid
4		Thyroid cartilage Cricothyroid muscle CN X, superior laryngeal nerve	Superior parathyroids	Left aortic arch Right subclavian
5			Parafollicular cells	
6		Cricoid & arytenoid cartilage Larynx muscles CN X, inferior laryngeal nerve	Laryngeal ventricle	Proximal pulmonary artery Ductus arteriosus

II. Head

A. Headaches

1. Migraine headaches
   a. Most common in females, throbbing headache with nausea, vomiting, vertigo, & photophobia; can be associated with menses
   b. Classic migraines can worsen during pregnancy & common migraines may disappear during this time
   c. Classic migraine is unilateral & is preceded by an aura
   d. Common migraine is bilateral & not preceded by an aura
   e. Classic migraine auras
      (1) May shimmer or scintillate within visual field
      (2) **Consist of pathognomonic zigzag lines (teichopsia)**, flashing lights (photopsias), blind spots (scotoma), or colors (rhodopsins)
      (3) Treatment (Tx) = nonsteroidal anti-inflammatory drugs (NSAIDs), dihydroergotamine, methysergide, or sumatriptan
      (4) **Beware of retroperitoneal fibroplasia in patients (pts) treated with methysergide, a classic side effect**
      (5) Prophylaxis with β-blockers & avoidance of triggering factors
2. Cluster headaches
   a. Seen primarily in males, attacks of severe unilateral stabbing periorbital/retro-orbital pain, lasting 15 minutes to 3 hours
   b. Seasonal attacks occur in series lasting weeks to months
   c. Symptoms (sx) also include lacrimation, conjunctival congestion, rhinorrhea; may also see ptosis & miosis
   d. Tx = NSAIDs or ergotamine
3. Tension headache (muscle contraction headache)
   a. Pt describes feeling as if a band is squeezing his or her head
   b. **Most common headache type**
   c. Sx are nonpulsatile & not aggravated by activity
   d. Often accompanied by myofascial trigger points
   e. Tx = NSAIDs, stress reduction
4. Withdrawal headache
   a. Most common cause of chronic headache
   b. Can be withdrawal from any medication
   c. Tx = NSAIDs

5. Temporal arteritis (giant cell)
    a. Seen mostly in elderly women, uncommon in African Americans
    b. Constant boring, temporal headache, worse at night, ↑ by cold, **often associated with polymyalgia rheumatica** (severe muscle aches)
    c. **If not diagnosed early can lead to blindness**
    d. Diagnosis (Dx) by artery biopsy, screen by ↑ erythrocyte sedimentation rate
    e. Tx = steroids
6. Subarachnoid hemorrhage (see Neurology, Section II.D.4)
    a. Described by patient as "worst headache of my life"
    b. Sudden occurrence caused by ruptured berry aneurysm
    c. **This is a medical emergency**
    d. Tx = neurosurgical evaluation & nimodipine to reduce incidence of postrupture vasospasm & ischemia

III. Eyes

A. Classic syndromes

1. Bitemporal hemianopsia (see Figure 2.1)
    a. Unable to see in bilateral temporal fields
    b. Usually caused by a pituitary tumor
2. Internuclear ophthalmoplegia
    a. **Classically found in multiple sclerosis**
    b. Lesion of median longitudinal fasciculus
    c. Presents with an inability to adduct the ipsilateral eye past midline (inability to perform conjugate gaze)
    d. Caused by lack of communication between contralateral cranial nerve (CN) VI nucleus & the ipsilateral CN III nucleus
3. Parinaud's syndrome
    a. Midbrain tectum lesion = bilateral paralysis of upward gaze
    b. Commonly associated with pineal tumor
4. Hyphema = blood in anterior chamber of eye, often due to trauma
5. Marcus Gunn pupil
    a. Due to afferent defect of CN II, pupil will not react to direct light but will react consensually when light is directed at the normal contralateral eye

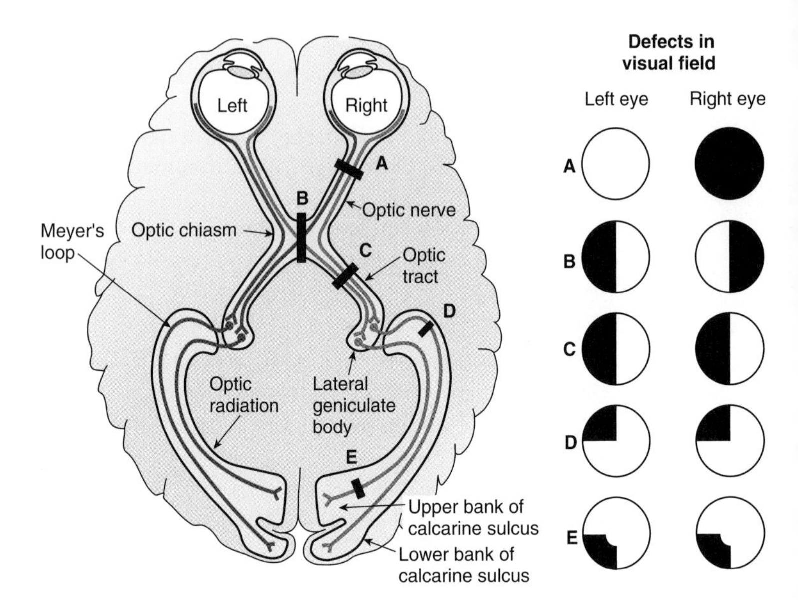

Figure 2.1 Visual Field Deficits
Lesions in the visual system are correlated with specific visual field deficits. **A.** Blindness in the right eye. **B.** Bitemporal heteronymous hemianopsia. **C.** Left homonymous hemianopsia. **D.** Superior quadrantic anopia. **E.** Inferior quadrantic anopsia with macular sparing. (Reproduced with permission from Pritchard TC, Alloway KD. *Medical Neuroscience*. Madison, CT: Fence Creek Publishing, 1999:307. © Fence Creek Publishing, LLC.)

b. **Characterized by ⊕ swinging flashlight test**
   (1) Swing penlight quickly back & forth between eyes
   (2) Denervated pupil will not constrict to direct light & **will actually dilate when light is shined in it** because it is dilating back to baseline when consensual light is removed from other eye

6. Argyll-Robertson pupil
   a. **Pathognomonic for tertiary syphilis (neurosyphilis)**
   b. Pupils constrict with accommodation, but do not constrict to direct light stimulation (pupils accommodate but do not react)
7. Lens dislocation
   a. Occurs in homocystinuria & Marfan's & Alport's syndromes
   b. Lens dislocates superiorly in Marfan's syndrome, inferiorly in homocystinuria, & variably in Alport's syndrome

8. Kayser-Fleischer ring
   a. **Pathognomonic for Wilson's disease** (see Neurology, Section VIII.E)
   b. Finding is a ring of golden pigment around the iris

B. Palpebra
   1. Chalazion = internal inflammation of meibomian sebaceous gland
   2. Hordeolum (stye) = inflammation of sebaceous glands of Zeiss or Moll
   3. Xanthelasma = painless yellow plaques occurring near inner canthi on eyelids, frequently associated with hypercholesterolemia

C. Conjunctiva
   1. Conjunctivitis (red eye) (see Table 2.2)
   2. Xerophthalmia (dry eyes)
      a. Vitamin A deficiency
         (1) Causes xerophthalmia and may be accompanied by **Bitot's spots, which represent areas of**

Table 2.2 Conjunctivitis

Type	Organisms	Sx	Tx
Bacterial	*Streptococcus pneumoniae*, *Staphylococcus* spp., *Haemophilus*, gonococcus, *Chlamydia trachomatis* (in neonates, sexually active adults)	**Purulent discharge, rarely itch,** conjunctival infection—gonococcus is only bacteria that causes preauricular adenopathy	Topical sulfacetamide or erythromycin
Viral ("pink eye")	Adenovirus most common, others = HSV, Varicella, EBV, Influenza, Echovirus, Coxsackie	**Preauricular adenopathy, rarely itch**, watery discharge (adenovirus → pharyngeal-conjunctival fever = fever ⊕ conjunctivitis ⊕ pharyngitis)	No treatment required, self-limiting disease
Allergic	n/a	**Marked pruritus**, bilateral watery eyes	antihistamine, steroid drops

desquamated, keratinized conjunctival cells, together with lipid material

(2) Tx = Vitamin A replacement & artificial tear drops

b. Sjögren's syndrome (see Musculoskeletal, Section IV.C)

(1) Causes **keratoconjunctivitis sicca (KS)**

(a) KS = lack of tears during Schirmer test

(b) Schirmer test = place filter paper over lower eyelid, if not wet in 15min confirms Dx of keratoconjunctivitis sicca

(2) Tx = apply artificial tear drops

D. Cornea

1. Corneal abrasion

a. Often results from direct trauma to eye

b. Eye is red, painful, tearing & photophobia are present

c. Dx = fluorescein to stain areas of corneal defect

d. Tx = topical antibiotics & oral analgesics

e. Cornea usually heals in 24–48 hours, should reexamine pt the next day

2. Corneal ulceration

a. Due to bacteria, fungi, amebae, or viruses

b. Often occurs in contact lens wearers

c. Lesion visible with fluorescein dye, pain/photophobia may be minimal

d. **Hypopyon (pus in anterior chamber) is a grave sign**

e. Healing of ulcer leads to fibrosis that can impair vision

f. **This is an emergency! Get ophthalmology consult now!**

3. Keratitis (inflammation of cornea)

a. Viral

(1) Acute keratitis usually caused by adenovirus or herpes simplex virus

(2) **Herpes shows characteristic dendritic branching on fluorescein staining**

(3) Multiple recurrences lead to corneal anesthesia, ulceration & permanent scar

(4) Tx = topical antiviral: vidarabine or idoxuridine

b. Bacterial

(1) Usually caused by extended wear contact lenses/corneal trauma

(2) Most common pathogens are *Pseudomonas aeruginosa*, *Streptococcus pneumonia*, *Moraxella* spp., & *Staphylococcus* spp.

(3) **This is an emergency! Get ophthalmology consult now!**

E. Scleritis/uveitis

1. Scleritis
   a. Extremely painful, often associated with collagen-vascular disease (dz)
   b. Risk of perforation of sclera, resulting in loss of the eye
   c. Tx = systemic cortisol ⊕ cyclophosphamide if underlying rheumatic condition is present
2. Uveitis
   a. Defined as inflammation of the iris, ciliary body, &/or choroid (all together = the uvea)
   b. Signs (Si)/Sx = hazy vision, black floating spots, can have pain & photophobia
   c. **This is an emergency**, as retinal detachment & acute glaucoma can rapidly onset
   d. 40% of time, uveitis is related to a systemic disease
   e. Associated systemic diseases
      (1) Autoinflammatory diseases = ankylosing spondylitis, Reiter's syndrome, Behçet's syndrome & sarcoidosis (see Musculoskeletal, Section IV.D, E, & I for these dzs)
      (2) Infections = toxoplasmosis, cytomegalovirus (CMV), toxocariasis, histoplasmosis, tuberculosis (TB), syphilis
      (3) Inflammatory bowel disease

F. Glaucoma

1. Major cause of blindness in the aging
2. Related to increased intraocular pressure (↑ 21 mm Hg) causing damage to retina & optic nerve
3. Can be open or closed type
   a. Open-angle glaucoma
      (1) Chronic condition caused by decreased permeability of trabeculae leading into canal of Schlemm
      (2) **Rarely causes pain or corneal edema**
      (3) Blindness begins at periphery of vision, gradually spans more of the visual field
      (4) Usually presents after 30 years of age
      (5) **On funduscopic examination, classic finding is increase in size of optic cup (> 1/2 size of disk)**
      (6) Tx = cholinomimetics, α-agonists, β-blockers, acetazolamide, or laser surgery to open additional spaces near Schlemm's canal to ease fluid outflow

b. Closed-angle glaucoma
   (1) Can be chronic or acute, the latter is an emergency
   (2) Typically idiopathic, can be drug induced (mydriatics)
   (3) Mydriatics cause the iris to move forward & occlude the aqueous fluid outflow tract (canal of Schlemm)
   (4) Prodromal Sx = sudden pain in eye & head, halos around light sources, ↓ vision
   (5) **Acute attack causes severe throbbing pain in eye,** radiating to CN V distribution, ↓ vision, nausea/vomiting, fixed, mid-dilated pupil
   (6) **This is considered an emergency because blindness can quickly occur**
   (7) Tx = IV mannitol & acetazolamide, & topical timolol, pilocarpine NOT recommended (can exacerbate condition)—surgery follows to prevent future occurrence

G. Retina
1. Retinal artery occlusion by emboli causes sudden, unilateral blindness (can also present in temporal arteritis)
   a. Pupil is sluggish to respond to direct light stimulation, but will respond normally to consensual light
   b. Fovea will often contain a cherry-red spot
2. Central retinal vein occlusion
   a. Associated with diabetes, glaucoma
   b. Physical finding = tortuous distended veins & numerous retinal hemorrhages
   c. Presents with painless, gradual loss of vision
3. Diabetic retinopathy
   a. Generally occurs after 10 year of diabetes, presents as background or proliferative type
   b. Background type
      (1) See flame hemorrhages, microaneurysms, & soft exudates (cotton wool spots)
      (2) Tx = strict glucose & hypertension control
   c. Proliferative type
      (1) More advanced disease, characterized by neovascularization easily visible around the fundus (hyperemia) & hard exudates
      (2) Tx = photocoagulation (laser ablation of retinal blood vessels), which slows disease progression but is not curative

4. Age-related macular degeneration (AMD)
   a. AMD causes painless loss of visual acuity
   b. Dx by altered pigmentation in macula
   c. Tx = ↓ sun exposure, antioxidants
   d. Pts tend to retain only peripheral vision
5. Retinal detachment
   a. Presents with painless, dark vitreous floaters, flashes of light (photopsias), blurry vision, eventually progressing to a curtain of blindness in vision as detachment worsens
   b. Tx = urgent surgical reattachment
6. Retinitis pigmentosa
   a. Slowly progressive defect in night vision (often starts in young children) with ring-shaped scotoma (blind spot) that gradually ↑ in size to obscure more vision
   b. Disease is hereditary with unclear transmission mode
   c. May be part of the Laurence-Moon-Biedl syndrome (see Endocrinology, Section IV.C.3)
   d. There is no treatment
7. Classic physical findings of retina
   a. **Leukocoria** = absent red reflex, actually appears white, seen in retinoblastoma
   b. **Roth spots** = small hemorrhagic spots in retina associated with endocarditis
   c. **Copper wiring, flame hemorrhages, A-V nicking** seen in subacute hypertension &/or atherosclerosis
   d. **Cotton wool spots** (soft exudates) seen in chronic hypertension
   e. Papilledema appears as disk hyperemia, blurring & elevation, associated with ↑ intracranial pressure
   f. Neovascularization in a "sea fan" formation seen in sickle cell anemia
   g. Wrinkles seen on retina/folding of retinal sheet seen in retinal detachment
   h. **Cherry-red spot on macula** seen in Tay-Sachs, Niemann-Pick's disease, central retinal artery occlusion
   i. Hollenhorst plaque = yellow cholesterol emboli in retinal artery
   j. Pigmented "freckle" on retina increasing in size over time = intraocular malignant melanoma

H. Neuritis
   1. Retrobulbar neuritis
      a. Caused by inflammation of the optic nerve, usuallyunilateral
      b. **Classically seen in multiple sclerosis, may be the initial sign**
      c. Presents with rapid loss of vision & pain upon moving eye, spontaneously remitting within 2 to 8 weeks
      d. Funduscopic examination is nonrevealing
      e. Each relapse damages the nerve more, until eventually blindness results
      f. Treatment is with corticosteroids
   2. Optic neuritis
      a. Inflammation of optic nerve within the eye
      b. Causes include viral infection, multiple sclerosis, vasculitis, methanol, meningitis, syphilis, tumor metastases
      c. Presents with variable loss of vision & loss of pupillary light reflex
      d. **Funduscopic examination reveals hyperemia**
      e. If patient is older than 60, strongly consider temporal arteritis as Dx, confirm with temporal artery biopsy
      f. Treatment is with corticosteroids

I. Eye colors
   1. **Red eye** seen in conjunctivitis, corneal abrasion, uveitis, foreign body, chemical burns, acute closed-angle glaucoma
   2. **Yellow eye** (icterus) from bilirubin staining of sclera (jaundice), yellow vision → digitalis toxicity
   3. **Blue sclera** classically found in osteogenesis imperfecta & Marfan's disease (see Musculoskeletal, Sections II.D & IV.G)
   4. **Opaque eye** due to cataract
      a. Opacity of lens severe enough to interfere with vision
      b. Causes = congenital, diabetes (sorbitol precipitation in lens), galactosemia (galactitol precipitation in lens), Hurler's disease (defect in iduronidase → mucopolysaccharide precipitation in lens) (see Appendix B: Hurler's dz)

IV. Ears

A. Otitis
   1. Otitis externa
      a. Defined as infection of external auditory meatus
      b. Usually caused by *Pseudomonas* infection

c. **Dx = pulling on pinna/pushing on tragus causes pain**
d. Differential diagnosis (DDx) = Ramsay Hunt syndrome (herpes zoster otiticus)
   (1) Herpes infection of geniculate ganglia (CN VII)
   (2) Si/Sx = painful vesicles in external auditory meatus

2. Otitis media
   a. Defined as inflammation of middle ear space
   b. Dx = fever, erythema of tympanic membrane (TM), bulging of the pars flaccida portion of the TM, opacity of the TM, otalgia
   c. Effusions can also be seen as meniscus of fluid behind the TM
      (1) Indicative of poor drainage of eustachian tubes
      (2) Otitis media with effusion common in young children due to their eustachian tubes being smaller & more horizontal, making drainage more difficult
   d. Pathogens = *S. pneumoniae, Haemophilus influenzae, Moraxella catarrhalis*
   e. Often due to viral infection
   f. Tx = amoxicillin (first line), amoxicillin/clavulanate potassium (Augmentin), or trimethoprim/sulfamethoxazole (Bactrim; second line)
   g. If chronic effusions are present, surgical placement of pressure equalization tubes used as a last resort

3. Bullous myringitis
   a. Associated with *Mycoplasma* infection of inner ear
   b. Presents with large, bulging tympanic membrane
   c. Tx = erythromycin

4. Unilateral serous otitis media
   a. Presents in adults, caused by nasopharyngeal carcinoma obstructing the eustachian tube
   b. Dx = magnetic resonance imaging of head
   c. Tx = surgical resection &/or radiation therapy

B. Tumors

1. Cholesteatoma
   a. Most common growth in middle ear
   b. Can be congenital or acquired
   c. It is an epithelial cyst that contains desquamated keratin & is often associated with inflammation (typically presents after chronic otitis media episodes)
   d. *Pseudomonas* can infect the keratin debris

e. If left untreated it can destroy bone & cause deafness & unilateral facial nerve paralysis
f. Tx = surgical removal

2. Glomus tumors (paragangliomas)
a. Most common true neoplasm of middle ear (glomus tympanicum)
b. Present with pulsatile tinnitus, lateral neck mass
c. Usually benign, can be associated with catecholamine release

3. Cholesterol granuloma
a. **Diagnostic dark bluish color of tympanic membrane without any prior trauma** (idiopathic hemotympanum)
b. Bluish color due to foreign body reaction to cholesterol crystals

C. Inner ear disease

1. Tinnitus (ringing in the ears)
a. Can be objective (heard by observer) or subjective (heard only by patient)
b. Can be caused by foreign bodies in external canal, pulsating vascular tumors, or medications

2. Vertigo
a. Defined as feeling as though surroundings are spinning when the eyes are open
b. Different from dizziness (dizziness = pt feels as if he/she is spinning, not the surroundings)
c. Causes of vertigo
(1) **Benign paroxysmal positional vertigo**
(a) Sudden episode of vertigo with head movement
(b) Episodes may only **last for seconds**
(c) May be related to otolith displacement in inner ear
(2) **Ménière's disease** (see Figure 2.2)
(a) Dilation of membranous labyrinth of ear, related to excess endolymph
(b) **Classic triad = hearing loss, tinnitus, & episodic vertigo lasting several hours**
(c) No cure, Tx is medical (anticholinergics, antihistamines, barbiturates, or diazepam) or surgical (labyrinthectomy or vestibular neurectomy)
(3) **Viral labyrinthitis**
(a) Preceded by viral illness
(b) Symptoms of vertigo **lasting days to weeks**
(c) Tx = meclizine

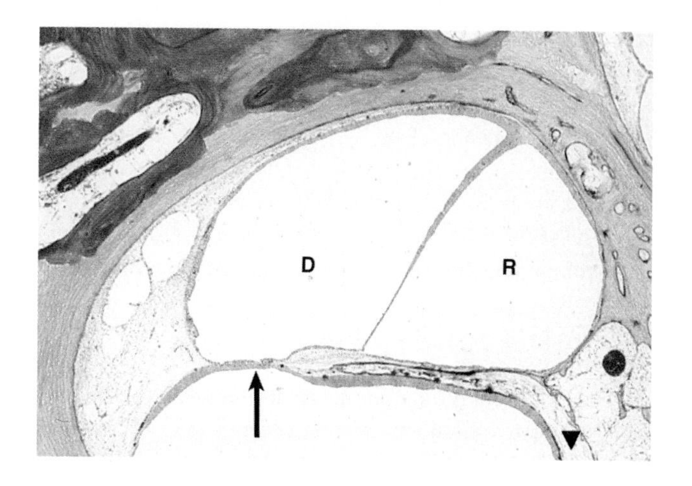

Figure 2.2 Ménière Disease
The cochlear duct (D) is markedly distended and the Reissner membrane (R) is pushed back by endolymphatic hydrops. Neither the organ of Corti (*arrow*) nor the spiral ganglion (*arrowhead*) is in its usual location. (From Rubin E, Gorstein F, Rubin R, et al. *Rubin's Pathology: Clinicopathologic Foundations of Medicine.* 4th ed. Baltimore: Lippincott Williams & Wilkins, 2005.)

(4) Acoustic neuroma
  (a) Benign tumor of the cerebellopontine angle (CN VIII) commonly arising from sheath of Schwann (schwannoma)
  (b) More commonly affects vestibular portion of CN VIII, but can also affect cochlear portion
  (c) Sx = vertigo, deafness, tinnitus, asymmetric hearing loss; also asymptomatic initially in some patients
  (d) Common in neurofibromatosis

D. Hearing loss
  1. Sensorineural hearing loss
    a. Due to damage beyond oval window (internal ear), affecting hair cells in cochlea or nerve fibers of CN VIII
    b. Alport's syndrome (see Table 7.4)
      (1) Sx = Sensorineural hearing loss, lens dislocation, hematuria
      (2) Disease related to thinning glomerular basement membrane in glomerulonephritis

c. Congenital: caused by exposure of fetus to rubella or syphilis
d. Elderly: bilateral high frequency sensorineural hearing loss

2. Conductive hearing loss
   a. Due to damage affecting middle ear or external ear
   b. Examples include otitis media, excess cerumen, otosclerosis, or perforated tympanic membrane
3. Combined hearing loss can be seen in chronic middle ear infection
4. 2 tests of hearing on physical examination
   a. Weber's test
      (1) Vibrating tuning fork is placed midline on top of head
      (2) Lateralization of hearing to one ear more than the other indicates ipsilateral conductive loss or contralateral sensorineural loss
   b. Rinne's test
      (1) Vibrating tuning fork placed next to ear, then when no longer heard placed against mastoid process until no longer heard
      (2) Normally air conduction should persist twice as long as bone conduction
      (3) Positive Rinne = the patient cannot hear the tuning fork placed against bone (this is the normal finding)
      (4) Negative Rinne = bone conduction is heard longer than air conduction, indicating a conductive hearing loss in that ear

V. Nose, Sinus, Face

A. Congenital disorders

1. Choanal atresia
   a. Caused by lack of orifice connecting external naris & nasopharynx
   b. **Classic presentation = cyanotic newborn whose hypoxia abates only during crying** (babies are involuntary nose breathers, but crying forces mouth breathing)
   c. Tx = surgery
2. Kartagener's syndrome
   a. Immotile cilia syndrome due to absence of dynein arms
   b. Patients infertile (sperm do not work without dynein), with ↓ olfaction, sinusitis, bronchiectasis, & situs inversus

c. Frequent respiratory infections due to lack of mucociliary escalator

3. Osler-Weber-Rendu syndrome (hereditary hemorrhagic telangiectasia)
   a. Autosomal dominant disorder of diffuse telangiectasias on lips, skin & mucous membranes, & internal organs
   b. Sx = severe nosebleed, hemoptysis, massive GI bleeds
   c. Dx = unexplained GI bleeds ⊕ typical red/violet telangiectasias
   d. Tx is supportive, e.g., blood transfusions
4. Cystic fibrosis
   a. Can present with chronic & severe pansinusitis in children (*Pseudomonas* sp.)
   b. Dx by sweat chloride test in older children
   c. In infants & toddlers (up to 1–2 years) chloride sweat test is unreliable, Dx by genetic screening

B. Trauma

1. Epistaxis (nosebleed)
   a. 90% of bleeds occur at Kiesselbach's plexus (the arterial anastomosis at anterior nasal septum)
   b. **#1 cause of epistaxis in children is trauma (induced by exploring digits)**
   c. Also a classic presentation in children with bleeding disorders
2. Facial fractures
   a. LeFort fractures are the classic facial trauma fractures
   b. Look for mobile palate, fractures always involve the pterygoid plates
   c. 3 types of LeFort fractures
      (1) LeFort 1 = maxilla fracture
      (2) LeFort 2 = pyramidal fracture on nasofrontal suture line
      (3) LeFort 3 = total craniofacial dysjunction
3. Basilar skull fractures
   a. **Present with 4 classic physical findings: raccoon's eyes & Battle's sign, hemotympanum, cerebrospinal fluid rhinorrhea, and otorrhea**
   b. Raccoon's eyes are dark circles (bruising) around the eyes, signifying orbital fractures
   c. Battle's sign is ecchymoses over the mastoid process, indicating a fracture there

C. Tumors
   1. Juvenile angiofibroma
      a. Benign vascular tumor causing unilateral epistaxis, usually seen in teenage boys
      b. Tx = radiation therapy or embolization & excision
   2. Polyps
      a. Nasal & sinus polyps are commonly caused by allergy, asthma, & infection
      b. These polyps can obstruct airway & also cause chronic sinus infections
      c. Tx = steroid nasal sprays &/or surgical excision

D. Facial nerve disorders
   1. Bell's palsy
      a. Idiopathic acute facial nerve paralysis, usually unilateral & self-limiting
      b. Can cause exposure keratitis
         (1) Inflammation secondary (2°) to dry eyes caused by inability to close eyelids
         (2) Tx = artificial tears or surgical closure of the eyelids
   2. Bilateral facial paralysis
      a. An unusual disorder with a limited differential diagnosis
      b. DDx = Lyme disease, sarcoidosis, temporal bone fractures, or Möbius syndrome (congenital facial paralysis & cranial nerve agenesis), Guillain-Barré, basilar meningitis, Wegener's

E. Sinusitis
   1. Maxillary sinuses most commonly involved
   2. Acute (< 4 weeks)
      a. Most common organisms are *S. pneumoniae, H. influenzae, M. catarrhalis*
      b. Sx = purulent rhinorrhea, headache, pain on sinus palpation, pressure, fever, halitosis, anosmia, periorbital edema, tooth pain
      c. Trimethoprim/sulfamethoxazole vs. amoxicillin/clavulanate potassium, decongestants
   3. Chronic (> 3 months)
      a. Most common organisms are *Bacteroides, Streptococcus* spp., *S. aureus, Pseudomonas*
      b. Sx = same as for acute but last longer, also look for otitis media in children

c. Tx = surgical correction of any meatal obstruction, nasal steroids, antibiotics only for acute exacerbations

4. Fungal
   a. Most common organisms are *Aspergillus* spp., **& in diabetics think Mucormycosis!**
   b. Usually seen in the immunocompromised
   c. Tx = surgery and amphotericin
5. Other causes: nasogastric tube, allergic rhinitis, rhinitis 2° to pregnancy, rhinitis medicamentosa (overuse of decongestants), & cocaine
6. Potential complications of sinusitis include meningitis, abscess formation, orbital infection, osteomyelitis

VI. Oromaxillary Disease

A. Congenital disorders

1. Hutchinson's teeth
   a. Notching of the permanent upper 2 incisors
   b. **Pathognomonic for congenital syphilis**
   c. **Part of Hutchinson's triad = notched teeth, keratitis, & deafness**
2. Cleft lip
   a. Can occur unilaterally or bilaterally
   b. **Unilateral cleft lip is the most common malformation of the head & neck**
   c. Caused by failure of fusion of maxillary prominences
3. Cleft palate
   a. Can be anterior or posterior (determined by position relative to incisive foramen)
   b. Anterior cleft palate due to failure of palatine shelves to fuse with primary palate
   c. Posterior cleft palate due to failure of palatine shelves to fuse with nasal septum
4. Macroglossia
   a. Congenitally enlarged tongue
   b. Occurs in amyloidosis, acromegaly, hypothyroidism, Down's syndrome
   c. This is different from glossitis (redness & swelling, with burning sensation), which is seen in vitamin B deficiencies

B. Infection/inflammation
   1. Herpes labialis (cold sores) usually due to herpes simplex virus type 1
   2. Aphthous stomatitis (canker sore) caused by iron, vitamin B12, or folate deficiency
   3. Oral candidiasis occurs in diabetics, immunocompromised, & is seen normally in young children
   4. Acute necrotizing gingivitis = "trench mouth" or "Vincent's infection"
      a. Caused by fusiform bacilli & spirochetes
      b. Sx/Si = malaise, ⊕/⊕ fever, painful/bleeding gingiva, fetid breath
      c. Dx = **punched-out lesion, gray membrane, bleed easily to touch is pathognomonic**
      d. Tx = débridement, analgesic, salt water rinse, penicillin if acute
   5. Ludwig's angina
      a. Cellulitis spreading from tooth infection
      b. Sx = edema/erythema of upper neck under the chin, can cause airway compromise due to swelling of tongue
      c. Tx = IV antibiotics, airway protection
   6. Fetor oris = foul-smelling breath, common in dental/tonsillar infections (peritonsillar abscess) & lung or sinus infections
   7. Trismus (lockjaw)
      a. Caused by spasm of muscles of mastication, so person has difficulty opening mouth
      b. Seen in tetanus & in other dzs that cause local or widespread muscle spasms: rabies, scleroderma, or tonsillar infection

C. Tumors
   1. Papilloma = most common tumor of oral mucosa, occurs in mouth
   2. Fibroma results from chronic irritation
   3. Epulis = benign tumor of gingivae, usually is reparative growth
   4. Leukoplakia = irregular white patches caused by hyperkeratosis 2° to chronic irritation
      a. Usually benign, rarely may be precancerous dysplasia
      b. **Note, oral hairy leukoplakia (OHL) is seen virtually exclusively in patients with human immunodeficiency virus**

   c. OHL = raised, white, patch with tiny hair-like spikes, caused by Epstein-Barr virus (EBV) or possibly other herpes
   d. Dx OHL = cannot scrape off with tongue blade, no response to antifungals, biopsy shows EBV⊕
5. Ameloblastoma = enamel precursor tumor, appears before age 35
6. **Most common oral cancer is squamous cell carcinoma, involves tongue in 50% cases, risks = smoking, alcohol,** chewing betel nuts

D. Salivary glands
1. Sialadenitis = inflammation of glands due to infection, inflammation, or sialolithiasis
2. Acute parotitis = mumps or other infection
   a. Mumps = paramyxovirus, spread by saliva droplet, more communicable than measles or chickenpox
      (1) Gland swelling lasts 5–9 days, incidence peaks in winter & early spring, usually in 5–15 year olds
      (2) Sx/Si = chills, anorexia, malaise, headache, low-moderate fever 12–24 hours before parotitis
      (3) During parotitis, temperature increases, painful chewing & swallowing
      (4) Prognosis excellent, Tx = symptomatic
      (5) Rare sequelae = orchitis, meningoencephalitis, Bell's palsy, pancreatitis
      (6) DDx = suppurative (strep/diphtheria/typhus), Mikulicz's syndrome, tumor, stone
   b. Mikulicz's syndrome = chronic, painless, parotid/lacrimal swelling, unknown etiology but occurs during TB, sarcoid, systemic lupus erythematosus, leukemia, & lymphosarcoma
3. Sjögren's syndrome can cause xerostomia & parotid swelling
4. Mucocele
   a. Cystic pool of mucus lined by granulation tissue, not epithelium, near salivary gland
   b. Results from leakage of damaged mucous ducts
5. Ranula = large mucocele of salivary gland at floor of the mouth
6. Salivary tumors usually occur in parotid gland
   a. **Most common salivary tumor is pleomorphic adenoma** (see Figure 2.3)
   b. Its proximity to facial nerve makes it difficult to remove

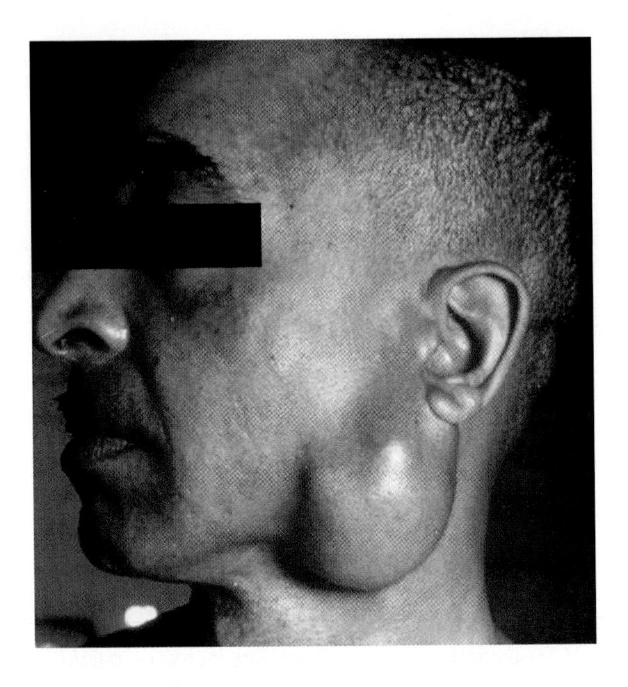

Figure 2.3 Pleomorphic Adenoma of the Parotid
A conspicuous tumor mass is seen at the angle of the jaw. (From Rubin E, Gorstein F, Rubin R, et al. *Rubin's Pathology: Clinicopathologic Foundations of Medicine*. 4th ed. Baltimore: Lippincott Williams & Wilkins, 2005.)

VII. Neck/Throat

A. Congenital disorders

1. Torticollis
   a. Lateral deviation of head due to hypertrophy of unilateral sternocleidomastoid
   b. Presents with rock hard knot in the sternocleidomastoid that is easy to confuse with the hyoid bone upon palpation
   c. Can be congenital or caused by neoplasm, infection, trauma, degenerative disease, or drug toxicity (particularly D_2 blockers = phenothiazines)
2. Thyroglossal duct cysts (see Endocrinology, Section V.B)
   a. **Midline** congenital cysts **usually present in childhood**
   b. **Dx by elevation of cysts upon swallowing**

3. Branchial cleft cysts
    a. **Lateral** congenital cysts **usually do not present until adult life** (they are present at birth, but are not noticed until they become infected or inflamed)
    b. Do NOT elevate upon swallowing
    c. Aspirate of cysts may contain cholesterol crystals, which is diagnostic
4. Cystic hygroma
    a. Occluded lymphatics that usually presents within first 2 years of life
    b. Presents as translucent, benign mass that is painless, soft, & compressible
5. Dermoid cyst
    a. Soft, fluctuant mass composed of an overgrowth of epithelium
    b. **No elevation with swallowing**
6. Carotid body tumor (paraganglioma)
    a. Not a vascular tumor, but originates from neural crest cells in the carotid body within the carotid sheath
    b. Palpable mass at bifurcation of common carotid artery
    c. Pressure on tumor can cause bradycardia & dizziness
    d. Vasoactive amines can occasionally be released from tumor causing hypertension & pupillary dilation
    e. Metastasis can occur upward along carotid sheath
    f. **Rule of 10: 10% malignant, 10% familial, 10% secrete catecholamines**

B. Pharyngitis/tonsillitis (sore throat)
1. Waldeyer's ring
    a. Oropharyngeal lymphoid tissue comprised of adenoids, lateral pharyngeal bands, palatine tonsil, lingual tonsils
    b. Common sites of inflammation
2. Bacterial
    a. *S. pyogenes* (group A strep) & *Staphylococcus* most common organisms
    b. Presents with severe pain in throat, temperatures of 103°F or more, mucosa is bright red, edematous, white or yellow exudate can be seen on tonsils
    c. Tx = penicillin
3. Membranous (diphtheria)
    a. Caused by *Corynebacterium diphtheriae*

b. **Pathognomonic physical finding = a patch of gray membrane on the tonsils extending down into the throat**
c. Potential consequences include airway occlusion by membrane & myocarditis
d. **Tx is antitoxin as quickly as possible!!!**
e. Antibiotics (erythromycin) are given to reduce bacterial load

4. Fungal
    a. Oral thrush or moniliasis, caused by *Candida* spp.
    b. Presents with white, cheesy patches on pharynx, tongue, & buccal mucosa (see Figure 2.4)
    c. Common in AIDS patients
    d. Tx = nystatin liquid, swish around mouth & swallow

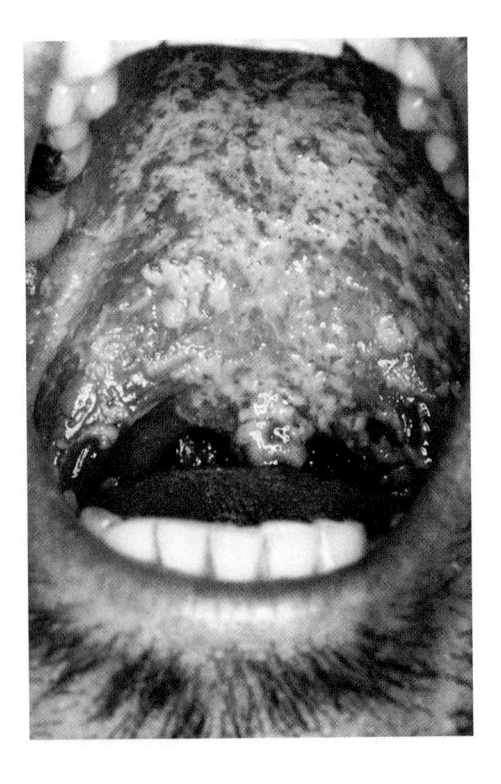

Figure 2.4 Candidiasis
The oral cavity of a patient with AIDS is covered by a white, curdlike exudate containing numerous fungal organisms. (From Rubin E, Gorstein F, Rubin R, et al. *Rubin's Pathology: Clinicopathologic Foundations of Medicine*. 4th ed. Baltimore: Lippincott Williams & Wilkins, 2005.)

5. Viral
   a. Adenovirus
      (1) Infects mucosa of respiratory tract, gastrointestinal tract, & conjunctiva
      (2) Causes pharyngoconjunctival fever, a self-limiting dz
   b. EBV
      (1) Infectious mononucleosis is difficult to distinguish from strep throat
      (2) More systemic findings are typically seen in mononucleosis
         (a) Si = generalized lymphadenopathy, exudative tonsillitis, palatal petechiae, & splenomegaly, **atypical lymphocytes** seen on blood smear (see Figure 2.5)
         (b) Lab testing shows ⊕ **heterophile antibody** in contrast to mononucleosis caused by CMV, which is heterophile antibody–negative
         (c) **Skin rash** commonly occurs in patients mistakenly treated with antibiotics (penicillin, ampicillin)
   c. Parainfluenza virus
      (1) The major cause of laryngotracheobronchitis (croup)
      (2) Seen mostly in children younger than 5 years

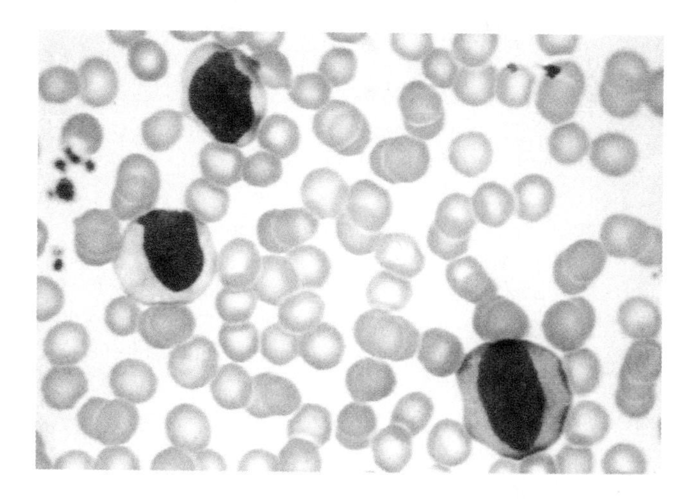

Figure 2.5 Infectious Mononucleosis
Atypical lymphocytes are characteristic. (From Rubin E, Gorstein F, Rubin R, et al. *Rubin's Pathology: Clinicopathologic Foundations of Medicine.* 4th ed. Baltimore: Lippincott Williams & Wilkins, 2005.)

(3) **Presents with barking cough worse at night**, pharyngitis, inspiratory stridor
(4) **Classic x-ray finding is a steeple sign on anterior x-ray of neck**

d. Coxsackie A virus
(1) Causes herpangina
(a) Classic presentation is sudden fever, pharyngitis, & body ache
(b) 2 days after onset, tender vesicles erupt along tonsillar pillars, uvula, & soft palate
(c) Vesicles ulcerate after several days
(2) Occurs in epidemics in infants & children
(3) Self-limiting disease, Tx = symptomatic

C. Epiglottitis
1. Presents in children, caused by *H. influenzae* type B
2. Rare now due to efficacy of HiB vaccine
3. Presents with acute airway obstruction, stridor, drooling, fever, dysphagia
4. Rarely seen in adults, usually caused by *S. pneumonia*
5. Classic x-ray finding is "**thumb sign**" on lateral neck film
6. Tx = immediate airway intubation, antibiotics

D. Quinsy peritonsillar abscess
1. Loculation of pus in the space that surrounds a tonsil
2. May be related to previous tonsillar infection, dental caries, or allergies
3. May be caused by anaerobic bacteria, but mostly caused by same agents seen in pharyngitis & tonsillitis
4. Physical examination
a. Pts have fever, drooling, odynophagia, trismus, & a muffled voice
b. Soft palate & uvula are displaced and a peritonsillar fluctuant swelling that is extremely painful to touch is noted
5. Tx = Ear, nose and throat specialist consult, incision & drainage, antibiotic treatment

E. Cervical lymphadenitis
1. Enlarged lymph nodes in neck
2. Bilateral lymphadenopathy is usually viral
3. Unilateral lymphadenopathy is usually bacterial
a. Common organisms include *S. aureus* & group A & B strep (*pyogenes* & *agalactiae*)

   b. Differentiate from cat scratch fever, often caused by *Bartonella henselae*, which is inoculated into patient after scratch by young cats
4. Hodgkin's lymphoma can also present unilaterally
5. Scrofula = localized lymphadenopathy related to TB infection
6. ***Actinomyces israelii* → localized cervical nodes that have bright red sinuses & drain pus containing "sulfur granules"**
7. Kawasaki's syndrome also causes cervical lymphadenopathy (see Dermatology, Section VIII.B)

3. CARDIOVASCULAR

I. Atherosclerosis

A. Pathologic characteristics
   1. Affects medium & large arteries, arteriosclerosis affects end-arterioles
   2. Subintima thickens & encroaches upon vessel lumen, plaque develops in the media
   3. Plaque has specific pathologic structure
      a. Core contains lipids, necrotic debris, macrophages (foam cells), lymphocytes
      b. Core covered by a fibrous cap made of smooth muscle (SM) cells & collagen
      c. Rupture of debris through cap exposes subendothelial layer of vessels to coagulation cascade, allowing acute thrombus to occur in already narrowed vessel

B. Etiology
   1. Etiology unknown, but at least 2 mechanisms likely
   2. Low-density lipoprotein (LDL) hypothesis
      a. LDL within the media is oxidized by endothelial cells
      b. Oxidized LDL (ox-LDL) activates macrophages that secrete inflammatory mediators causing tissue damage
      c. ox-LDL also stimulates SM cell proliferation
   3. Endothelial cell (EC) damage hypothesis
      a. A priori damage to ECs exposing vessel wall to blood
      b. Platelets adhere to denuded vessel wall, secrete factors causing inflammation & SM proliferation
   4. Models likely coexist, e.g., ox-LDL is known to damage ECs

C. Cholesterol
   1. LDL levels are directly related to risk of coronary artery disease (CAD), while high-density lipoproteins (HDLs) are inversely related **(HDL is protective)**
   2. HDL ↓ by smoking, obesity, inactivity (exercise ↑ HDL), steroids
   3. Saturated fat intake correlates with ↑ serum LDL much better than cholesterol intake
   4. Coronary risk ratio = total cholesterol/HDL, ratio > 5.0 indicates ↑ risk of heart disease

II. Hypertension

A. Definition

BP ≥ 140/90 mm Hg measured on 3 separate days

B. Causes

1. 95% of all hypertension (HTN) is idiopathic, called **"essential HTN"**
2. The remainder are called "secondary (2°) HTN"
3. Most of 2° HTN causes can be divided into 3 organ systems
   a. Cardiovascular
      (1) Aortic regurgitation & patent ductus arteriosus cause a **wide pulse pressure** (systolic–diastolic)
      (2) Coarctation of the aorta characterized by HTN in upper extremities with **weak lower extremity pulses & normal-to-low BP in lower extremities**
   b. Renal causes (see Nephrology, Sections IV & V)
      (1) **Glomerular disease (dz)** (diabetic nephropathy, focal segmental glomerulosclerosis, & any glomerulonephritis) **that commonly present with proteinuria**
      (2) **Renal artery stenosis**, suspect in **refractory HTN** in older men due to atherosclerosis or young women due to fibromuscular dysplasia
      (3) Polycystic kidneys (see Nephrology, Section VIII)
   c. Endocrine causes (see Endocrinology, Sections III.B,D,E)
      (1) Any disorder of ↑ steroids, typically **Cushing's & Conn's syndromes, which should be suspected if HTN is accompanied by significant hypokalemia** due to excess aldosterone activity
      (2) Pheochromocytoma, which is accompanied by episodic, severe autonomic symptoms
      (3) Acromegaly
      (4) Hyperthyroidism, which **can present with isolated systolic HTN** (wide pulse pressure)
4. 2° HTN also may be iatrogenic
   a. Medications that cause HTN include oral contraceptives, glucocorticoids, phenylephrine, nonsteroidal anti-inflammatory drugs (NSAIDs)
   b. "White coat HTN" is a common cause of factitious HTN, where patient's BP ↑ in doctor's office 2° to anxiety

C. Malignant hypertension
  1. Can be hypertensive urgency or emergency
  2. Hypertensive urgency
     a. High blood pressure (BP) (e.g., systolic > 200 mm Hg or diastolic > 110 mm Hg, but numbers vary depending upon source) **without evidence of end-organ damage**
     b. Treatment (Tx) = oral BP medications with goal of slowly reducing BP over several days
  3. Hypertensive emergency
     a. Defined as severe HTN with evidence of end organ compromise (e.g., encephalopathy, renal failure, congestive heart failure [CHF]/ischemia)
     b. Signs/symptoms (Si/Sx) = mental status changes, papilledema, focal neurologic findings, anuria, chest pain or evidence of CHF (e.g., lower extremity edema, elevated jugular venous pressure, rales on pulmonary examination)
     c. **This is a medical emergency and immediate therapy is needed**
     d. Tx = Nitroprusside or labetalol, **but do NOT lower blood pressure too quickly, or patient will have a stroke**

D. Hypertension treatment
  1. Lifestyle modifications first line in all patients who do not have comorbid conditions & whose HTN is not urgent or emergent
     a. Weight loss can significantly lower BP
     b. Exercise can lower BP independent of weight loss
     c. Eliminating alcohol & smoking can lower BP
     d. ↓ fat intake to ↓ risk of CAD; HTN is a cofactor for CAD
     e. Salt restriction helps lower BP in patients (pts) with fluid overload states (e.g., renal failure, CHF)
  2. Medications
     a. Indications
        (1) Failure of lifestyle modifications to control HTN in 6 months to 1 year (depending upon severity of HTN)
        (2) Immediate use necessary if comorbid organ disease present (e.g., stroke, angina, renal disease)
        (3) Immediate use in emergent or urgent hypertensive states
     b. First line choices
        (1) **No comorbid conditions: diuretics or β-blockers** (proven to ↓ mortality in HTN)
        (2) **Diabetes: angiotensin-converting enzyme (ACE)**

inhibitors, because these are proven to ↓ vascular, neurologic & retinal complications

(3) ↓ **left ventricular ejection fraction (HTN or not): ACE inhibitors** (proven to ↓ mortality)

(4) **Status post myocardial infarct: β-blockers & ACE inhibitors** (proven to ↓ mortality)

(5) **Osteoporosis**: thiazide diuretics (↓ Ca^{++} excretion)

(6) **Benign prostatic hypertrophy (BPH)**: α-blockers, will treat HTN & BPH concurrently

(7) **Pheochromocytoma**: α-blockers & excision of tumor

c. Contraindications

(1) **β-blockers in chronic obstructive pulmonary disease** due to associated bronchospasm

(2) **β-blockers relatively contraindicated in diabetes**, due to alteration in insulin/glucose homeostasis & blockade of autonomic response to hypoglycemia (which diabetics depend on to sense when they need a dose of glucose)

(3) **β-blockers in hyperkalemia**, due to propensity for ↑ serum potassium levels, particularly in diabetics

(4) **ACE inhibitors in pregnancy** due to teratogenicity

(5) **ACE inhibitors in renal artery stenosis** due to precipitation of acute renal failure (glomerular pressure dependent upon angiotensin-mediated constriction of efferent arteriole)

(6) **Diuretics in gout** due to causation of hyperuricemia

(7) **K^+-sparing diuretics & ACE inhibitors in renal failure (creatinine > 1.5)** due to hyperkalemia morbidity

(8) **Thiazide diuretics in diabetes** due to hyperglycemia

III. Ischemic Heart Disease (Coronary Artery Disease)

A. Risk factors for coronary artery disease

1. **Major risk factors (memorize these!!!)**
   a. Diabetes (may be the most important)
   b. Smoking
   c. Hypertension
   d. Hypercholesterolemia
   e. Family history

2. Minor risk factors: obesity, age, lack of estrogen (males or postmenopausal women not on estrogen replacement), homocystinuria
3. Smoking is the #1 preventable risk factor
4. Unlike diabetic microvascular disease (e.g., retinopathy, nephropathy, etc.) **there is no evidence that tight glucose control can diminish onset of CAD in diabetics**

B. Angina pectoris

1. Sx due to not enough blood flow to meet O_2 demand of heart
   a. Myocardial O_2 consumption depends on heart rate, BP, contractility
   b. Most common cause is CAD secondary to atherosclerosis
   c. Poor arterial supply leads to myocardial **ischemia, which on electrocardiography (ECG) appears as ST depression & T wave inversion**
   d. Cellular consequences of ischemia
      (1) ATP production ceases immediately ⇒ ↑ ADP & P_i, blocking actin-myosin cross-bridge relaxation
      (2) ↓ pH & ↑ P_i inhibit Ca binding to troponin, blocking force development
      (3) K^+ leaks out of ATP-K channel → ST ↓ on ECG & eventual conduction block 2° to cell hypopolarization
2. Classic Sx = precordial pain radiating to left arm, relieved by rest & nitroglycerin
   a. **Classic Sx often not present in elderly & diabetics who have neuropathies**
   b. Pain may radiate to a number of places, including jaw, back, abdomen, fingers, or right arm
   c. **↑ Sx frequency, progressive ↓ in exertion causing onset of pain & pain not relieved by rest are poor prognostic factors, indicating unstable angina, which presages myocardial infarct (MI)**
3. Prinzmetal's (variant) angina = **pain at rest, due to vasospasm, ECG shows ST elevation**
4. Differential diagnosis (DDx) = peptic ulcer disease, hiatal hernia, gastroesophageal spasm, cholecystitis, achalasia
5. Tx
   a. Give aspirin and β-blockers, and other medications as needed to control BP
   b. Quit smoking! (2 years after quitting, MI risk is the same as that in the general population)

c. ↓ LDL levels, ↑ HDL levels effective in MI prophylaxis
d. Achieve above by ↓ saturated fat intake (more important than actual cholesterol intake), ↑ exercise, ↑ fiber intake, stop smoking, lose weight, HMG-CoA reductase inhibitors
e. Folate
(1) ↑ serum homocysteine recently linked to MI, but link not universally agreed upon (may not be causal)
(2) Folate lowers homocysteine levels; however, in light of above its use is not yet generally recommended
f. Endovascular intervention
(1) Percutaneous transluminal coronary angioplasty (PTCA)
(2) Indicated with failure of medical management
(3) Lower risk morbidity than surgery but associated with up to 50% restenosis of artery within 6 months
(4) Placement of stent during angioplasty reduces restenosis rate to 20%–30%
g. Surgery
(1) Procedure is coronary artery bypass graft (CABG)
(2) Indications = failure of medical management & concurrent stenosis of right coronary artery, left anterior descending artery & left circumflex artery (3-vessel disease)
(3) Comparable mortality rates after several years with PTCA, except diabetic patients (do better with CABG)

C. Myocardial infarct
1. Infarct usually 2° to acute thrombosis in atherosclerotic vessel
2. Area of supply by each vessel determines extent of infarct
a. Left anterior descending artery supplies anterior wall of left ventricle (LV) & anterior 2/3 of septum
b. Left circumflex artery supplies lateral free wall
c. Right coronary artery (RCA) supplies right ventricle (RV), inferior wall of LV & posterior 1/3 of septum
d. Sinoatrial & atrioventricular nodes usually supplied by RCA, so RCA infarcts tend to cause bradycardia secondary to heart block
3. Pathologic consequences of ischemia/infarct
a. Myocyte death begins within 20–40 minutes of occlusion
b. Damaged tissue blocks electrical conduction → arrhythmia
c. Infarction of papillary muscles → valvular regurgitation
d. By 4–12 hours, polymorphonuclear neutrophils (PMNs) infiltrate & destroy dead tissue

e. Coagulation necrosis is visible at 12–18 hours
f. Macrophages & fibroblasts replace PMNs starting at 24–48 hours, & the fibrotic phase begins
g. Myocyte replacement by collagen → weakening of ventricular wall by day 4–5→ ventricular aneurysm
h. After 1 week, infarcted tissue changes from hyperemic to pale yellow, soft, well demarcated
i. Ventricular aneurysm (systolic bulge) develops from scar tissue replacing heart wall in 10–20% of pts with anterior MI
   (1) Diagnosis (Dx) = ST elevation on ECG days to weeks post MI
   (2) Sequelae = arrhythmia or aneurysmal rupture → sudden death

4. Diagnosis of infarct
   a. **ECG → ST elevation & Q waves (beware, non–Q-wave subendocardial infarcts → T-wave inversion ± ST depression)**
   b. CK-MB & myoglobin were standard of diagnosis, but now troponins are replacing them—**troponin I is more specific and as sensitive as CK-MB**
5. Treatment is to reestablish vessel patency
   a. Medical Tx = thrombolysis within 6 hours of the infarct by using **tissue plasminogen activator (TPA)** + **heparin** (first line) or streptokinase
   b. PTCA may be more effective, can open vessels mechanically or with local administration of thrombolytics
   c. CABG is longer term Tx, rarely used for acute process
   d. Adjuvant medical therapies
      (1) **#1 priority is aspirin! (proven to ↓ mortality)**
      (2) **#2 priority is β-blocker (proven to ↓ mortality)**
      (3) Statin drugs to lower cholesterol are essential **(LDL must be < 100 postinfarct**, proven to ↓ mortality)
      (4) Heparin should be given for 48 hours postinfarct **if TPA was used to lyse the clot** (heparin has no proven benefit if streptokinase was used or if no lysis was performed)
      (5) O_2 & morphine for pain control
      (6) Nitroglycerin dilates occluded artery, reducing both pre- & afterloads → ↓ myocardial O_2 demand
      (7) ACE inhibitors are excellent late/long-term therapy, ↓ afterload & prevent remodeling

(8) Exercise strengthens heart, develops collateral circulation, raises HDLs
(9) STOP SMOKING!!!!!!!!!!!!!!!!

IV. Selected Arrhythmias

A. Reentry

1. Requirements are 1) unidirectional block, 2) slow conduction, 3) retrograde conduction (some people combine #2 & #3)
2. Tissue damage causes the above requirements to be met
3. Macroreentry causes ventricular tachycardia
4. Microreentry causes ventricular fibrillation

B. Basic heart blocks (see Table 3.1)

1. Primary (1°) block
   a. **ECG → PR interval > 0.20 sec**
   b. Implies a conduction delay at the AV node

Table 3.1 Bradyarrhythmias

Complete (Third Degree) AV Block:	
First Degree AV Block:	
Mobitz Type II:	
Mobitz Type I: (Wenckebach Phenomenon)	
Sinus Bradycardia:	
2:1 AV Block:	

2. 2° block has 2 subtypes
   a. Mobitz type I ("Wenckebach block")
      (1) **ECG → PR intervals progressively ↑ from beat to beat**, until finally they become so long that beat cannot be conducted across AV node → beat is dropped
      (2) Following the dropped beat, the PR interval resets to baseline & then begins to progressively lengthen again from beat to beat until the next beat is dropped
   b. Mobitz type II
      (1) **EKG → PR interval fixed at > 0.20 seconds & there is a fixed ratio of dropped beats**
      (2) Described by number of QRS complexes occurring before each dropped beat
      (3) Example: pattern = 3:1 block when 3 QRS complexes occur before each dropped beat (3 QRS, skip beat, 3 QRS, skip beat, 3 QRS, skip beat, etc.)
3. Tertiary (3°) block
   a. This is a complete heart block
   b. **ECG → absolutely no relationship between the P–P intervals & the QRS intervals**
   c. The atrial rate is totally distinct from the ventricular rate

C. Atrial fibrillation (A-FIB) (see Table 3.2)
1. Pulse is **irregularly irregular, classic descriptor of a-fib**
2. Patient often perceives a-fib as chest discomfort/palpitations
3. A-fib results in stasis of blood in the atrium, predisposing to thrombus formation & subsequent collateral embolization
4. All patients with a-fib lasting 24–48 hours should be anticoagulated with warfarin (first line) (do this before electrical cardioversion to prevent embolization during cardioversion)
5. Rapid ventricular rate is prevented by medications that delay AV node conduction—e.g., digoxin, Ca-channel/β blockers
6. Conversion of a-fib to normal rhythm may be spontaneous, medically induced, induced by electrical cardioversion, or impossible depending on disease severity

D. Supraventricular tachycardia (SVT)
1. Supraventricular tachycardia (SVT) is a grab-bag of tachyarrhythmias originating "above the ventricle"
2. Pacer can be in atrium or at AV junction, & multiple pacers can be active at any one time (multifocal atrial tachycardia)

Table 3.2 Tachydysrhythmias

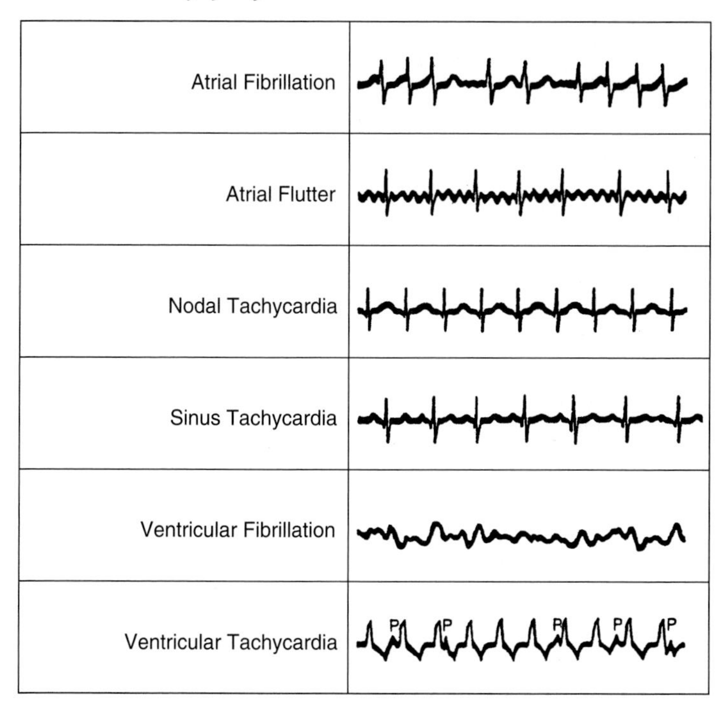

3. Differentiation of SVT from ventricular tachycardia requires careful ECG analysis; they cannot be distinguished clinically
4. Tx = resolution of underlying etiology (e.g., electrolyte imbalance), ventricular rate control (digoxin, Ca^{2++}-channel blocker, β-blocker) & electrical cardioversion in unstable pts

E. Ventricular tachycardia (V-TACH) (see Table 3.2)
   1. Defined as ≥ 3 consecutive premature ventricular contractions (PVCs)
   2. Sustained v-tach lasts minimum of 30 seconds, requires immediate intervention due to risk of onset of ventricular fibrillation (v-fib) (see below)
   3. First-line medical Tx is amiodarone or lidocaine, which can convert rhythm to normal; however, if pt unstable or hypotensive (obviously including those without pulses!), Tx is immediate electrical defibrillation

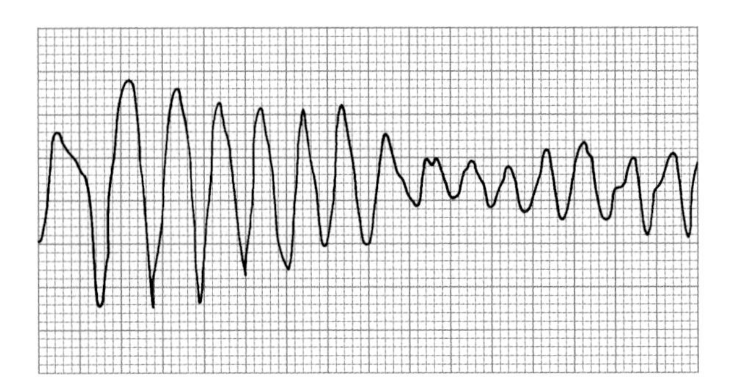

Figure 3.1 Torsades des Pointes

F. Torsades des pointes ("twisting of the points") (see Figure 3.1)
   1. A special ventricular tachyarrhythmia characterized by shifting sinusoidal waveforms on ECG, can progress to v-fib (see below)
   2. Anything that prolongs the QT interval predisposes to torsades
   3. This may be secondary to congenital long QT syndrome, but far more commonly is iatrogenic, due to drug toxicity
      a. Tricyclic antidepressants prolong the QT → torsades
      b. Quinidine (& other antiarrhythmics) may cause it
      c. Erythromycin causes it secondary to P450 interactions with other drugs, particularly antihistamines
      d. Can also be caused by electrolyte imbalances, including hypocalcemia & hypokalemia (can be diuretic induced)

G. Ventricular fibrillation (V-FIB)
   1. **Emergent electric countershock is the primary therapy** (very rarely precordial chest thump is effective), converts rhythm 95% of the time
   2. Second line is lidocaine or amiodarone
   3. Without Tx, natural course = total failure of cardiac output → death

V. Congestive Heart Failure

A. Etiologies and definition
   1. Definition = cardiac output insufficient to meet systemic demand, can have right, left, or both-sided failure

2. Causes = valve dz, MI (acute & chronic), HTN, anemia, pulmonary embolism, cardiomyopathy, thyrotoxicosis, endocarditis

B. Signs and symptoms are multiorgan
   1. Left-sided failure leads to pulmonary edema, **dyspnea on exertion, orthopnea, paroxysmal nocturnal dyspnea**
   2. Mitral regurgitation, due to heart dilation, worsens the ↓ in cardiac output
   3. Renal hypoperfusion → activation of renin-angiotensin axis → ↑ aldosterone → Na retention → ↑ in total body fluid load (see Figure 3.2)

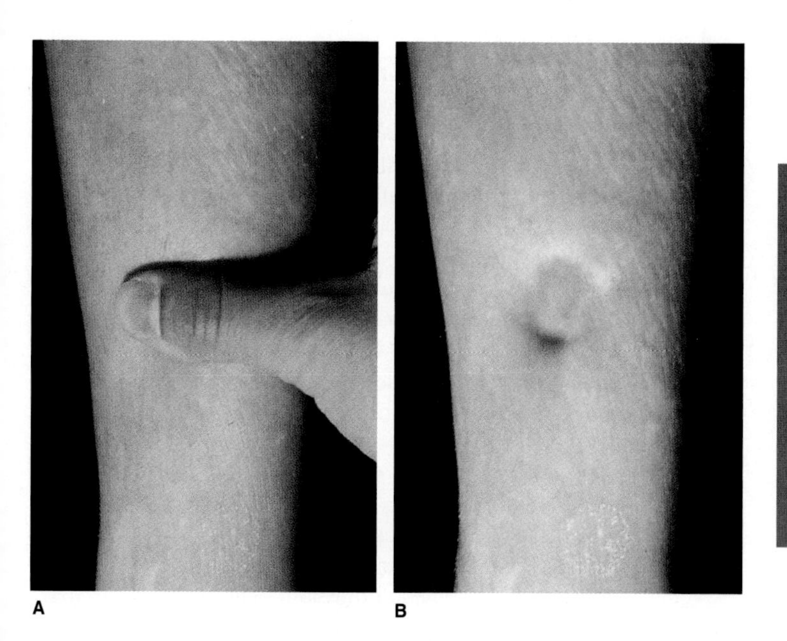

Figure 3.2 Pitting Edema of the Leg
A. In a patient with CHF, severe edema of the leg is demonstrated by applying pressure with a finger. **B.** The resulting "pitting" reflects the inelasticity of the fluid-filled tissue. (From Rubin E, Gorstein F, Rubin R, et al. *Rubin's Pathology: Clinicopathologic Foundations of Medicine*. 4th ed. Baltimore: Lippincott Williams & Wilkins, 2005.)

4. In right-sided failure (#1 cause is prior left-sided failure) lack of forward venous flow leads to liver engorgement with elevated transaminases (cardiac cirrhosis) & lower extremity edema
5. A-fib common in CHF, possibly due to dilated atria
   a. **Patients with a-fib lasting ≥48 hours should receive anticoagulant therapy unless contraindicated (coumadin first line, aspirin second line)**
   b. Beware of cerebrovascular accidents in these patients!!!
6. Myocardial failure leads to genetic transcriptional changes, including production of novel forms of myosin subunits ("**remodeling**")—this maladaptive response exacerbates disease but seems to be inhibited by ACE inhibitors & β-blockers

C. Treatment
1. Reduce physical activity
2. **ACE inhibitors (first line for CHF) & β-blockers** at least partially inhibit cardiac remodeling, improving long-term outcome, both also reduce afterload
3. Digitalis used in pts with a-fib, as the drug's cholinomimetic effects protect ventricular rate by slowing AV nodal conduction
4. **ACE inhibitors, β-blockers, and spironolactone have been proven to improve survival, while digitalis and loop diuretics palliate symptoms and decrease hospitalizations but have not been proven to increase survival**
5. Beware of giving loop/thiazide diuretics with digitalis—diuretics → hypokalemia, which can induce lethal digitalis toxicity, monitor K^+ levels carefully & give oral K^+ tablets to maintain K^+ within normal range
   a. Digitalis toxicity presents as supraventricular tachycardia with AV block & can cause yellow vision
   b. Tx acutely with antidigitalis FAB antibodies as well as correction of underlying potassium deficit
6. Aspirin or warfarin is used for thrombus prophylaxis

VI. Cardiomyopathy

A. Dilated cardiomyopathy
1. Can be diffuse (involving all 4 chambers) or nondiffuse

2. Causes are many & variable
    a. Ischemia due to CAD is common cause of diffuse disease
    b. Myocarditis can cause cardiomyopathy
        (1) **Coxsackievirus is most common infectious cause of myocarditis in US—presents suddenly after flu-like illness**
        (2) Chagas' disease (*Trypanosoma cruzi*) common in Central & South America
        (3) HIV causes it independent of other infection
        (4) Spirochetes (particularly Lyme disease)
        (5) *Bordetella pertussis* is a rare cause today
        (6) Granulomatous dz (sarcoid, Wegener's)
    c. Metabolic disorders
        (1) Malnutrition (kwashiorkor)
        (2) Genetic storage disorders
        (3) Uremia
        (4) Acromegaly
    d. Drugs can cause (**alcohol**, doxorubicin, adriamycin, azathioprine)
3. Dilation → ↓ ventricular function, with ↓ ejection fraction & cardiac output

B. Hypertrophic cardiomyopathy
1. Genetic disorder of myelin subunits, autosomal dominant
2. Results in stiff ventricle that does not stretch with increased preload, **this is a diastolic disease in contrast to dilated cardiomyopathy, which is a systolic disease**
3. ↓ compliance → ↑ coronary artery resistance (coronary flow maximal during diastole, when intraventricular pressure is lowest)
4. Causes angina due to inability of coronary arteries to meet demands of hypertrophied muscle
5. Sudden death often occurs in young people due to arrhythmias Tx with implantable defibrillator

C. Restrictive (fibrotic) cardiomyopathy
1. Caused by amyloidosis, scleroderma, hemochromatosis, Fabry's, Gaucher's & Loeffler's dz (eosinophilic pneumonia), sarcoidosis
2. Cell death → fibrosis → rigid, noncompliant ventricle
3. Like hypertrophic cardiomyopathy, it is a **diastolic disease**

D. Comparison of cardiomyopathies (see Table 3.3)

Table 3.3 Cardiomyopathy

	Dilated	Hypertrophic	Restrictive
Cause	Ischemic, infectious, metabolic, toxic	Genetic myosin disorder	Metabolic, autoimmune
Si/Sx	R & L heart failure, a-fib, S3 gallop, mitral regurgitation	Exertional syncope, angina, ECG → LVH, CXR → NI-sized heart (hypertrophy of ventricle walls comes at expense of chamber size)	Pulmonary HTN, S4 gallop, pulsus paradoxus (≥10 mm Hg drop in BP during inspiration), ECG shows low QRS voltage
Px	30% survival at 5 yr	5% annual mortality usually due to sudden death	30% survival at 5 yr
Tx	ACE inhibitors, vasodilators, diuretics	β-blockers (↓ HR & contractility → ↑ diastolic flow)	None

VII. Valvular Diseases

A. Mitral valve prolapse
   1. Seen in 7% of population, in vast majority is a benign finding in young people that is asymptomatic & eventually disappears
   2. Seen in Marfan's patients, but also in people who have normal variant laxity of connective tissue, e.g., double-jointed
   3. **Murmur: pathologic prolapse → late systolic murmur with midsystolic click (Barlow's syndrome)**, predisposing to regurgitation

B. Mitral valve regurgitation
   1. Seen in severe mitral valve prolapse, rheumatic fever, papillary muscle dysfunction (often 2° to MI) & endocarditis
   2. Results in dilation of left atrium, ↑ in LA pressure, leading to pulmonary edema/dyspnea
   3. See Table 3.4 for physical findings
   4. ECG
      a. 1 × 1 mm depression in P wave in V_1 indicative of left atrial enlargement
      b. Left ventricular hypertrophy (LVH) indicated by AVL ≥ 11mm tall &/or (S wave in V_1 + R wave in V_5) ≥ 35 mm

5. **Ortner's syndrome** is impingement of recurrent laryngeal nerve by the enlarging atrium, leading to hoarseness
6. Treatment with ACE inhibitors, vasodilators, diuretics, digoxin, consider surgery in severe cases

C. Mitral stenosis
1. Almost always due to prior rheumatic fever
2. Mitral valve restricted by commissural fusion
3. Decreased flow across the mitral valve leads to left atrial enlargement (LAE) & eventually to right heart failure
4. A-fib commonly present, beware of mural thrombus
5. Si/Sx = exertional dyspnea, orthopnea, hemoptysis, pulmonary edema, a-fib, Ortner's syndrome
6. See Table 3.4 for physical findings
7. ECG → LAE by voltage (see Section VII.B.4.a)
8. Tx = β-blockers to slow HR, digitalis for patients in a-fib to block ventricular response, anticoagulants for embolus prophylaxis, valve replacement for uncontrollable dz
9. Although mitral stenosis (MS) causes a ↓↓↓ in cardiac output, it is not the result of ventricular failure & therefore its Tx is unique among disorders of ↓ cardiac output—**NEVER give ⊕ inotropic agents for mitral stenosis as are given for other ↓ cardiac output dzs**

D. Aortic regurgitation
1. Seen in endocarditis, rheumatic fever, VS defect (children), congenital bicuspid aorta, 3° syphilis, aortic dissection, Marfan's syndrome, trauma
2. **There are 3 murmurs in aortic regurgitation (AR)** (see Table 3.4)
3. AR has numerous classic signs
   a. **Water-hammer pulse** = wide pulse pressure presenting with forceful arterial pulse upswing with rapid fall-off
   b. **Traube's sign** = pistol-shot bruit over femoral pulse
   c. **Corrigan's pulse** = unusually large carotid pulsations
   d. **Quincke's sign** = pulsatile blanching & reddening of fingernails upon light pressure
   e. **de Musset's sign** = head-bobbing caused by carotid pulsations
   f. **Muller's sign** = pulsatile bobbing of the uvula
   g. **Duroziez's sign** = to-and-fro murmur over femoral artery heard best with mild pressure applied to the artery

Table 3.4 Major Murmurs*

Disease	Murmur	Physical Examination
Mitral stenosis	Low-pitched **mid-to-late diastolic rumble** at apex, opening snap & loud S1: use bell	Feel for RV lift 2° to RVH
Mitral valve prolapse	**Late systolic murmur with midsystolic click (Barlow's syndrome)**	Valsalva → click earlier in systole, murmur prolonged
Mitral regurgitation	High-pitched **apical blowing holosystolic murmur radiate to axilla**, S3: use diaphragm	Laterally displaced PMI, systolic thrill
Tricuspid stenosis	Low-pitched **diastolic rumble** often confused with MS: use bell	**Murmur louder with inspiration**—differentiates it from MS
Tricuspid regurgitation	High-pitched **blowing holosystolic** murmur at left sternal border: use diaphragm	**Jugular & hepatic pulsations, murmur louder with inspiration**
Aortic stenosis	**Midsystolic crescendo-decrescendo murmur at second right interspace, radiates to carotids & apex, with S4 due to atrial kick**, systolic ejection click	**Pulsus parvus et tardus** = peripheral pulses are weak & late compared to heart sounds, systolic thrill second interspace
Aortic sclerosis	Very similar to AS but peaks earlier in systole due to minimal pressure gradient across valve	None

Table 3.4 *Continued*

Disease	Murmur	Physical Examination
Aortic regurgitation	**3 murmurs:** • High pitched **blowing early diastolic** at aorta & left sternal border • **Austin Flint** = **apical diastolic rumble** due to mitral valve flutter, sounds similar to mitral stenosis but no opening snap • Midsystolic flow murmur at base	Laterally displaced PMI, **wide pulse pressure, pulsus bisferiens** (double-peaked arterial pulse): see text for classic eponym physical findings
Atrial septal defect	Loud S1, **wide fixed-split S2**, midsystolic ejection murmur, tricuspid rumble	Acyanotic until Eisenmenger syndrome develops
Ventricular septal defect	Harsh **holosystolic** murmur heard diffusely over entire precordium, maximally at fourth LICS	Typically acyanotic, see text for maladie de Roger
Hypertrophic subaortic stenosis	Brisk carotid upstroke, loud S4, mid-to-late systolic murmur at apex & left sternal border that is poorly transmitted to carotids	**Murmur increases with standing & Valsalva**
Coarctation of the aorta	**Continuous murmur heard over collateral vessels in back**, & late systolic murmur heard between scapulae	↑↑ **pulses in upper extremities with delayed & weak pulses in lower extremities**
Tetralogy of Fallot	Aortic ejection click, subpulmonic systolic ejection murmur whose intensity is inversely proportional to disease severity	Cyanosis, clubbing, classic squatting posture adopted during "Tet spells"
Patent ductus arteriosus	**Continuous machinery murmur heard best at second left interspace**	Wide pulse pressure, pulmonary vasculature visible on CXR

*The authors thank Dr. J. Michael Criley & Dr. Richard D. Spellberg for assistance with creation of this table.

4. ECG → LVH by voltage (see Section VII.B.4.b)
5. Tx = afterload reduction with ACE inhibitors or vasodilators, antibiotic prophylaxis prior to procedures (e.g., dental work), consider valve replacement if necessary

E. Aortic stenosis
   1. Frequently congenital, also seen in rheumatic fever
   2. Very mild degenerative calcification is called "aortic sclerosis" & seems to be a normal part of aging
   3. Pathology is due to first, fibrotic thickening of valve, & second, subsequent calcification
   4. Obstructive hypertrophic subaortic stenosis
      a. Also called "hypertrophic obstructive cardiomyopathy"
      b. Ventricular septum hypertrophies inferior to the valve
      c. Stenosis due to septal wall impinging upon anterior leaflet (rarely posterior leaflet) of mitral valve during systole
   5. **Classic triad of Sx = syncope, angina, exertional dyspnea**
   6. See Table 3.4 for physical findings
   7. ECG → LVH by voltage (see Section VII.B.4.b)
   8. Dx = echocardiography (gold standard)
   9. Tx = digitalis, effective only in mild disease
   10. Severe disease demands surgical intervention
   11. Patients need endocarditis prophylaxis prior to procedures
   12. **NEVER give aortic stenosis patients b-blockers or afterload reducers (vasodilators & ACE inhibitors)**—due to ↓↓ cardiac output, these pts have maximally constricted peripheral vessels to maintain BP; therefore, such drugs will cause them to go into shock

F. Tricuspid and pulmonary valves (see Figure 3.3)
   1. Both undergo fibrosis in carcinoid syndrome
   2. Endocarditis prophylaxis required prior to procedures (e.g., dental work)
   3. Tricuspid stenosis
      a. **Diastolic rumble easily confused with mitral stenosis**
      b. **Differentiate from MS by ↑ loud with inspiration** (see Table 3.4)
      c. ECG → P wave in lead II ≥ 2.5mm tall, indicative of right atrial enlargement (RAE)

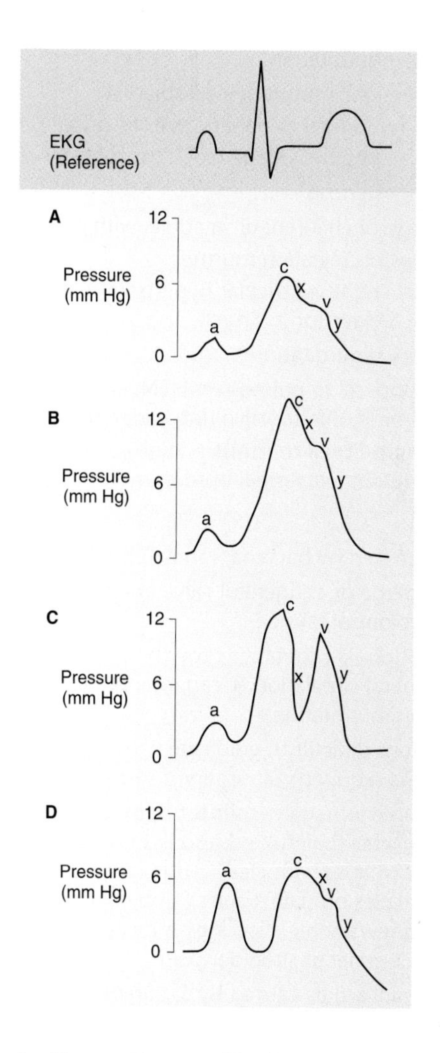

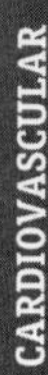

Figure 3.3 Jugular Venous Pressure Tracing
A. Normal: *a* wave, atrial contraction; *c* wave, bulging of tricuspid cusps into the right atrium at the beginning of each systole; *x* descent, relaxation of the right atrium; *v* wave, volume of blood that enters the right atrium during ventricular systole; *y* descent, rapid flow of blood into the right ventricle upon opening of the tricuspid valve. **B.** Right ventricular failure: overall increase in jugular venous pulsations and merging of *c* and *v* waves. **C.** Tricuspid regurgitation: overall increase in pressure and marked increase in the magnitude of the *x* descent, resulting in separate *c* and *v* waves. **D.** Canon *a* waves: marked increase in a wave intensity with no increase in jugular venous pulsations (found in AV dissociation). (Adapted from Berg D. *Advanced Clinical Skills and Physical Diagnosis*. Oxford: Blackwell Science, 1999.)

4. Tricuspid regurgitation
   a. Holosystolic murmur (see Table 3.4)
   b. Look for jugular & hepatic systolic pulsations
   c. ECG → RAE by voltage (see Tricuspid stenosis)
5. Pulmonary stenosis
   a. Disease of children, or in adults with carcinoid syndrome
   b. Midsystolic ejection murmur
   c. ECG → right ventricular hypertrophy (RVH) by R wave in V1 > S wave (or ≥ 5mm)
6. Pulmonary regurgitation
   a. Develops 2° to pulmonary HTN, endocarditis, or carcinoid syndrome, due to valve ring widening
   b. **Graham Steell murmur** = high-pitched diastolic blowing murmur at left sternal border, mimicking AR murmur

G. Endocarditis
1. Usually caused by bacteria, rarely fungi (*Candida, Aspergillus*)
2. Prior damage or congenital valve anomaly predisposes to microbial colonization
3. Colonization → vegetative growth → septic thrombi to brain or peripheral circulation & can interfere with valve function (causing regurgitation)
4. Vegetations difficult to eradicate with IV antibiotics (minimum 4–6 weeks required) & surgery is sometimes necessary
5. Si/Sx = splenomegaly, **splinter hemorrhages** in fingernails, **Osler's nodes** (painful red nodules on digits), **Roth spots** (retinal hemorrhages with clear central areas), **Janeway lesions** (dark macules on palms/soles), conjunctival petechiae, brain/kidney/splenic abscesses→ focal neuro findings/hematuria/abdominal or shoulder pain
6. Acute endocarditis caused by *S. aureus, S. pneumoniae, N. gonorrhea*
7. Subacute disease (slower onset, symptoms less severe) caused by *Enterococcus, S. viridans, S. epidermidis*
8. ***S. bovis & Clostridium septicum* endocarditis commonly seen with GI cancer, always search for malignancy in these pts!**
9. HACEK organisms
   a. **Cause culture-negative endocarditis** (organisms are fastidious, difficult to culture)
   b. *Hemophilus aphrophilus, paraphilias, parainfluenza*
   c. *Actinobacillus actinomycetemcomitans*

d. ***C**ardiobacterium hominis*
e. ***E**ikenella corrodens*
f. ***K**ingella kingae*

10. Nonbacterial thrombotic endocarditis
    a. Nonseptic platelets & fibrin vegetations on heart valves
    b. Caused by mechanical injury to valve (e.g., catheters)
11. Marantic endocarditis
    a. Cancer seeding of heart valves during metastasis
    b. Very poor prognosis (Px), malignant emboli → cerebral infarcts
12. SLE causes **Libman-Sacks endocarditis,** may be due to autoantibody damage of valves—usually endocarditis is a Sx, but murmur can be heard

H. Rheumatic fever/heart disease
   1. Presents usually in 5–15 year olds after group A strep infection
   2. Dx = Jones criteria (2 major & 1 minor)
   3. Major criteria (**mnemonic: J♥NES**)
      a. **J**oints (migratory polyarthritis), responds to nonsteroidal anti-inflammatory drugs
      b. **♥**carditis (pancarditis, Carey-Coombs murmur = mid-diastolic)
      c. **N**odules (subcutaneous)
      d. **E**rythema marginatum (serpiginous skin rash)
      e. **S**ydenham's chorea (face, tongue, upper-limb chorea)
   4. Minor criteria = fever, ↑ erythrocyte sedimentation rate, arthralgia, long ECG PR interval
   5. In addition to Jones criteria, need evidence of prior strep infection by either culture or ⊕ antistreptolysin O antibody titers
   6. Tx = penicillin

VIII. Pericardial Disease

A. Pericardial fluid (see Figure 3.4)
   1. Hydropericardium is serous accumulation within pericardial sac; can result from any disease causing systemic edema
   2. Hemopericardium is blood in the pericardial sack, often 2° to trauma, metastatic cancer, viral/bacterial infections
   3. Both can lead to cardiac tamponade
      a. Compression of heart by pericardial fluid → ↓ cardiac output
      b. **Look for pulsus paradoxus, which is ≥ 10 mm Hg fall in BP during inspiration**

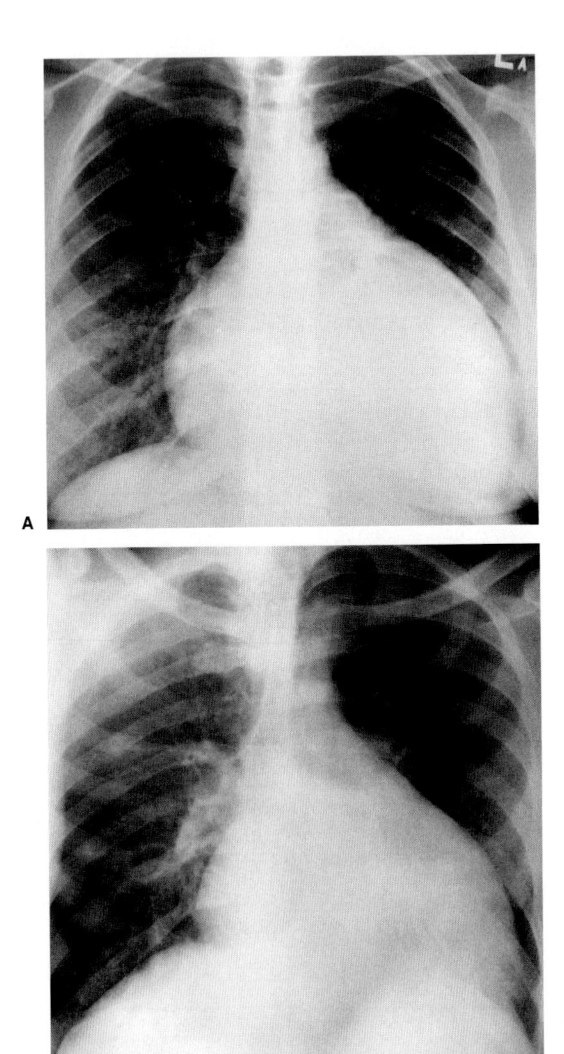

Figure 3.4
A. Pericardial effusion. The heart is greatly enlarged. (Three weeks before, the heart had been normal in shape and size.) The outline is well defined and the shape globular. The lungs are normal. The cause in this case was a viral pericarditis. This appearance of the heart, though highly suggestive of, is not specific to pericardial effusion. (Compare with **B.**) **B.** Congestive cardiomyopathy causing generalized cardiac dilatation. This appearance can easily be confused radiologically with a pericardial effusion. (From Armstrong P, Wastie M. *Diagnostic Imaging*. 4th ed. Oxford: Blackwell Science, 1998.)

c. ECG shows **electrical alternans**, which is beat-to-beat alternating height of QRS complex
4. Tx = immediate pericardiocentesis in tamponade, otherwise treat the underlying condition & allow the fluid to resorb

B. Pericarditis

1. Caused by bacterial, viral, or fungal infections, also in generalized serositis 2° to rheumatoid arthritis, systemic lupus erythematosus, scleroderma, uremia
2. **Dressler's syndrome** develops within 2–4 weeks after acute MI or heart surgery, may be due to autoimmune reaction to antigens exposed when myocardial tissue is damaged
3. Pericardial effusions can result from pericarditis, may be fibrinous, serous, sanguinous, or purulent, can cause cardiac tamponade if accumulates rapidly
4. **Dx by classic triad: distant heart sounds, distended jugular veins, hypotension**
5. Listen for pleural friction rub
6. **ECG → ST elevation in all leads**, also see PR depression

IX. Aortic Dissection

A. Characteristics

1. Dissection of vessel wall along tunica media, forming false lumen
2. Commonly & mistakenly referred to as "dissecting aortic aneurysm"—it is not an aneurysm
3. Associated with syphilis, Marfan's, & hypertension
4. Syphilis causes thoracic aortic dissections
5. Si/Sx = abrupt onset, severe "tearing" or "ripping" anterior chest pain radiating to back, lower BP in one arm, absent pulses, aortic insufficiency, widened mediastinum on chest x-ray
6. Tx = emergently ↓ BP followed by surgical repair

X. Congenital Heart Diseases

A. Causes

1. Genetic (Down's syndrome, etc.), infections (rubella, etc.), drugs (thalidomide, etc.), metabolic (diabetes, etc.)

B. Fetal circulation—a review (see Figure 3.5)

1. Foramen ovale (FO) permits flow from RA to LA so blood can bypass the useless lungs & go directly to systemic circulation

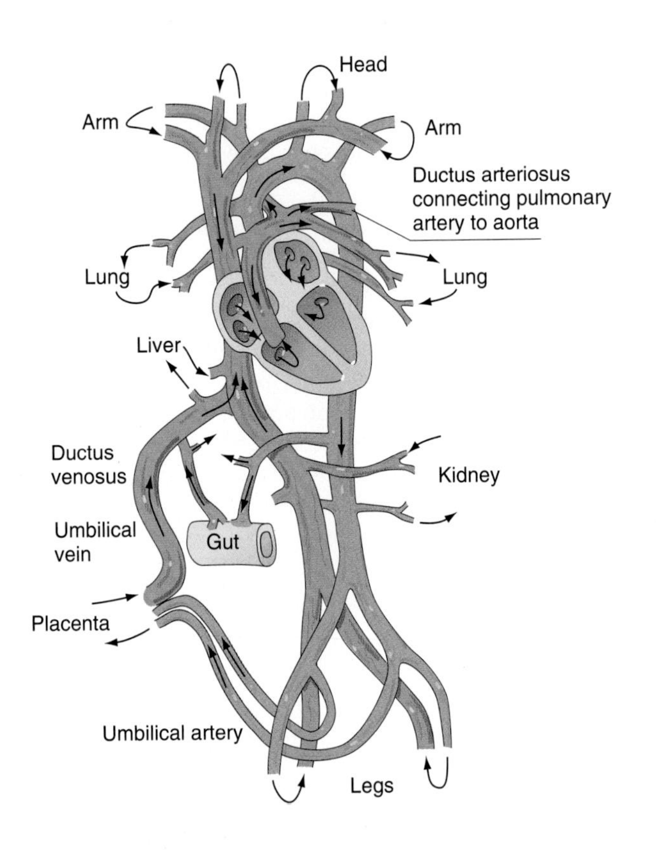

Figure 3.5 Fetal Circulation in Utero
The relative oxygenation of the blood is indicated by the colors and the direction of blood flow is indicated by the arrows. Note: (i) the ductus venosus carrying blood from the placenta and (ii) the ductus arteriosus carrying blood from the pulmonary artery to the aorta and so bypassing the lungs. (Adapted from Axford JS. *Medicine*. Oxford: Blackwell Science, 1998.)

2. Ductus arteriosus (DA) is second bypass route, allowing blood in pulmonary arteries to transfer directly to aorta
3. Fetal RV is hypertrophied since it supplies the lung & the periphery via both the FO & DA
4. At birth lungs expand, pulmonary vascular resistance falls, LA pressure rises, closing the FO
5. DA persists for hours to days, however, & is finally shut off due to inhibition of prostaglandin signals that keep it patent

6. As lung perfusion ↑ & peripheral bypass tracts are shut off, the workload on the LV ↑ & the RV workload ↓
7. Eventually, over years, the RV shrinks & LV hypertrophies

C. Ventricular septal defect
1. **Most common congenital heart defect** (excluding bicuspid aortic valve, which is usually clinically insignificant)
2. Small defects may be completely asymptomatic throughout entire life
3. 30% of small-to-medium defects close spontaneously by age 2
4. Maladie de Roger
    a. Si/Sx = small ventricular septal defect (VSD), left parasternal thrill with loud holosystolic murmur at fourth left intercostal interspace
    b. Course is benign, endocarditis prophylaxis necessary
5. Large defects lead to CHF, impaired development/growth, frequent pulmonary infections
6. Eisenmenger's complex = R → L shunt 2° to pulmonary HTN
    a. Normal shunt in VSD is L → R
    b. Eventually pulmonary HTN develops 2° ↑ pulmonic flow
    c. In months to years, pulmonary HTN → RV hypertrophy
    d. RV hypertrophy eventually leads to a flow reversal through the shunt, so that a R → L shunt develops
    e. Causes cyanosis 2° to lack of blood flow to lung
    f. Allows venous thrombi (e.g., deep venous thrombosis) to bypass lung, causing systemic embolization
    g. These emboli are known as **paradoxical emboli**, because they are venous emboli that bypass the lung via the shunt & enter the systemic arterial circulation
7. See Table 3.4 for physical findings
8. Tx = complete closure for simple defects

D. Patent ductus arteriosus
1. Tied with atrial septal defects for second most common congenital heart dz
2. Increased incidence with premature births, predispose to endocarditis & pulmonary vascular disease
3. See Table 3.4 for physical findings
4. **Tx = indomethacin** (block prostaglandins, induce closure) for infants, otherwise surgery

5. In infants with cyanosis refractory to O_2 therapy, PDA can be kept open to ↑ pulmonary blood flow by **Tx with prostaglandin**

E. Atrial septal defect
1. Tied with PDA for second most common congenital heart defect
2. Usually asymptomatic, often found on routine preschool physicals
3. Predispose to CHF in second & third decades, also predispose to stroke due to embolus bypass tract (Eisenmenger's complex)
4. See Table 3.4 for physical findings
5. Tx = surgical patching of bypass, more important for females due to eventual increased cardiovascular stress of pregnancy

F. Tetralogy of fallot
1. Four physical defects comprising the tetralogy are
   a. Ventricular septal defect
   b. Pulmonary outflow obstruction
   c. Right ventricular hypertrophy
   d. Overriding aorta (aorta inlet spans both ventricles)
2. Child acyanotic at birth, increasing cyanosis over first 6mo
3. **"Tet spell"** = acute cyanosis & panic in child, child adopts a squatting posture to improve blood flow to lungs
4. See Table 3.4 for physical findings
5. **Chest x-ray (CXR) shows classic boot-shaped contour** due to RV enlargement
6. Tx = surgical repair of VSD, repair of pulmonary outflow tracts

G. Transposition of the great arteries
1. Aorta comes off right ventricle, pulmonary artery off left ventricle
2. Must have persistent arteriovenous communication or dz is incompatible with life (can be via patent ductus arteriosus or persistent foramen ovale)
3. Si/Sx = marked cyanosis at birth, early digital clubbing, often no murmur
4. **CXR → enlarged egg-shaped heart**, ↑ pulmonary vasculature
5. Invariably fatal within several months of birth without Tx
6. Tx = surgical switching of arterial roots to normal positions with repair of communication defect

H. Coarctation of the aorta
1. Aortic narrowing, often asymptomatic in young child, see Table 3.4 for physical findings

Table 3.5 Differential Diagnosis for Murmurs*

Timing	Possible Disease: Differentiating Characteristics			
Midsystolic ("ejection")	***Aortic stenosis/sclerosis***: crescendo-decrescendo, second right interspace	***Pulmonic stenosis***: second left interspace, ECG → RVH	**Any high flow state** → "flow murmur": ***aortic regurgitation*** (listen for other AR murmurs), ***A-S defect*** (fixed split S2), ***anemia, pregnancy, adolescence***	
Late systolic	***Aortic stenosis***: Worse dz → later peak	***Mitral valve prolapse***: apical murmur	***Hypertrophic subaortic stenosis***: murmur louder with Valsalva	
Holosystolic	***Mitral regurgitation***: radiates to axilla	***V-S defect***: diffuse across precordium	***Tricuspid regurgitation***: louder with inspiration	
Early diastolic	***Aortic regurgitation***: blowing aortic murmur		***Pulmonic regurgitation***: Graham Steell murmur	
Mid-diastolic	***Mitral stenosis***: opening snap, no change with inspiration	***Aortic regurgitation*** (Austin Flint murmur): apical, resembles MS	***A-S Defect***: listen for fixed split S2, diastolic rumble	***Tricuspid stenosis***: louder with inspiration
Continuous	***Patent ductus***: machinery murmur loudest in back	***Mammary souffle***: harmless, heard in pregnancy due to ↑ flow in mammary artery	***Coarctation of aorta***: upper/lower extremity pulse discrepancy	***A-V fistula***

*The authors thank Dr. J. Michael Criley & Dr. Richard D. Spellberg for their assistance with creation of this table.

2. **Classic CXR sign → rib-notching**
3. Often presents with circle of Willis aneurysms, in Turner's syndrome, or with congenital bicuspid aortic valve
4. Tx = surgical resection of coarctation & reanastomosis

XI. Murmurs

A. Summary of major murmurs (see Table 3.4)

B. Physical examination differential diagnosis for murmurs (see Table 3.5)

4. PULMONARY

I. Respiratory Physiology (The Big Picture)

A. Chemoreceptors

1. Central chemoreceptors located in brain stem medulla
   a. Respond to ↓ pH & ↑ PCO_2
   b. Do not respond to O_2 at all
2. Peripheral chemoreceptors located in carotid & aortic bodies
   a. Respond to ↓ PO_2 (<60 mm Hg) & ↑ PCO_2 & ↓ pH
   b. **NOTE: In chronically hypercapnic patients, both central & peripheral receptors become refractory to ↑ CO_2 drive.** In these patients, the ONLY drive to maintain respiration is due to hypoxia recorded by peripheral receptors. Therefore, **be very careful administering high fraction of inspired oxygen (FIO_2) to correct hypoxemia in chronically hypercapnic patients**. Since the hypoxia is the only stimulus for their respiration, correcting it can lead ultimately to respiratory failure.

B. Spirometry in disease (see Figures 4.1 and 4.2)

1. Obstructive disease: ↓ forced expiratory volume (FEV), ↓ **FEV/forced expiratory vital capacity (FVC)**, ↑ TLC
   a. Differential diagnosis (DDx) = emphysema, asthma, chronic bronchitis
   b. **Emphysema has ↓ diffusion limited carbon monoxide (DLCO)** (marker of diffusion capacity, ↓ in emphysema due to alveolar destruction), **blood gas → adequate oxygenation ("pink puffer")**
   c. **Asthma has a pathognomonic >12% ↑ in FEV after administration of bronchodilators**
   d. **Chronic bronchitis blood gas → hypoxia ("blue bloater")**
2. Restrictive disease: N/↓ FEV, N/↑ FEV/FVC, ↓ **total lung capacity (TLC)**
   a. DDx = parenchymal (sarcoidosis, interstitial fibrosis), neuromuscular, skeletal
   b. Parenchymal diseases characterized by ↓ DLCO
   c. Neuromuscular & skeletal (scoliosis/thoracic cage) diseases have normal DLCO
   d. **Note: Emphysema is NOT a restrictive disease, even though it IS a parenchymal disease & has ↓ DLCO!!!**

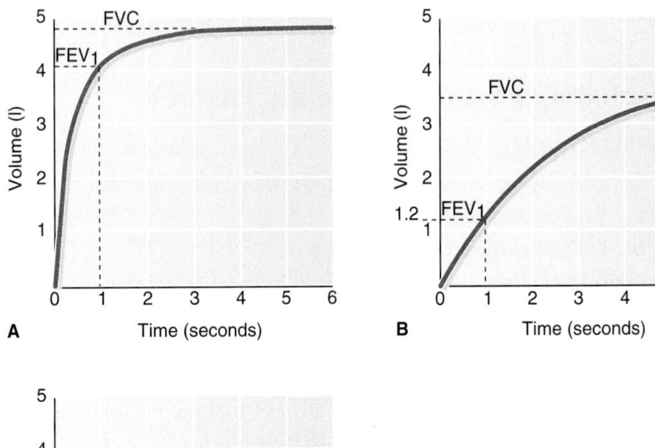

Figure 4.1 Lung Spirometry
A. Spirogram trace of a normal adult male: FEV_1 4.1 L; FVC 4.91 L; FEV_1/FEC 84%. **B.** Spirogram tracing of a person with airways obstruction (e.g., emphysema, chronic bronchitis): FEV_1 1.2 L; FVC 3.5 L; FEV_1/FVC 32%. **C.** Spirogram tracing of a person with a restrictive defect (e.g., fibrosing alveolitis): FEV_1 1.9 liters; FVC 2.1 liters; FEV_1/FVC 90%.

3. Combined diseases: ↓ FEV, ↓ FEV/FVC, ↓ DLCO
4. Diseases with normal spirometry
   a. ↓ DLCO can be due to anemia (slow O_2 diffusion because few RBCs to pick up the O_2), pulmonary emboli (lack of blood flow), early parenchymal disease, liver disease (pulmonary edema), primary pulmonary hypertension—**anything that interferes with blood flow through the lungs causes ↓ DLCO with normal spirometry**

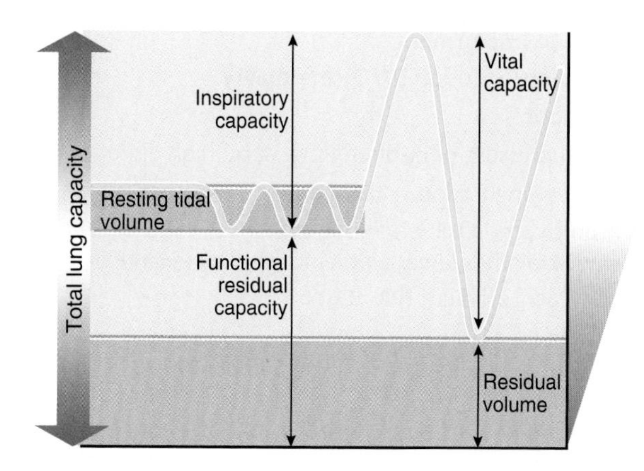

Figure 4.2 Lung Volumes
Spirogram tracing showing static lung volumes. (Adapted from Axford JS. Medicine. Oxford : Blackwell Science, 1998.)

b. ↑ DLCO due to pulmonary hemorrhage (**free blood in the lung parenchyma takes up O_2, whereas in emboli, blood supply is cut off**), Goodpasture's syndrome (due to pulmonary hemorrhage), idiopathic pulmonary hemosiderosis, chest trauma, polycythemia, ventricular septal defect (VSD) with L → R shunt—**things that ↑ blood content of the lung cause ↑ DLCO with normal spirometry**

II. Hypoxemia—5 Mechanisms (see Table 4.1)

1. **Low inspired PO_2**
2. **Hypoventilation**

Table 4.1 Differential Diagnosis of Hypoxemia

	PCO_2	$PA\text{-}aO_2$ Gradient	Response to O_2	DLCO
↓ FIO_2	Nml	Nml	⊕	Nml
Hypoventilation	↑	Nml	⊕	Nml
Diffusion impairment	Nml	↑	⊕	↓
V/Q mismatch	↑/Nml	↑	⊕	Nml
Shunt	↑/Nml	↑	–	Nml

3. **Diffusion Impairment**
4. Ventilation/perfusion **(V/Q) Inequality**
5. **R–L Shunt**

A. Low partial pressure of inspired PO_2—e.g., high altitude
1. Acute compensation = tachypnea
2. Chronic compensation = polycythemia, ↑ 2,3-BPG → hemoglobin has lower affinity for O_2 at a given PO_2
3. PAO_2-PaO_2 gradient (PA-aO_2)
    a. Defined as difference between PO_2 in alveoli & arteries
    b. Normal gradient = 10, ↑ by 5–6 per decade above 50 years
    c. **Gradient normal in hypoxemia caused by low inspired PO_2**
    d. Clinically, PAO_2 is calculated (see formula below) & PaO_2 is measured by laboratory analysis of arterial blood

    $$PAO_2 = FIO_2(P_{breath} - P_{H2O}) - (PaCO_2/R)$$

    At sea level: $FIO_2 = 0.21$, $P_{H2O} = 47$, $P_{breath} = 760$: $\mathbf{PAO_2 = 150 - (PaCO_2/R)}$

    $PaCO_2$ is measured by laboratory analysis of arterial blood, $R = 0.8$

B. Hypoventilation (↑ PCO_2)
1. Defined as low air flow, not low respiratory rate (hypopnea)
2. Can be due to hypopnea (slow respiration rate) or ↓ flow from equivalent rate (neuromuscular weakness, chest wall, etc.)
3. $PaCO_2$ is inversely proportional to ventilation
4. **Hypoventilation thus causes both hypoxemia & hypercapnia**
5. **Small ↑ in FIO_2 WILL correct hypoventilatory hypoxemia**
6. PA-aO_2 is normal
7. Causes
    a. With normal lungs: 2 types
        (1) Primary (1°) = CNS dysfunction
            (a) Causes = sleep, hypercapnia, alkalosis, drugs (narcotics), myxedema, brain damage, trauma, infection, neoplasm
            (b) Central hypoventilation (Ondine's curse), often seen in obese people (Obesity Hypoventilation Syndrome)

(2) Secondary (2°) = peripheral nervous system (PNS)/neuromuscular (NM) dysfunction, anatomic
(a) Causes = polio, Guillain-Barré, myasthenia gravis, Duchenne's muscular dystrophy, diaphragm paralysis
(b) Also kyphoscoliosis, obesity, tracheal stenosis, obstructive sleep apnea

b. With damaged lungs, can be due to any obstructive or restrictive lung disease

C. Diffusion impairment

1. This is the rarest of the 5 potential causes of hypoxemia
2. O_2 equilibrium normally occurs in 0.75 seconds = one third transit time through capillaries
3. Causes of impairment = increased diffusion path (fibrosis), decreased transit time (↑ cardiac output, anemia)
4. **PA-aO_2 is elevated** (O_2 cannot get from alveoli to capillaries)
5. DLCO
   a. A test of diffusion capacity
   b. DLCO ↓ in diffusion impairment
6. **Diffusion impaired hypoxemia CAN be overcome by ↑ FIO_2**

D. V/Q inequality

1. Causes hypoxemia but not necessarily hypercapnia (due to reflexive ↑ ventilation)
2. **PA-aO_2 is elevated**
3. Increased alveolar dead space, normal = 30%
4. Increased shunt, normal = 5% or less
5. **V/Q inequality hypoxemia CAN be improved by ↑ FIO_2**

E. R–L shunt

1. Occurs in pulmonary edema, pneumonia, atelectasis, atrial & ventricular septal defects, & chronic liver disease
2. **PA-aO_2 is elevated**
3. **R–L shunt hypoxemia CANNOT be overcome by ↑ FIO_2**
4. Do NOT see hypercapnia due to the reflexive ↑ in ventilation
   a. ↑ ventilation corrects hypercapnia but not hypoxia
   b. This is because of the sigmoid Hb-O_2 curve, since O_2 already at upper end of **sigmoid** saturation curve, cannot saturate the blood any further
   c. However, since CO_2 exhalation is **linear** with ventilation, excess CO_2 is blown off

Algorithm 4.1

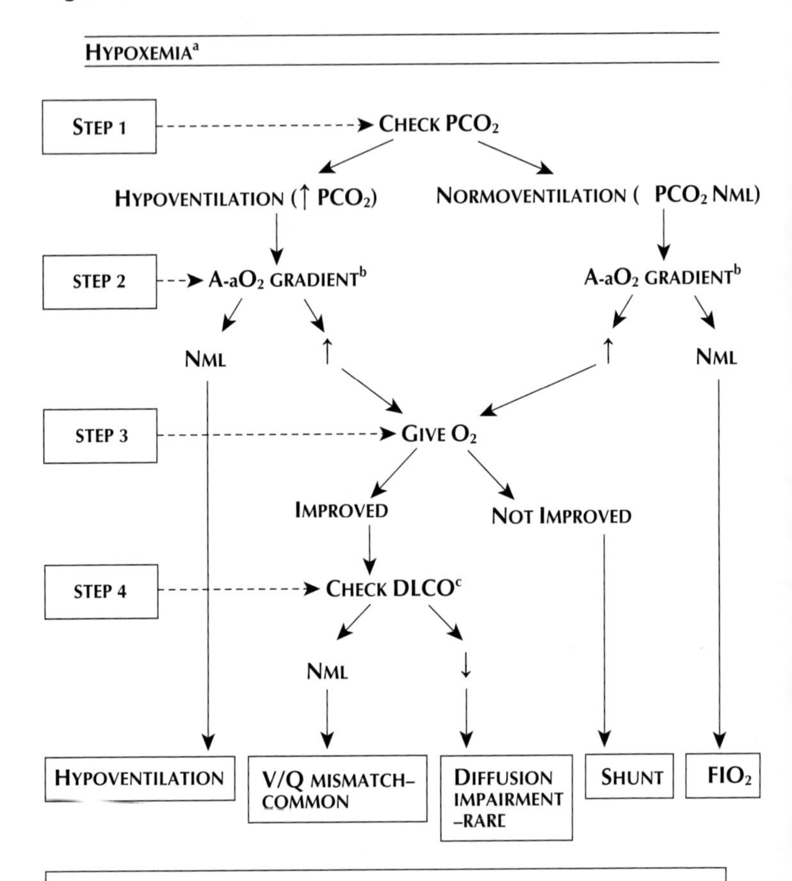

[a] The authors thank Dr. Arian Torbati for his assistance with this algorithm.
[b] A-a O_2 gradient = difference in alveolar and arterial O_2 concentrations.
[c] DLCO = diffusion limited carbon monoxide, a measurement of diffusion capacity.

III. Chronic Obstructive Pulmonary Disease

A. General characteristics

1. 3 major causes are emphysema, chronic bronchitis, & asthma: also seen in bronchiectasis
2. **Chief mechanism of hypoxemia is V/Q mismatch**
3. 80% airway resistance due to small airways & bronchospasm

4. Hypoxemia during sleep is more severe during rapid eye movement because of hypoventilation secondary to skeletal muscle paralysis

B. Emphysema ("pink puffer")
   1. Due to dilation of air spaces with destruction of alveolar walls
   2. Centriacinar type is caused by smoking & coal dust
   3. Centrilobular type is specific for smokers
   4. **Panacinar is pathognomonic for α-1-antitrypsin deficiency (chromosome 14)**
      a. PiZZ allele homozygotes have ↑ risk due to ↓↓ in enzyme
      b. Will also see hepatic cirrhosis in these patients
   5. Paraseptal or distal acinar disease results in spontaneous pneumothorax, associated with blebs or bullae

C. Chronic bronchitis ("blue bloater")
   1. Defined as expectoration on most days during at least 3 consecutive months for at least 2 consecutive years
   2. Pathology → mucous gland hypertrophy & loss of ciliated bronchial epithelium
   3. Diagnosis (Dx) by ↑ Reid index (>50%), which is the ratio of the thickness of gland layer to total bronchial wall
   4. Leading cause is smoking
   5. Signs/symptoms (Si/Sx) = wheezing crackles, cyanosis

D. Asthma
   1. Bronchial hyperresponsiveness causes reversible bronchoconstriction due to airway smooth muscle contraction
   2. Pathologically see thickening of basement membrane of bronchial epithelium, as well as mucous plugs, bronchial smooth muscular hypertrophy & destruction of cilia
   3. Status asthmaticus is a major complication
      a. Prolonged attack lasting for days & refractory to Tx
      b. Can result in death
      c. Tx = emergent β_2-agonists (e.g., albuterol)
   4. Extrinsic asthma
      a. Due to type 1 hypersensitivity response
      b. Mast cells activated by IgE cross-linked by an allergen
      c. Begins in childhood, usually with family history
   5. Intrinsic asthma
      a. Begins in adult life, not associated with history of asthma, complicated by chronic bronchitis

b. Early phase reaction mediated by nerves & inflammatory cells already present in airway, causing interstitial edema, vasodilation, & bronchospasm
c. Late phase reaction (3–8 hours after challenge) mediated by new inflammatory cells (neutrophils, eosinophils) → bronchospasm, activated T cells & mast cells may persist long after the challenge

E. Bronchiectasis
1. Permanent abnormal dilation of bronchioles
2. See inflammation & necrosis of bronchial walls
3. Si/Sx = foul breath, purulent sputum, recurrent infections, hemoptysis
4. Most commonly due to scarring from chronic infections (e.g., tuberculosis [TB] and granulomatous diseases), recurrent pneumonia (often in patients with congenital deficiency), also with cystic fibrosis or immotile ciliary syndrome (see Head and Neck, Section V.A.2)

IV. Restrictive Lung Disease

A. Loss of functional lung tissue—FEV/FVC = normal
1. Surgical resection, atelectasis, foreign body/tumor airway obstruction

B. Parenchymal diseases—↑ FEV/FVC (↑ elastic recoil)
1. Collagen-vascular disease (dz) (e.g., rheumatoid arthritis, systemic lupus erythematosus [SLE], scleroderma)
2. Hereditary = familial idiopathic pulmonary fibrosis (IPF), lipid storage disease, neurofibromatosis, tuberous sclerosis
3. Drugs/iatrogenic = chemotherapy (the B's, **b**usulfan & **b**leomycin), amiodarone, radiation, chemical poisoning
4. Hypersensitivity pneumonitis = farmer's lung, bagassosis (sugar cane), byssinosis (cotton)
5. Infections = TB, *Coccidioides, Histoplasmosis*, cytomegalovirus (CMV), *Pneumocystis*
6. Pneumoconiosis = asbestosis, silicosis, talc lung
7. Inflammatory = Goodpasture's, Wegener's, Churg-Strauss, sarcoidosis, IPF

C. Interstitial fibrosis
1. Nonspecific reaction to chronic injury

2. Insidious progression with few inflammatory cells but many fibroblasts
3. Precipitants include silica, asbestos, oxygen toxicity, sulfur dioxide, organic dusts, CMV, TB, fungi, *Pneumocystis carinii* pneumonia (PCP), sarcoidosis, IPF, collagen-vascular disease
4. **Classic chest x-ray (CXR) finding is "honeycomb" lung**
5. IPF (Hamman-Rich syndrome is a rapid onset variant) leads to death in 2–5 years from cor pulmonale 2° to hypoxemia-induced pulmonary hypertension (HTN)
6. Dx IPF by clinical progression, biopsy & exclusion of other dz
7. Pathology → pulmonary vascular hypertrophy, bacterial pneumonia

D. Pleural effusions
1. Pleural space normally contains between 7 and 14 mL of fluid
2. An effusion (↑ fluid) can be due to ↓ oncotic pressure (transudate) or ↑ permeability of pleural vessels & ↑ hydrostatic pressure (exudate)
3. Transudate = plasma ultrafiltrate with **a low protein content** compared to serum (see Table 4.2)
4. Exudate = escape of fluid/proteins/cells from the vessels into the tissues or body cavities, fluid has **a high protein content** with cellular debris
5. Transudate causes = congestive heart failure, nephrotic syndrome, hepatic cirrhosis
6. Exudative causes = malignancy, pneumonia ("parapneumonic effusion"), collagen vascular (CV) dz, trauma, pulmonary embolism, radiation Tx & chylothorax
7. Thoracentesis
   a. Fluid withdrawal from the chest cavity with a needle for Dx & treatment (Tx) purposes
   b. Laboratory studies for fluid
      (1) Standard = protein, lactate dehydrogenase (LDH), cytology, cell count, specific gravity, pH, amylase, glucose, Gram's stain, bacterial/fungal cultures
      (2) Always concurrently send blood for LDH & protein
      (3) If TB suspected send for acid-fast bacillus stain & culture
      (4) If CV dz suspected, send for rheumatoid factor & antinuclear antibodies

Table 4.2 Summary of Transudate versus Exudate Findings

Study	Transudate	Exudate
Fluid quality	Serous	Cloudy, serous/ serosanguinous, blood
Protein	Effusion ≤3.0 g/dL Effusion/serum ratio ≤0.5	Effusion >3.0 g/dL* Effusion/serum ratio >0.5*
LDH	Effusion ≤200 IU/L Effusion/serum ratio ≤0.6	Effusion >200 IU/L* Effusion/serum ratio >0.6*
Specific gravity	≤1.015	>1.015
pH	≥7.2	<7.2 → parapneumonic effusion (PPE)
Gram's stain	No organisms	ANY organism → PPE
Cell count	WBC ≤1000	WBC >1000 (lymphocytes → TB)
Glucose	≥50 mg/dL	<50 mg/dL → infxn, neoplasm, collagen-vascular (≤10 → rheumatoid arthritis)
Amylase	↑ in pancreatitis, esophageal rupture, malignancy	
RF	Titer > 1:320 → virtually pathognomonic for rheumatoid arthritis (pH often <7.2)	
ANA	Titer > 1:160 → highly indicative for systemic lupus erythematosus (pH often >7.4)	

*Any one of these findings rules out transudative effusion, rules in exudative effusion.

E. Nonpulmonary diseases
   1. Chest wall disease
      a. FEV/FVC = normal for wall disease, ↓ in neuromuscular
      b. Causes include kyphoscoliosis, ankylosing spondylitis, myasthenia gravis, multiple sclerosis, amyotrophic lateral sclerosis, Guillain-Barré, trauma to cord
   2. Extrapulmonary diseases → pregnancy, obesity, ascites (due to pressure upward on diaphragm)
   3. Systemic disease involving lung—see Table 4.3

Table 4.3 Lung Presentation of Systemic Diseases

Disease	Signs/Symptoms	Dx	Tx/Other
Inflammatory			
Goodpasture's	90% present with hemoptysis, look for proteinuria, iron deficiency anemia common, ↑ **DLCO** (lung hemorrhage)	Renal biopsy (Bx) → acute glomerulonephritis & linear anti-GBM IgG deposits	Steroids, Cytoxan, **Emergent!**
Wegener's	>50% have sinusitis or epistaxis, systemic vasculitis → fever, Sx in eye, cutaneous nodules, arthritis, neuropathy	**C ANCA is specific but Bx of vasculitic lesion necessary for Dx**	Cytoxan & Steroids
Churg-Strauss	A polyarteritis nodosa variant occurring in asthmatics with lung Sx (e.g., asthma) & **systemic Sx = fever, tachycardia, MI**	Bx → vessel inflammation (↑ in lung), **eosinophilia in lung & blood, P-ANCA highly sensitive**	Steroids if not self-limiting
Sarcoidosis	More common in African Americans in third–fourth decade, 50% have lung Sx like dry cough/dyspnea, CXR → bilateral hilar nodes [see Musculoskeletal, Section IV.I]	Bronchoalveolar lavage shows CD4:CD8 ratio = 2:1 to 10:1 Dx = exclude infection ⊕ **Bx → noncaseating granulomas**	aSx no Tx Sx get NSAIDs or steroids
Lymphoid interstitial pneumonitis	30% have Sjögren's, also seen in AIDS, Sx = insidious exertional dyspnea, anorexia, fatigue, can → lymphoma	CXR → mostly lower lobe disease Bx → massive lymphocyte infiltrate, but alveolar architecture preserved	Variable response to steroids

(Continued)

Table 4.3 *Continued*

Disease	Signs/Symptoms	Dx	Tx/Other
Histiocytosis X (eosinophilic granuloma)	**Spontaneous pneumothorax is classic presentation**, occurs in young adults with bone & lung lesions, 90% pts smoke [see Musculoskeletal, Section II.G]	CXR → honeycomb, hilar nodes Bx → eosinophilic granulomas, fibrosis, histiocytosis X bodies	If not self-limited, Tx = surgical excision
Asbestosis	Pleurisy, insidious exertional dyspnea, if a smoker will see bronchitis, COPD	**CXR → pleural plaques, diffuse fibrosis—watch for mesothelioma!**	Prophylaxis: no Tx
Silicosis	Shortness of breath, cough, late → orthopnea, exertional dyspnea (cor pulmonale), pulmonary HTN	**CXR → eggshell calcifications in hilar lymph nodes**, Dx = Bx	Prophylaxis: no Tx postexposure!
Idiopathic pulmonary fibrosis	Autosomal dominant dz presents earlier than acquired (30s–40s), Sx = insidious, progressive exertional dyspnea, non-productive cough, weight loss, arthralgia	Dx = compatible history, other etiologies ruled out, Bx nonspecific fibrosis—Px better if Bx → lymphocyte predominance	Steroids & Cytoxan
Collagen Vascular Diseases [See Musculoskeletal, Section IV for individual diseases]			
Rheumatoid Lung	Pleural effusion, nodules in lung, dyspnea, ⊕ arthritis, & usual Sx findings	High titer rheumatoid factor & low glucose in pleural effusion	Steroids
SLE	Pleural effusion, pulmonary edema, dyspnea, usual Sx findings	⊕ anti-ds-DNA Ab (99% specific), + ANA (>95% sensitive)	Steroids

Polymyositis	Symmetric muscle weakness, skin rash, acute onset preceded by infection (can be insidious), polyarthralgias, Raynaud's	1) Proximal muscle weakness 2) ↑ CPK, aldolase, 3) muscle Bx (definitive)	Steroids, ↓ dose as Sx subside
Scleroderma	Pulmonary fibrosis, exertional dyspnea, cutaneous thickening, polyarthralgia, GE reflux, chronic, slowly progressive	Dx = anti-SCL Ab (specific but not sensitive), otherwise Dx is clinical	Tx each organ separately
Hypersensitivity			
Hypersensitivity pneumonitis	Acute fever, dyspnea, cough 4–6 hrs postexposure, resolves spontaneously when exposure ends, **no eosinophilia**	Bx → noncaseating granulomas in lung, **distinguish from sarcoid by CD4:CD8 ratio < 1:2 on BAL**	Steroids
Eosinophilic pneumonia (simple variant = Loeffler's	Loeffler's = low fever, can be minimal respiratory Sx, moderate eosinophilia, chronic Sx → asthma, eosinophilia, but neither have systemic involvement	**Peripheral eosinophilia** in 2/3 of patients, as well as elevated IgE, CXR shows classic reverse butterfly peripheral infiltrates	Steroids

V. Pulmonary Vascular Disease

A. Brief review of pulmonary vascular physiology

1. 3 zones: V/Q ratio ↓ & perfusion ↑ from zone 1 to 3
    a. Zone 1 = furthest from ground, minimal perfusion
    b. Zone 2 = pressure lower than right ventricle but higher than left atrium
    c. Zone 3 = capillary dilation, greatest flow, flow depends on pulmonary artery–left atrial pressure (PAP–LAP) difference
2. Normal blood flow stops at end of diastole, when PAP = LAP

B. Pulmonary edema—adult respiratory distress syndrome (also can be 2° to cardiogenic shock)

1. 2 stages: exudative vs. proliferative
    a. Exudative due to endothelial injury, biopsy → hyaline membrane, type II pneumocyte proliferation, fibroblast proliferation, inflammation
    b. Proliferative → interstitial fibrosis (can be within 3 days to a week), alveolar destruction, increased angiogenesis, & organization of exudate
2. Leads to obliteration of alveoli & bronchi following resolution
3. Edema is due to capillary leak, as opposed to pulmonary hypertension in cardiogenic pulmonary edema
4. Differential for pulmonary edema
    a. If pulmonary capillary wedge pressure <12 = noncardiogenic (adult respiratory distress syndrome)
    b. If pulmonary capillary wedge pressure >15 = cardiogenic
5. Si/Sx = dyspnea, tachypnea, stiff/small lungs, resistant hypoxemia, diffuse alveolar infiltrate
6. Causes = sepsis, GI aspiration, trauma, toxic gas inhalation
7. Tx = O_2, diuretics, positive end-expiratory pressure (PEEP) ventilation
8. Purpose of PEEP
    a. Helps prevent airway collapse in a failing lung
    b. ↑ functional residual capacity (maintain lung volume)
    c. ↓ shunting
    d. Expands alveoli for better diffusion

C. Pulmonary embolism
   1. 95% of emboli are from leg deep venous thrombi (DVT) **(DVT histology → lines of Zahn = alternating red/white stripes)**
   2. Si/Sx = swollen, painful leg, sudden dyspnea/tachypnea, tachycardia, hemoptysis—often are no peripheral Sx at all
   3. Local V/Q goes to infinity
   4. Patient (pt) will be hypocapnic due to reflex hyperventilation
   5. Risk factors
      a. **Virchow's triad = endothelial cell trauma, stasis, hypercoagulable states**
      b. Hypercoagulation causes = nephrosis, disseminated intravascular coagulation, tumor, postpartum amniotic fluid exposure, antithrombin III deficiency, protein C or S deficiency, factor V Leiden deficiency, oral contraceptives, smoking [see Hematology, Section IV.E.4]
   6. Most emboli are clinically silent (60–80%)
   7. PE can cause lung infarctions
      a. 75% occur in lower lobes
      b. **Classic CXR finding is "Hampton's hump,"** a wedge-shaped opacification at distal edges of lung fields, but most common CXR finding is normal or mild atelectasis (see Figure 4.3)
   8. Electrocardiograph (ECG) findings
      a. Classically (but rarely) → S wave in lead I, Q wave in III, inverted T wave in III ($S_IQ_{III}T_{III}$), large R wave in V1
      b. **Most common finding is simply sinus tachycardia**
   9. Dx = leg Utz to check for DVT, **spiral computed tomography of chest, & V/Q scan best to rule out PE** & pulmonary angiography (gold standard)
   10. Tx = prevention with heparin, inferior vena cava (IVC) filter, or Coumadin, use tPA thrombolysis in massive PE or hemodynamic compromise

D. Pulmonary hypertension
   1. Defined as pulmonary pressure $\geq ^1/_4$ systemic (should be 1/8)
   2. Si/Sx: ECG → right atrial enlargement, CXR → large hilar shadows, loud S_2, tricuspid regurgitation murmur, crackles heard due to fibrosis, ↓ breath sounds, cyanosis, pulsatile liver

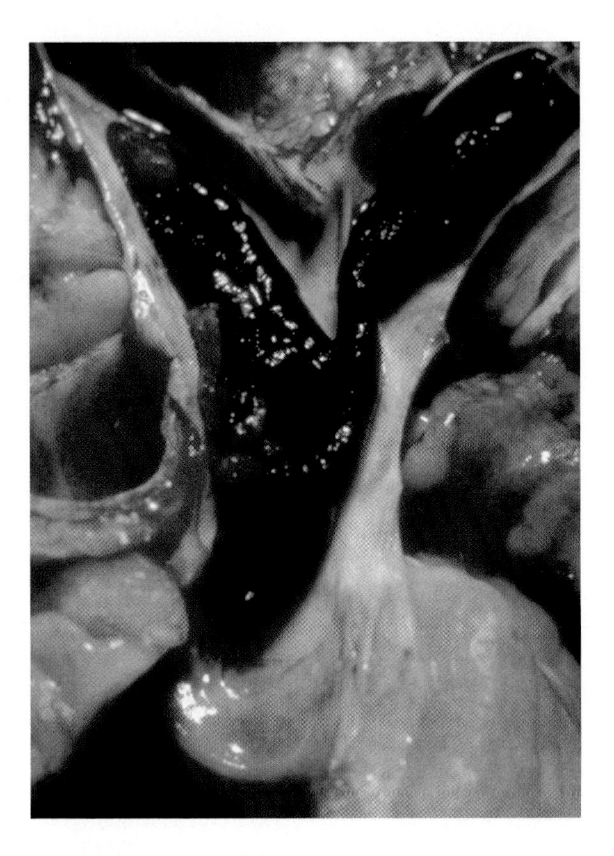

Figure 4.3 Pulmonary Embolism
The main pulmonary artery and its bifurcation have been opened to reveal a large saddle embolus. (From Rubin E, Gorstein F, Rubin R, et al. Rubin's Pathology: Clinicopathologic Foundations of Medicine. 4th ed. Baltimore: Lippincott Williams & Wilkins, 2005.)

3. Can be active (1° pulmonary dz) or passive (2° to heart dz)
   a. 1° dz includes idiopathic pulmonary HTN (rare, occurs in young women), chronic obstructive pulmonary disease (COPD), & interstitial restrictive diseases
   b. 2° dz seen in any heart disease, **commonly seen in HIV**
4. Hypoxemia → reflex vasoconstriction to shunt blood away from V/Q mismatches
5. Long term leads to hypertension with vascular smooth muscle thickening & intimal fibrosis

VI. Neuromuscular Disease

A. Normal functions of respiratory muscles

1. Diaphragm contracts, ↑ P_{abd} ↓ P_{pleura} → lower rib expansion & inspiration
2. Parasternal intercostals are 1° inspiratory muscles
3. External intercostals are 2° inspiratory muscles, internals are 2° expiration
4. Scalenes are 1° inspiratory muscles, elevate sternum during quiet breathing, abdominal muscles are expiratory
5. However, if abdominals fully contract → forced expiration of functional residual capacity → deeper subsequent inspiration, particularly useful in COPD

B. Pulmonary function tests (PFTs) in muscle deficits

1. 1° hypoventilation = ↓ neuronal response to hypoxemia
   a. Dx by voluntary ↑ in ventilation normalizing hypoxemia
   b. Patients have normal function testing, but resting hypoxemia
2. Quadriplegia
   a. Cord section above C_3 leads to total diaphragm paralysis, below C_3 = partial paralysis
   b. **If intercostals paralyzed but diaphragm is preserved, abdomen moves out & chest moves in with inspiration**
3. Isolated diaphragm paralysis mimics congestive heart failure (CHF) orthopnea
   a. Can be caused by viral infection or trauma
   b. Leads to dysjunction of thoracoabdominal wall motion
   c. **On inspiration, abdomen moves in as chest moves out, so is opposite of quadriplegia above**
   d. Bilateral paralysis leads to drop in mean inspiratory pressure (MIP) & can cause orthopnea-like CHF
4. Kyphoscoliosis → ↓ lung volumes, restrictive hypoxemia, hypercapnia, pulmonary hypertension, right ventricular hypertrophy, & cor pulmonale

VII. Respiratory Tract Cancers

A. Epidemiology

1. **Lung cancers are #1 cause of cancer deaths & second most frequent cancers in both males & females**
2. Although numbers have dropped in males, female deaths related to lung cancer are increasing

3. Lung cancer can only be seen on x-rays once they are >1 cm in size, by that time they have usually already metastasized, so x-rays not a good screening tool
4. Etiology: smoking, radon, asbestos, uranium, arsenic, radiation, chromates, vinyl chlorides & genetic predisposition
5. Staging important to guide Tx & to establish prognosis (Px) of disease
6. Associated Sx = cough, hemoptysis, hoarseness (recurrent laryngeal nerve paralysis), superior vena cava syndrome (obstructed SVC → facial swelling, cyanosis & dilation of veins of head & neck) & paraneoplastic syndromes

B. Asbestos
   1. Asbestos-related conditions
      a. Asbestosis, characterized by pleural plaques extending to costophrenic angles, with pleural effusions
      b. **Malignant mesothelioma is pathognomonic for asbestos exposure**
      c. Mesothelioma histology → **psammoma bodies** (other psammoma body dz = serous papillary cystadenocarcinoma of ovary, papillary adenocarcinoma of thyroid & meningioma)
   2. **Pathognomonic histology → ferruginous bodies: iron-coated asbestos particles**

C. Parenchymal lung cancers (see Table 4.4)

D. Other cancer syndromes
   1. **Superior sulcus tumor (Pancoast tumor): classic lung tumor causes Horner's syndrome** (ptosis, miosis, anhydrosis) by damaging the sympathetic cervical ganglion in the lower neck
   2. Small-cell carcinoma (CA) can cause a **myasthenia gravis–like condition known as the Lambert Eaton syndrome** [see Musculoskeletal, Section V.F.8.a] due to induction of Abs to tumor that cross-react with presynaptic Ca channel
   3. Renal cell CA metastatic to lung can cause 2° polycythemia by ectopic production of erythropoietin

VIII. Mediastinal Tumors (see Table 4.5)

IX. Sleep Apnea

A. Sleep apnea probability
   1. ↑ likelihood with ↑ neck size, hypertension, loud snoring, witnessed apneas/choking/gasping

Table 4.4 Summary of Parenchymal Lung Cancers

Cancer	Characteristics	Histology
Adenocarcinoma	• **Most frequent lung CA in nonsmokers** • **Presents in subpleura & lung periphery** • Presents in preexisting scars, "scar cancer" • Carcinoembryonic antigen (CEA) ⊕, used to follow Tx, not for screening due to ↓ specificity • Characterized by mutated K-ras oncogenes	Glandular (acinar) or papillary formations, often containing mucin
Bronchoalveolar carcinoma	• Subtype of adenocarcinoma not **related to smoking** • **Presents in lung periphery** • Reacts with antisurfactant antibodies	Arises in bronchiolar Clara cells or type II pneumocytes
Large cell carcinoma	• **Presents in lung periphery** • Highly anaplastic, undifferentiated cancer • Poor prognosis	Emperipolesis: pleomorphic giant cells with leukocyte fragments in cytoplasm
Squamous cell carcinoma (bronchogenic carcinoma)	• **Central hilar masses arising from bronchus** • **Strong link to smoking** • **Causes hypercalcemia due to secretion of PTHrp** (parathyroid hormone related peptide)	**Classic finding is keratin pearls** & intercellular bridges (desmosomes), frequently masses cavitate

(Continued)

Table 4.4 *Continued*

Cancer	Characteristics	Histology
Small cell (oat cell) carcinoma	• **Usually has central hilar location** • **Often already metastatic at Dx**, ↑↑ **poor Px** • **Strong link to smoking (99% are smokers)** • Causes numerous endocrine syndromes • ACTH secretion (cushingoid) • Secretes ADH, causing SIADH	Neoplasm of neuroendocrine Kulchitsky cells, histology → **small**, **dark blue cells like lymphocytes**, highly undifferentiated
Bronchial carcinoid tumors	• Carcinoid syndrome caused by tumor secretion of serotonin (5-HT) • **Si/Sx = recurrent diarrhea, skin flushing, asthmatic wheezing & carcinoid heart dz** • Dx by ↑ 5-HIAA metabolite in urine • Tx = methysergide, a 5-HT antagonist	Also neoplasms of neuroendocrine Kulchitsky cells, histologically → small, **uniform, dark blue cells arranged in nests**
Lymphangi-oleiomyomatosis	• Neoplasm of lung smooth muscle • Leads to cystic obstructions of bronchioles, vascular system, & lymphatics • **Almost always seen in menstruating women** • Estrogen may be involved in pathogenesis • Si/Sx = dyspnea, hemoptysis, **pneumothorax** • Tx = progesterone or lung transplant	Immature smooth muscle cells

Table 4.5 Summary of Mediastinal Tumors

Anterior*	Middle	Posterior†
Thymoma	Lymphoma	Neuroblastoma
Thyroid tumor	Pericardial cyst	Schwannoma
Teratoma Terrible lymphoma	Bronchial cyst	Neurofibroma

*The four Ts.
†Neural tumors.

2. All pts with unexplained daytime sleepiness should be evaluated
3. Increased frequency in patients with hypothyroidism

B. Apnea types
   1. Apnea ≡ absent air flow for 10sec
   2. Hypopnea ≡ ↓ airflow for 10sec
   3. Central apnea ≡ no effort to breathe is made
      a. Patient has no arousals, usually **REM related**
      b. Short apneas can be normal & can occur at sleep onset
      c. Very common, CO_2 threshold dependent
      d. Often seen in obese people, known as Obesity Hypoventilation Syndrome, often accompanied by Obstructive Sleep Apnea
   4. Obstructive Sleep Apnea ≡ ⊕ ventilatory effort but no airflow because airway is closed
      a. Apnea terminated by arousal from sleep
      b. **Called "Pickwickian syndrome,"** pts have daytime sleepiness
      c. Most commonly found in obese persons, site of obstruction is usually abnormal pharyngeal passageway
      d. Tx = weight loss, continuous positive airway pressure (CPAP) worn while patient sleeps, surgical resection of neck tissue
   5. Mixed apnea ≡ no initial effort & obstruction when effort resumes

X. Occupational & Environmental Diseases

A. General characteristics
   1. Usually affects preexisting illness rather than causing new dz

2. Early recognition & removal from environment essential for positive long-term prognosis

B. Pneumoconiosis ("dust disease")
   1. Caused by coal dust (**anthracosis**), asbestos, crystalline silica, iron oxide & barium
   2. **See noncongruence between radiographic & clinical signs**
      a. Iron has significant x-ray findings but is not of significance physiologically
      b. Important to consider if dust is fibrogenic or not
      c. Coal dust & silica → small opacities known as "simple pneumoconiosis," & patient may not exhibit symptoms
      d. Others exposed to same substances may suffer from progressive massive fibrosis

C. Allergic occupational asthma
   1. Most commonly recognized occupational dz, can be fatal
   2. One form involves allergic sensitization to a specific work place chemical (e.g., dilocyanates in auto spray paints/polyurethane, also red cedar wood)
   3. These patients will always continue to have airway hyperresponsiveness after they develop allergic sensitization
   4. Permanent changes occur in over 50% of those affected
   5. Only Tx = early recognition & removal from exposure

D. Nonallergic occupational asthma
   1. Reactive airway dysfunction syndrome (RADS)
   2. Due to single high-level exposure to a highly toxic material (often chlorine) & the patient thereafter develops asthma
   3. This doesn't involve allergic sensitization to the agent but develops as a result of direct mucosal injury

E. Hypersensitive pneumonitis
   1. Farmer's lung disease, acute & chronic
   2. Acute disease due to high level exposure to inhaled fungal or protein antigens
      a. Si/Sx = fever, chills, lung infiltrates, leukocytosis, dyspnea
      b. Lasts 24–48 hours
   3. Chronic disease: prolonged exposure to lower antigen levels
      a. Clinically indistinguishable from idiopathic pulmonary fibrosis
      b. Much worse prognosis than acute disease

F. Other disorders
  1. Chronic beryllium disease causes granulomatous & fibrotic response, looks like sarcoidosis
  2. Cobalt exposure: giant cell pneumonitis, **giant cells are virtually pathognomonic**
  3. Inhalation fevers
     a. Nonallergic response, usually occurs in welders
     b. Si/Sx = fever, dyspnea, pulmonary infiltrates in short-lived episodes
     c. Steel workers exposed to zinc fumes, causing zinc fever or galvanized fever
     d. Teflon & certain mycotoxins produced by fungal outgrowth can also cause this condition
  4. Acute gassing seen in fires burning carbon, cyanide, acroleic & structural materials in indoor fires, chlorine gas, oil refinery sulfur gas, all of which lead to RADS

XI. Pulmonary Defenses

A. Physical defenses
  1. Anatomic barriers
     a. Particle size & site of deposit
        (1) Particles >20 μm deposit in nasal turbinates
        (2) Particles 15–20 μm deposit in the larynx
        (3) Particles <10 μm deposit in the carina & major airways
        (4) Particles <2 μm reach the alveoli
     b. Impaction begins on the posterior wall of pharynx, where tonsils & adenoids are located
     c. Sedimentation due to gravitational forces in regions of low flow & is single most important determinant of deposition from fifth bronchial division to terminal lung units
     d. Brownian motion
        (1) Important for very small particles <0.01 μm, which can readily enter peripheral alveoli
        (2) Important in acquiring *Mycobacterium tuberculosis* & in pharmacotherapy (bronchodilator administration)
  2. Mucociliary escalator
     a. Particles of 10–12 μm are deposited in the upper part of airway (larynx to the terminal bronchioles) where they are rapidly removed by ciliary transport

   b. Particles of 3μm are deposited in nonciliated areas lower down & therefore removal is slower
3. Cough reflexes
   a. Airway reflexes result in bronchoconstriction to prevent deeper penetration of irritants
   b. Coughing removes excess secretions & foreign bodies
   c. Starts with a deep inspiration, followed by a forced expiration against a closed glottis
4. Secretions
   a. Airways lined by high levels of IgA & complement system components
   b. Surfactant may also have bacteriostatic properties
5. Result of above is that the lung is normally sterile from first bronchial division to terminal lung units

XII. Pneumonia (see Figures 4.4 and 4.5 and Table 4.6)

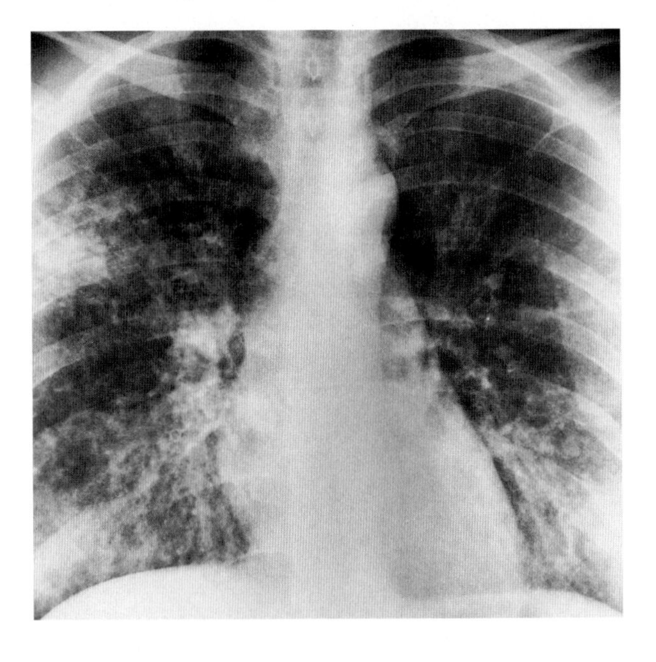

Figure 4.4 Mycoplasma Pneumonia
Widespread ill-defined consolidation is seen in both lungs. (From Armstrong P, Wastie M. Diagnostic Imaging. 4th edition. Oxford: Blackwell Science, 1998.)

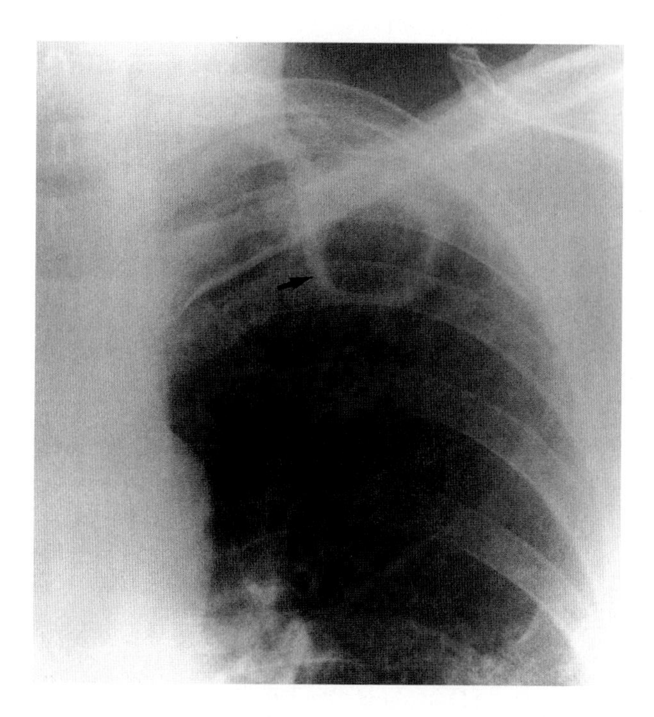

Figure 4.5 Fungus Infection
The cavity (arrow) in this patient from southeastern United States was due to North American blastomycosis. Note the similarity to tuberculosis. Other fungi, e.g., histoplasmosis, can give an identical appearance. (From Armstrong P, Wastie M. Diagnostic Imaging. 4th edition. Oxford: Blackwell Science, 1998.)

XIII. Tuberculosis

A. Characteristics

1. Chronic infection with *Mycobacterium tuberculosis*, an acid-fast bacilli, which can grow on Lowenstein-Jensen agar (see Figure 4.6)
2. Spread via inhalation of respiratory droplets
3. Rising incidence in the US due to HIV & multidrug resistance
4. Affects elderly, urban poor/homeless & immigrants from endemic areas

Table 4.6 Summary of Pneumonia

Organism	Characteristics	Tx
	Typical Bacterial Pneumonia	
Streptococcus pneumonia	Children, elderly, immunosuppressed pts, acute onset with rigors, can rapidly progress, #1 cause of CAP* (70%) ↑ frequency in asplenic and AIDS pts	Ceftriaxone, macrolide, or fluoroquinolone (resistance to all increasing)
Haemophilus	*H. influenzae* causes 10% CAP*, same patients as *S. pneumonia*	Ceftriaxone, macrolide, or fluoroquinolone (resistance to all increasing)
Moraxella catarrhalis	Causes 5% CAP*, common in COPD & immunosuppressed	Ceftriaxone, macrolide, or fluoroquinolone (resistance to all increasing)
Staphylococcus aureus	2° infects after influenza virus, commonly → pleural effusion	Oxacillin†
Gram-negative rods	Often nosocomial infections	3rd generation cephalosporin
Pseudomonas	Often in cystic fibrosis, commonly nosocomial, cavitates, rapid antibiotic resistance (use 2 antibiotics!)	3rd generation cephalosporin + fluoroquinolone
Klebsiella	Seen in alcoholics, diabetics, nosocomial, classically sputum is "currant jelly" bloody red, antibiotic resistant	3rd generation cephalosporin + fluoroquinolone
Anaerobes	Aspiration pneumonia seen in loss of consciousness, dementia, alcoholic, → abscess, foul sputum, dz in dependent lung lobes	Metronidazole/Clindamycin

Atypical Pneumonia		
Mycoplasma pneumonia	Classically young adults (college), causes 10% of CAP*, after 2–4wk incubation → tracheobronchitis & nocturnal cough	Doxycycline, macrolide, or quinolone
Legionella pneumophila	Seen in alcoholic, transplant pts, COPD, malignancy, diabetes, water exposure (e.g., air conditioner): 25% lethal with Tx, classic Si/Sx = hyponatremia, CNS changes, LDH > 700, diarrhea	Doxycycline, macrolide, or quinolone
Chlamydia pneumonia	Seen in elderly pts, Sx = sore throat, hoarse voice, sinusitis	Doxycycline, macrolide, or quinolone
Chlamydia psittaci	Contracted from birds (often parrots), bird may show signs of illness also (e.g., ruffled feathers)	Doxycycline, macrolide, or quinolone
Coxiella burnetii	Called "Q-fever," contracted from farm animals (e.g., cattle, goats), inhalation or ingestion of milk, etc.	Doxycycline, macrolide, or quinolone
Francisella tularensis	Found in hunters, butchers, etc., classically contracted from rabbits, but other animals & ticks as well	Streptomycin
Actinomyces israelii	50% → empyema, crosses tissue planes (e.g., pericardium, spine), look for sinus tract drainage through anterior chest wall	Penicillin (6–12 mo)
Nocardia asteroides	Gm ⊕ acid fast aerobe, mimics TB, Si/Sx = fever, night sweats, ***eosinophilia***, seen in AIDS as opportunistic infection	Bactrim

(Continued)

Table 4.6 *Continued*

Organism	Characteristics	Tx
	Fungal Pneumonia	
Pneumocystis carinii	Insidious onset of dry cough/dyspnea, bilateral infiltrates, not pleural effusions (very rare), Dx → bronchoscopy, ↑ LDH: AIDS pts with CD4 < 200 get prophylaxis with Bactrim	Bactrim
Coccidioides immitis	"San Joaquin Valley Fever," major risks = travel to SW desert (e.g., California, Arizona, New Mexico, Texas), imprisonment, ↑ incidence after earthquakes, Filipinos & African Americans have ↑ rate	Amphotericin (ampB) or fluconazole (flucon) disseminated dz, Dx best by serology
Histoplasma	Exposure to Ohio/Mississippi River valleys, bat or bird dung	AmpB/flucon
Aspergillus	Seen in neutropenic pts, CXR → "fungus-ball" with cavitation	AmpB/itracon‡
Cryptococcus	Seen in AIDS patients or any immunosuppressed	AmpB/flucon
	Viral Pneumonia	
Influenza	Present in patients > 65 yr, can be deadly	Amantadine/oseltamivir/ zanamivir
Hantavirus	Children/young adults exposed to SW desert rodents, 50% fatal with Tx, 3–6 day prodromal fever & myalgias → acute ARDS	Supportive (intubation)
Other	RSV, adenovirus, parainfluenza, less severe than influenza	Supportive

*CAP = community acquired pneumonia.
†Vancomycin if resistant to oxacillin.

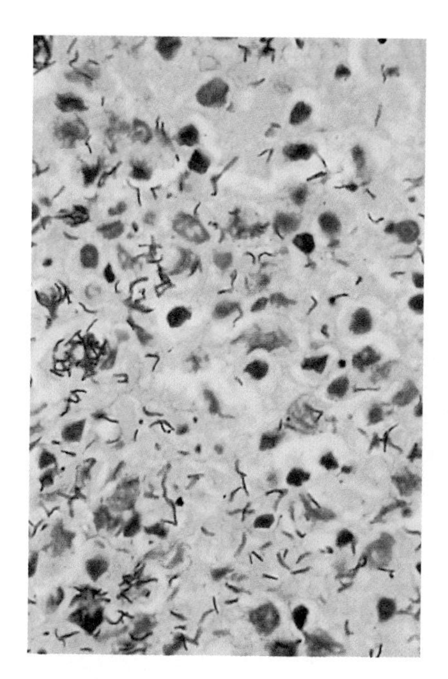

Figure 4.6 Ziehl-Neelsen-stained Material Obtained from a Caseating Mediastinal Lymph Nodes
Many acid-alcohol-fast bacteria are seen, with the typical red cording or clustering appearance of *M. tuberculsosis*. (From Bannister BA, Begg NT, Gillespie SH. Clinical Surgery. Oxford: Blackwell Science, 1996.)

B. Primary TB

1. Classically disease of lower lung lobes (bacilli deposited in dependent portion of lung during inspiration)
2. Usually asymptomatic
3. After inhalation of mycobacteria, macrophages engulf the bacilli that survive intracellularly
4. **Classic histopathologic finding is the "caseating granuloma"**
5. **Classic radiologic finding is "Ghon complex"** = calcified nodule at primary focus ⊕ calcified hilar lymph nodes (see Figure 4.7)

C. Secondary (Reactivation) TB

1. Reactivation of bacilli in **apical lung segments** due to the ↑ oxygen tension in upper lobes (see Figure 4.8)

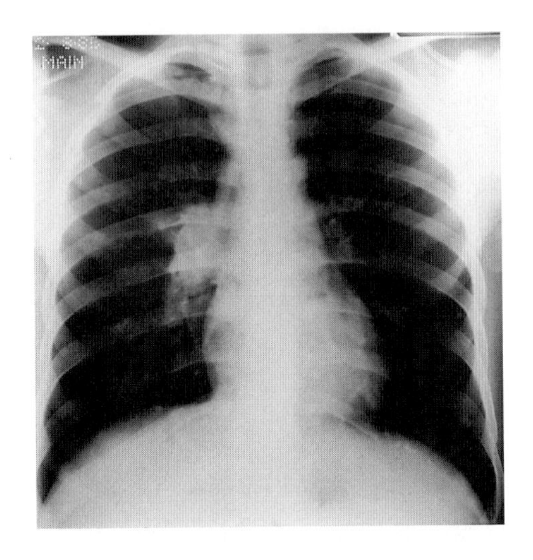

Figure 4.7 Primary Pulmonary TB
Chest radiograph showing unilateral hilar lymphadenopathy. The Ghon focus is often not visible on the radiograph. (From Axford JS. Medicine. Oxford: Blackwell Science, 1998.)

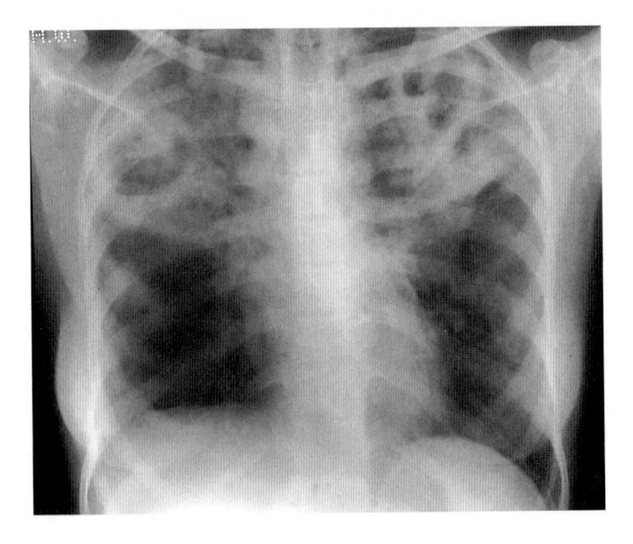

Figure 4.8 Postprimary TB
Chest radiograph showing bilateral apical cavitating pneumonia. (From Axford JS. Medicine. Oxford: Blackwell Science, 1998.)

2. Si/Sx = insidious onset, fevers, chills, night sweats, weight loss, cough, hemoptysis, upper lobe infiltrate or scarring on CXR
3. Risk factors = HIV, imprisonment, homeless, malnourished

D. Miliary (disseminated) TB (see Figure 4.9)
1. Hematogenous **dissemination involving any organ**, often the liver, spleen, bone, kidneys, pericardium, spine, meninges
2. Presents in any patient with immune deficiency
3. Classic syndromes
   a. Potts disease = TB of spine, presents with multiple compression fractures
   b. Scrofula = TB causing massive cervical lymphadenopathy
   c. Gastroenteritis with profuse diarrhea & colitis

E. Diagnosis & treatment
1. Latent infection (new terminology and guidelines as of 2000)
   a. Latent infection is defined by positive PPD status with no Si/Sx of active disease and no active disease on CXR
   b. PPD test is a **screening test for latent infection**, it is **NOT** a diagnostic test for active tuberculosis
   c. Guidelines for interpretation of PPD
      (1) ≥5 mm induration is a positive test for latent infection if the patient:
         (a) has HIV

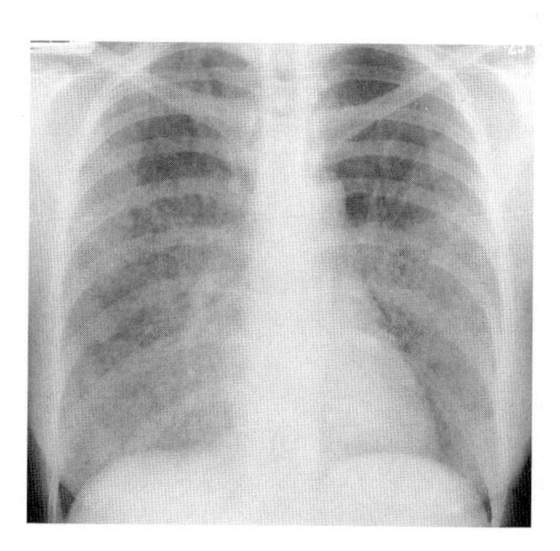

Figure 4.9 Miliary TB
Chest radiograph showing widespread small nodules throughout the lung fields. (From Axford JS. Medicine. Oxford: Blackwell Science, 1998.)

(b) has been in close contact with someone with active TB
(c) has fibrotic changes on CXR consistent with old TB
(d) is taking immunosuppressive medicines (e.g., >15 mg/d of prednisone for >1mo, cyclosporin, etc.)

(2) ≥10mm induration is a positive test for latent infection if the patient:
(a) is a recent immigrant from a high risk country (most developing countries)
(b) is an injection drug user
(c) works or resides in a prison/jail, nursing home, health care facility (that's you and us!), or a homeless shelter
(d) has a chronic debilitating illness such as renal failure, cancer, or diabetes mellitus

(3) ≥15 mm induration is a positive test for latent infection if the patient does not meet any of the above categories

d. Treatment of latent infection (formerly known as "prophylaxis")
(1) Since asymptomatic patients with positive PPDs are now considered to be latently infected, the term prophylaxis is not accurate
(2) Decision to treat patients with positive PPDs was formerly made based upon age, as risk of isoniazid-induced hepatitis increases with age
(3) However, the new guidelines specify that **all patients with positive PPDs as defined above should receive treatment for latent TB irrespective of age**
(4) The key is that you should only put a PPD on a person whom you would treat if they were positive—thus, think twice about putting a PPD on a person older than 35 unless you think they are truly at risk for having latent infection
(5) Isoniazid for 9 months is the 1st line therapy for all patients with latent TB (irrespective of HIV status)—alternative regimens are available but should only be given by very experienced providers

2. Active infection
a. To reiterate a point made above: **PPD is not intended as a diagnostic test for active TB**—it is commonly falsely negative in pts with active dz, and a positive test only indicates

latent infection, not active disease, thus it is neither sensitive nor specific for active disease

b. Active infection is diagnosed based on 3 components: clinical assessment, CXR, and sputum (or other body fluid if miliary disease is considered)
   (1) Clinical indicators of active dz include subacute/chronic cough, night-sweats, weight loss, hemoptysis, etc.
   (2) CXR indicators of active dz include upper lobe infiltrates or scarring, cavitary lesions in a patient with symptoms
   (3) Sputum for acid-fast staining is the diagnostic study of choice
c. Treatment
   (1) Start regimen with 4 drugs: isoniazid, rifampin, ethambutol, pyrazinamide
   (2) Narrow regimen based on sensitivities of culture organism
   (3) If culture negative, narrow to 2 drugs at 2 months (isoniazid & rifampin)
   (4) Treat for a minimum of 6 months
   (5) Treatment should be given by specialists in TB care

5. BREAST

I. General

A. Mastalgia
   1. Cyclical or noncyclical breast pain NOT due to lumps
   2. Treatment (Tx) = danazol, works by inducing amenorrhea (hirsutism & weight gain side effects)
   3. Pain worse with respiration may be due to Tietze syndrome (costochondritis)
   4. Mondor's disease = thoracoepigastric vein phlebitis → skin retraction along vein course

B. Gynecomastia
   1. Enlargement of male breast (unilateral or bilateral)
   2. Lobules not found in male breast as in the female breast
   3. Occurs as result of an imbalance in estrogen and androgen hormones usually occurring during puberty but can occur in old age
   4. Can also be seen in hyperestrogen states, such as cirrhosis of liver or use of drugs that inhibit liver breakdown of estrogen, ie, alcohol, marijuana, heroin, and psychoactive drugs
   5. Seen in Kleinfelter's syndrome and those with a testicular neoplasm

C. Cancer risks
   1. Risk increased by
      a. #1 factor is gender (1% of breast cancers are in men)
      b. Age (#1 factor in women)
      c. Young first menarche (<11 yr)
      d. Old first pregnancy (>30 yr)
      e. Late menopause (>50 yr)
      f. Family history
         (1) 95% of cancers are not familial
         (2) Increased incidence in patient with a first degree relative with history of breast cancer
         (3) Autosomal dominant (not 100% penetrance) conditions with increased risk; BRCA-1, BRCA-2, Li-Fraumeni syndrome, Cowden's disease, and Peutz-Jeghers
      g. Prior breast cancer in opposite breast
   2. Risk NOT increased by caffeine, sexual orientation

3. Risk NOT increased by fibroadenoma or fibrocystic disease
4. Cancer occurs most frequently in upper outer quadrant (Tail of Spencer)

D. Breast tumors

1. **Fibroadenoma (FA)** (see Figure 5.1)
    a. Most common tumor in teens & young women (peak in 20s)
    b. Histologic appearance: myxoid stroma & curvilinear, slit ducts
    c. FAs grow rapidly, no increase risk for developing cancer (CA)
    d. Tx NOT required, often will resorb within several weeks, reevaluation after a month is standard

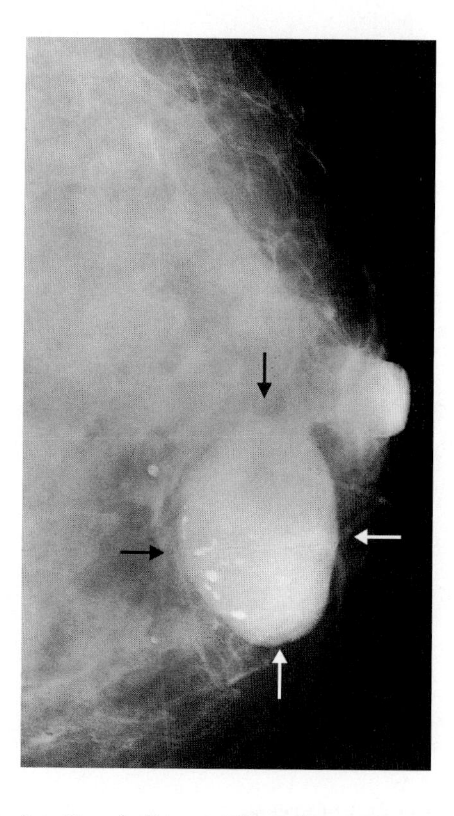

Figure 5.1 Benign Mass in Breast (Fibroadenoma)
Mammogram showing mass (arrows) with very well-defined borders and coarse structured calcification. (From Armstrong P, Wastie M. Diagnostic Imaging. 4th ed. Oxford: Blackwell Science, 1998.)

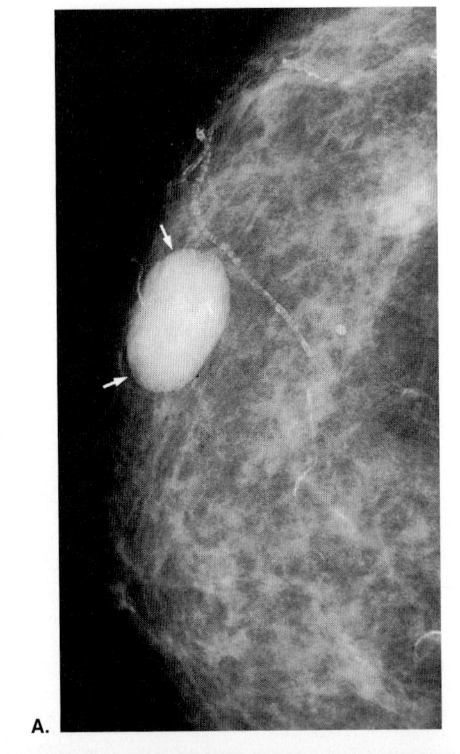

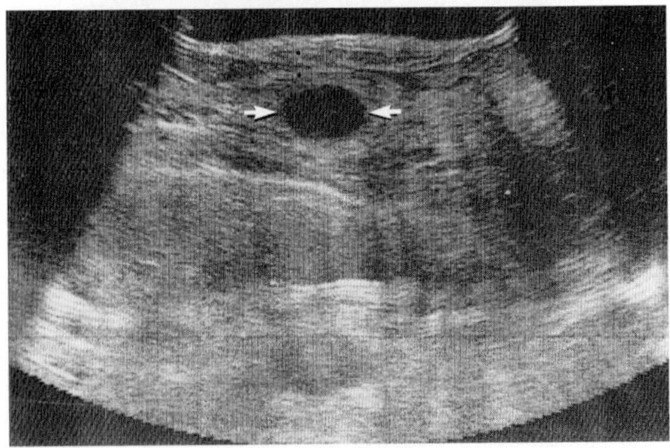

Figure 5.2 Benign Cyst of Breast
A. Mammogram showing oval, very well-defined mass without calcifications (arrows). **B.** The mass (arrows) was shown to be cystic on ultrasound; cyst aspiration was undertaken. (From Armstrong P, Wastie M. Diagnostic Imaging. 4th ed. Oxford: Blackwell Science, 1998.)

2. **Fibrocsytic Disease** (See Figure 5.2)
    a. Most common tumor in 35–50 year olds, rarely post-menopausal, arise in terminal ductal lobular unit
    b. Patients complain of multiple bilateral small lumps tender during menstrual cycle
    c. Cysts can arise overnight, of no clinical significance
    d. Not associated with increased risk of cancer unless biopsy specimen reveals epithelial (ductal or lobular) hyperplasia with atypia (see Figure 5.3)
    e. Diagnosis (Dx)/Tx = fine-needle aspiration (FNA), drainage of fluid
        (1) If aspirated fluid is bloody, send for cytology to rule out cystic malignancy
3. **Fibrous Pseudolump**
    a. Parenchymal atrophy in premenopausal breast, multiple nodules will be present
4. **Intraductal Papilloma**
    a. Often presents with serous/**bloody nipple discharge (guaiac-positive)**
    b. Will be solitary growth in perimenopause, but can have multiple nodules if younger
    c. **Solitary papillomas do not ↑ CA risk, but multiple papillomas DO**
5. **Intraductal Hyperplasia**
    a. Dx by biopsy, greater than 2 cell layers in ductal epithelium, either with or without atypia
    b. If atypia is present, increased risk for CA later developing in EITHER breast
    c. It is NOT premalignant; it is a MARKER for future malignancy, which won't be in the same place
6. **Ductal Carcinoma in Situ (DCIS)**
    a. Usually nonpalpable, seen as irregularly shaped ductal calcifications on mammography
    b. Unless comedonecrosis is present, not be visibly detectable
    c. Comedonecrosis common in *her2/neu* + (*c-erbB-2*+) disease
    d. This is a true premalignancy, will lead to invasive ductal CA
    e. Histologic appearance: haphazard cells along papillae (in contrast to hyperplasia, which is orderly), punched-out areas in ducts with "Roman bridge" pattern due to cells infiltrating open spaces

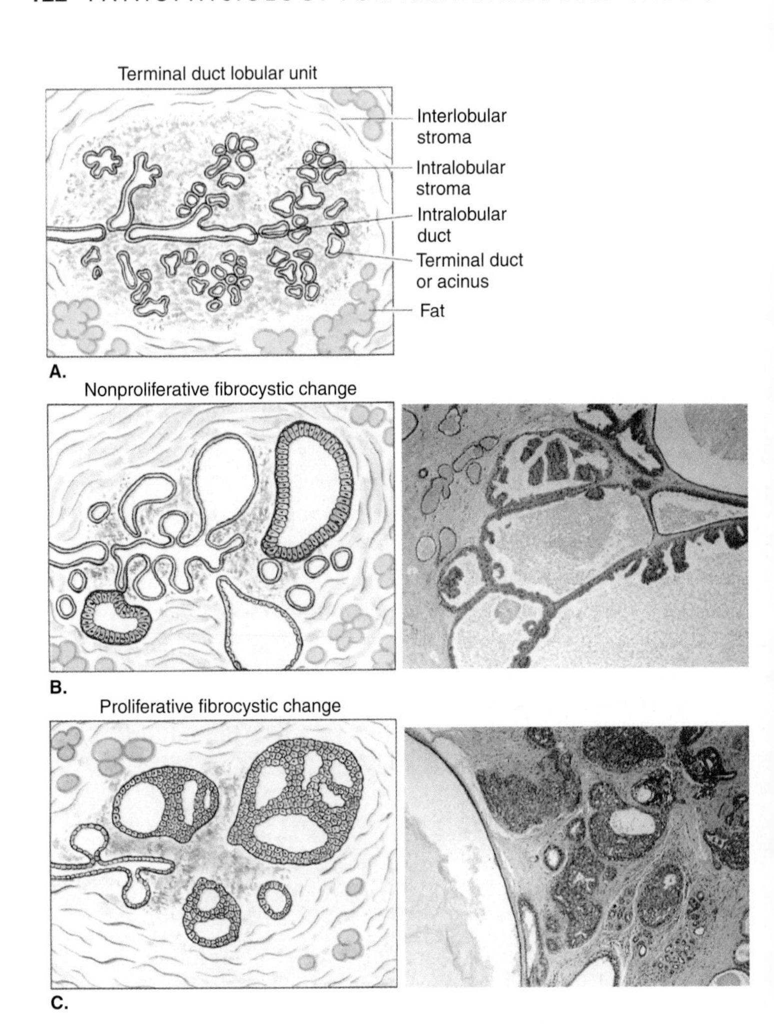

Figure 5.3 Histology of Fibrocystic Change
A.The normal terminal lobular unit. **B.** Nonproliferative fibrocystic change: this lesion combines cystic dilation of the terminal ducts with varying degrees of apocrine metaplasia of the epithelium and increased fibrous stroma. **C.** Proliferative fibrocystic change: terminal duct dilation and intraductal epithelial hyperplasia are present. (From Rubin E, Gorstein F, Rubin R, et al. Rubin's Pathology: Clinicopathologic Foundations of Medicine. 4th ed. Baltimore: Lippincott Williams & Wilkins, 2005.)

f. Tx = excision of mass, ensure clean margins on excision (if not excise again with wider margins) & add postop radiation to reduce rate of recurrence

7. **Lobular Carcinoma in Situ (LCIS)**
   a. Cannot be detected clinically or by gross examination, mammography is also a poor tool for diagnosing this disease

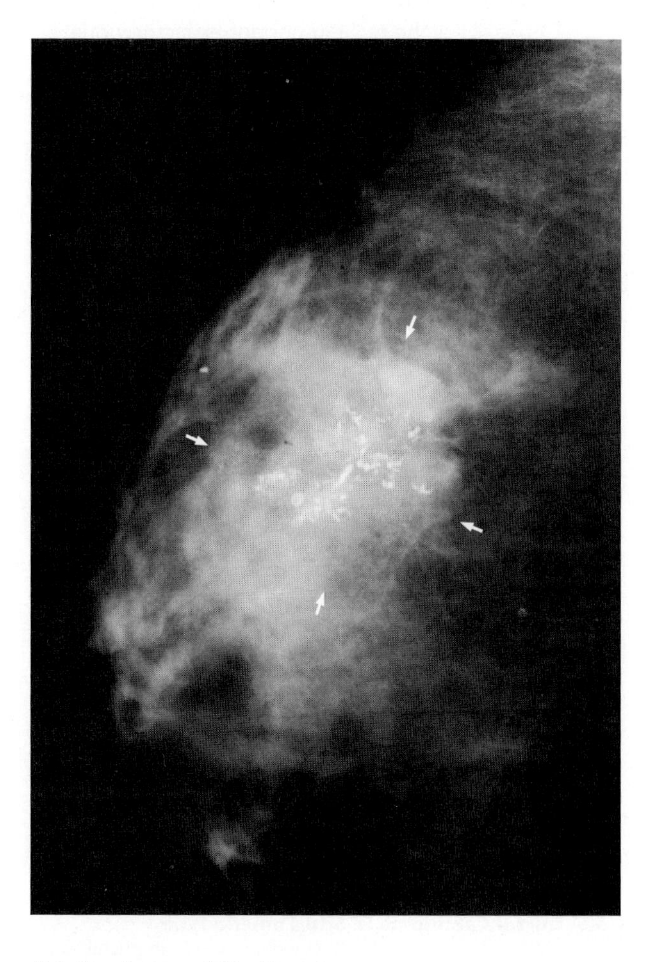

Figure 5.4 Carcinoma of the Breast
Mammogram showing ill-defined mass (arrows) containing numerous malignant linear and branching microcalcifications. (From Armstrong P, Wastie M. Diagnostic Imaging. 4th ed. Oxford: Blackwell Science, 1998.)

   b. It is NOT precancerous like DCIS is, but it IS a marker for future invasive ductal CA risk
   c. Histologic studies show mucinous cells almost always present, "saw-tooth" & clover-leaf configurations occur in the ducts
8. **Invasive Ductal Carcinoma (IDC)** (See Figures 5.4 and 5.5)
   a. Most common breast cancer, occurs commonly in mid 30s to late 50s, forms solid tumors
   b. Tumor size is the most important Px factor, node involvement is also an important prognostic factor
   c. Moderately differentiated IDC comes from cribriform or papillary intraductal originators
   d. Poorly differentiated IDC comes from intraductal comedo originator
   e. Forms solid tumor, there are many subtypes of this tumor (e.g., mucinous, medullary, etc.)
9. **Invasive Lobular Carcinoma** (See Figure 5.6)
   a. Only 3% to 5% of invasive CA is lobular, present at 45–56 years, vague appearance on mammogram

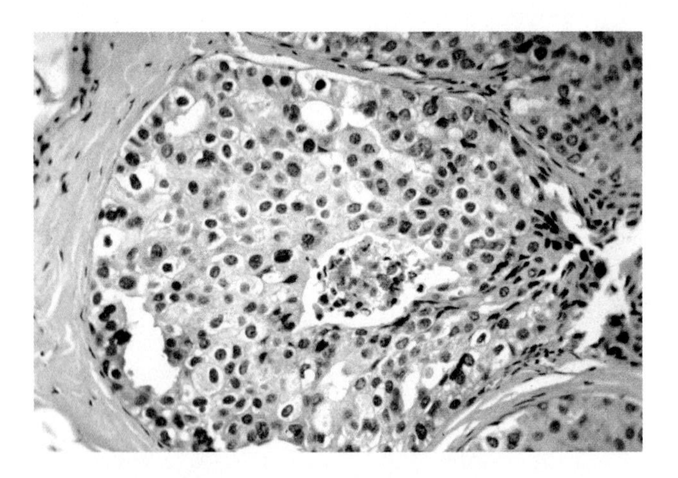

Figure 5.5 Ductal Carcinoma in Situ Comedo-type
The terminal ducts are distended by carcinoma in situ (intraductal carcinoma). The centers of the tumor masses are necrotic and display dystrophic calcification. (From Rubin E, Gorstein F, Rubin R, et al. Rubin's Pathology: Clinicopathologic Foundations of Medicine. 4th ed. Baltimore: Lippincott Williams & Wilkins, 2005.)

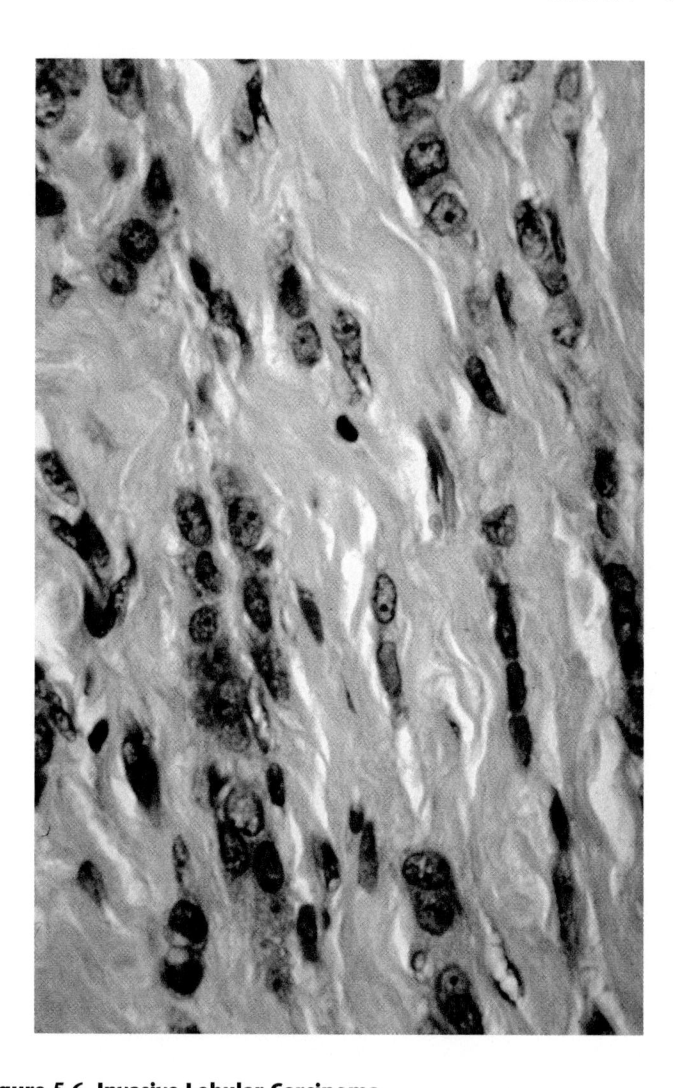

Figure 5.6 Invasive Lobular Carcinoma
In contrast to invasive ductal carcinoma, the cells of lobular carcinoma tend to form single strands that invade between collagen fibers in a single pattern. The tumor cells are similar to those seen in lobular carcinoma in situ. (From Rubin E, Gorstein F, Rubin R, et al. Rubin's Pathology: Clinicopathologic Foundations of Medicine. 4th ed. Baltimore: Lippincott Williams & Wilkins, 2005.)

b. Patients have increased frequency of bilateral cancer
c. **Exhibits single file growth pattern within a fibrous stroma**

10. **Paget's Breast Disease (NOT BONE DISEASE!)**
    a. Presents with dermatitis/macular rash over nipple or areola
    b. Underlying ductal CA almost always present
11. **Inflammatory Carcinoma**
    a. Breast has classic Sx of inflammation: redness, pain & heat
    b. Rapidly progressive breast cancer, almost always widely metastatic at presentation
    c. Prognosis poor

E. Mammography (see Figures 5.1 to 5.3)
1. Highly effective screening tool in all but young women
2. **Dense breast tissue found in young women interferes with the test's sensitivity & specificity**
3. All women older than 50 should have yearly mammograms (proven to ↓ mortality in these patients)
4. Women older than 40 recommended to have yearly or biannual mammograms (efficacy less clear in this group)
5. Women with first-degree relatives who have cancer should begin mammogram screenings **10 years before the age at which the relative developed cancer**

6. GASTROENTEROLOGY AND LIVER

I. Esophageal Disease

A. Normal esophageal physiology
   1. Upper & lower sphincters (UES, LES) tonically contracted to prevent reflux
   2. Recurrent laryngeal nerves carry the tonic excitation to the UES, myenteric plexus innervates LES
   3. The UES, but not LES, is under voluntary control
   4. Primary (1°) peristalsis triggered by swallowing, secondary (2°) by esophageal distension, inhibitory signals carried to LES by vagus

B. Achalasia
   1. Failure of esophageal smooth muscle function
   2. **Pathognomonic → no peristalsis, ↑ LES tone, no LES relaxation**
   3. Symptoms (Sx) = dysphagia, chest pain, vomiting, barium swallow shows classic rat tail appearance through the LES
   4. Over time the upper esophagus dilates, relieving some pain, but causing nocturnal regurgitation/aspiration
   5. Treatment (Tx) = LES ablation, nifedipine, botulinum toxin, or balloon sphincterotomy

C. Diffuse esophageal spasm
   1. Caused by intermittent, large amplitude peristalsis
   2. Sx = dysphagia, chest pain mimics angina (substernal, radiates to jaw, back, or arm)
   3. Pain can be associated with eating, but usually spontaneous
   4. Rarely leads to achalasia
   5. Causes 40% of chest pain cases if coronary artery disease not present (gastroesophageal [GE] reflux causes another 40%)

D. Neuromuscular disorders
   1. Causes = stroke, Parkinson's, amyotrophic lateral sclerosis, myasthenia, multiple sclerosis, polymyositis, Duchenne's
   2. Look for ↓ pharyngeal contraction & ↓ UES relaxation

E. Zenker's diverticulum
   1. Outpouching proximal to UES → food retention/regurgitation
   2. Diverticula can be at mid-esophagus or above LES (epiphrenic diverticula)
   3. Commonly involves cricopharyngeus & inferior constrictor muscle
F. Tracheoesophageal fistula (see Figure 6.1)
   1. Congenital, presents in newborn usually as 1 of 6 variants
   2. Usually esophageal atresia & tracheoesophageal fistula near bifurcation of trachea
   3. Associated with polyhydramnios due to inability of fetus to swallow amniotic fluid & associated with esophageal atresia
   4. Esophageal atresia = esophagus ends in blind pouch, fistula is necessary for the newborn to live
   5. Occasionally fistula can be between a completely patent esophagus and trachea
G. Gastroesophageal reflux disease (GERD)
   1. LES defect, ↑ abdominal pressure → burning substernal pain
   2. Reflux normally terminated by peristalsis & saliva, both may be defective in GERD
   3. Water brash = sudden salty fluid in mouth (salivary secretion)
   4. Beware of Barrett's esophagus = metaplasia from squamous to columnar epithelia near LES, due to chronic GE reflux
   5. Barrett's → 10% risk of developing adenocarcinoma (premalignant)
   6. Scleroderma causes dysphagia due to ↓ peristalsis/LES tone → reflux, erosive esophagitis
H. Esophageal carcinoma
   1. Most tumors are leiomyomas, totally benign
   2. Most cancers are squamous cell CA, **strongly associated with smoking & drinking alcohol**
   3. Adenocarcinoma is more rare, follows Barrett's esophagus
I. Hiatal hernia
   1. Sac-like herniation of stomach through diaphragm
   2. Can lead to reflux esophagitis
J. Esophageal injuries
   1. Mallory-Weiss tear = laceration at GE junction during vomiting, causing massive hemorrhage

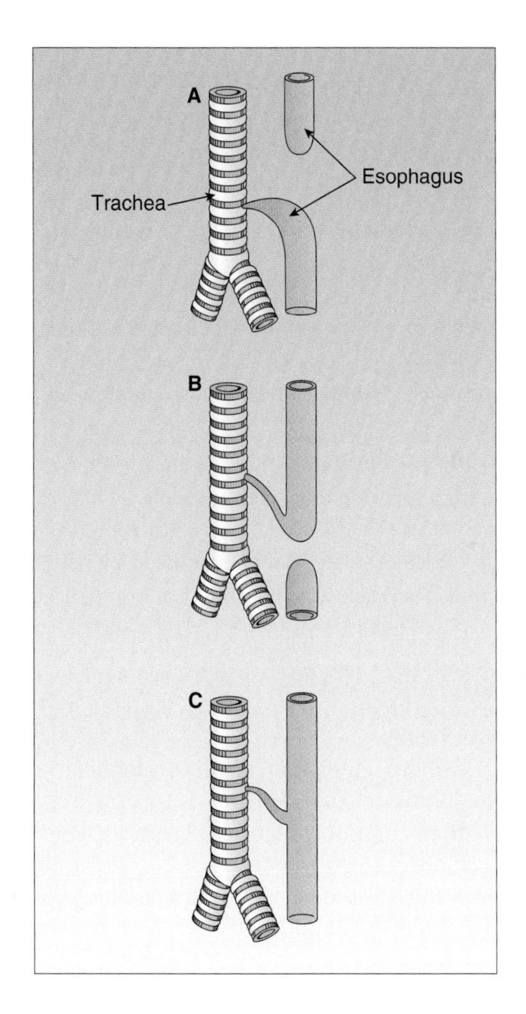

Figure 6.1 Congenital Tracheoesophageal Fistulas
A. The most common type is a communication between the trachea and the lower portion of the esophagus. The upper segment of the esophagus ends in a blind sac. **B.** In a few cases, the proximal esophagus communicates with the trachea. **C.** The least common anomaly, the H type, is a fistula between a continuous esophagus and trachea. (From Rubin E, Gorstein F, Rubin R, et al. Rubin's Pathology: Clinicopathologic Foundations of Medicine. 4th ed. Baltimore: Lippincott Williams & Wilkins, 2005.)

2. Boerhaave's syndrome = **complete esophageal rupture** 2° to forceful vomiting or instrumentation
3. Schatzki ring = mucosal indentation at GE junction, ring < 12 mm diameter leads to food lodging

K. Pathology of esophagitis
1. Reflux most common with hiatal hernia
2. Infectious most often due to cytomegalovirus (CMV), herpes, *Candida*
3. Diverticula can be pulsion (due to ↑ pressure) or traction (inflammation)
4. Pulsion usually at upper or lower end, traction can be in middle

L. Plummer-vinson syndrome
1. Classic triad = esophageal web, spoon nail, iron deficiency anemia
2. Webs produce dysphagia, may be missed by barium swallow
3. Webs may disappear with treatment of iron deficiency
4. Can also see glossitis

II. Stomach

A. Normal physiology
1. Proximal fundus has high pressure, controls fluid emptying from the stomach to duodenum
2. Distal antrum grinds solids into small particles, controls passage to duodenum
3. Parietal & chief cells are located in the fundus, most of antrum is goblet & mucosal production

B. Dumping syndrome
1. Occurs postvagotomy (can be autovagotomy, e.g., diabetic gastroparesis)
2. Sx/Si = postprandial nausea/vomiting, diaphoresis, palpitations, diarrhea
3. Vagotomy → rapid fluid transfer to duodenum, leading to rapid caloric uptake, but solid emptying is delayed
4. ↑↑ insulin after rapid caloric fluid uptake → reactive hypoglycemia
5. Tx = pyloric sphincterotomy so food can escape the stomach
6. Medical Tx for stasis = metoclopramide

C. Congenital pyloric stenosis
   1. Causes projectile vomiting in first **2 weeks to 2 months of life**
   2. More common in males & in first-born children
   3. **Pathognomonic physical finding is palpable "olive" nodule in mid-epigastrium**, representing hypertrophied pyloric sphincter
   4. If "olive" is not present, diagnosis made by ultrasound
   5. Tx = longitudinal surgical incision in hypertrophied muscle

D. Acute erosive gastritis
   1. Causes = nonsteroidal anti-inflammatory drugs (NSAIDs), smoking, alcohol, Curler's or Cushing's ulcer
   2. Curler's ulcer seen in burn patients (pts) (**mnemonic:** curling iron is hot! It burns!)
   3. Cushing's ulcer is postbrain injury, due to ↑ acid production 2° to ↑ steroid levels (**mnemonic:** think Cushing's disease (dz), elevated cortisol)
   4. Typically see in ICU posttrauma/burn/head injury/hemorrhage, first sign may be blood in nasogastric (NG) aspirate

E. Chronic (nonerosive) gastritis (atrophic gastritis)
   1. Type A = fundal gastritis = autoimmune (pernicious anemia), associated with thyroiditis, Addison's disease
   2. Type B = antral gastritis, associated with *Helicobacter pylori*, NSAIDs, herpes, CMV
   3. NSAIDs: most common cause of chronic gastritis (in antrum, not fundus)
   4. Menetrier's disease = giant hypertrophic gastritis
      a. Look for extreme enlargement of gastric rugae
      b. Can lose enough serum proteins through stomach to become hypoalbuminemic
   5. Gastritis is a risk factor for development of gastric CA

F. Gastric ulcers (GU)
   1. *H. pylori* found in 70% of gastric ulcers
   2. GU Sx = pain worsened by food, particularly if in antrum
   3. GU is NOT a cancer precursor, but can be caused by cancers
   4. 10% of GUs are caused by ulcerating malignancy
   5. **As opposed to duodenal ulcers, GUs are NOT caused by acid hypersecretion**—patients with GU have low-to-normal acid secretion, may have ↓ mucosal protection from acid
   6. Sequelae = bleeding, perforation, penetration, obstruction

G. Gastric cancer

1. Stomach CA most common after 50 years, ↑ incidence in men
2. Linked to blood group A (suggesting genetic predisposition), immunosuppression & environmental factors
3. Nitrosamines, excess salt intake, low fiber intake, *H. pylori*, achlorhydria, chronic gastritis are all risk factors
4. Almost always adenocarcinoma, usually involves antrum, rarely fundus, aggressive spread to nodes/liver
5. Rarer gastric tumors = lymphoma, leiomyosarcoma/leiomyoma
6. Several classic physical findings in metastatic gastric cancers
   a. **Virchow's node = large rock-hard supraclavicular node**
   b. **Krukenberg tumor = mucinous, signet-ring cells metastasize from gastric CA to bilateral ovaries, so palpate for ovarian masses in women**
   c. **Sister Mary Joseph sign = metastasis to umbilicus, feel for hard nodule there, associated with poor prognosis**
   d. **Blumer's shelf = palpable nodule superiorly on rectal exam, caused by metastasis of GI cancer**
7. Linitis plastica
   a. Infiltrating, diffuse CA, invariably fatal within months
   b. **This is the most deadly form of gastric cancer**
8. Lymphoma causes 4% of gastric cancers, better Px than adenocarcinoma

III. Small Intestine

A. Normal physiology

1. 4 phases of activity: 1) quiescent, 2) random motor, 3) migrating motor complex (MMC), 4) return to 1
2. MMC moves desquamated cells & bacteria out of gut
3. Food induces prolonged phase 2 to ↑ mixing time & ↑ absorption
4. Ileus (paralyzed bowel) follows distention due to obstruction, surgical handling, peritoneal irritation
5. Pseudoobstruction can be 2° to diabetes or scleroderma
6. Thyrotoxicosis & carcinoid syndrome cause prolonged MMC → diarrhea

B. Duodenal ulcer (DU)

1. Almost all DU patients have ↑ acid production, 80% have ↑ nocturnal secretion

2. *H. pylori* found in 90% of duodenal ulcers
3. **Acid protects against cancer, DU is not a cancer precursor!**
4. DU associated with blood type O, may be partially genetic (note: g**A**stric cancer associated with type A, du**O**denal ulcer associated with type O)
5. Acid in duodenum leads to gastric metaplasia there, allowing *H. pylori* to get a foothold, cause DU
6. Smoking & excessive alcohol intake ↑ risk for peptic ulcer
7. DU Sx/Si = epigastric pain 1–3hr postprandial, relieved by food/antacids, pain typically awakens patient at night
8. Bleeding from DU typically causes melena
9. Gastrinoma causes ulcers in atypical locations like the jejunum
10. Zollinger-Ellison syndrome
    a. Gastrinoma secretes ↑ gastrin → disseminated GI ulcers
    b. Dx by ↑ fasting gastrin, also Sx = diarrhea/steatorrhea
    c. Associated with multiendocrine neoplasia (MEN) type I [see Endocrinology, Section VII]

C. Crohn's disease (inflammatory bowel disease)
1. A GI inflammatory disease that may be infectious in nature
2. Affects any part of GI, most commonly small & large bowel
3. Lesions → transmural chronic inflammation, **noncaseating granulomas**, fibrous tracts (adhesions) between loops of bowel, **cobblestone mucosal morphology, skip lesions** (see Figures 6.2 and 6.3)
4. **Creeping fat on gross dissection is pathognomonic**
5. Si/Sx = abdominal pain, diarrhea, malabsorption, fever, stricture causing obstruction (see Figure 6.4), fistulae, calcium oxalate kidney stones/gallstones & other extraintestinal manifestations [see below, Section IV.D.2]

D. Meckel's diverticulum
1. Most common congenital anomaly of small bowel
2. It is a remnant of the embryonic vitelline duct
3. May contain ectopic gastric, duodenal, colonic, or pancreatic tissue
4. Usually aSx, may have bloody diarrhea, peptic ulceration, intussusception causing obstruction & volvulus
5. **Rule of 2s: 2% of population has them, located 2 ft from ileocecal valve, 2 inches long, usually presents within first 2 years of life**

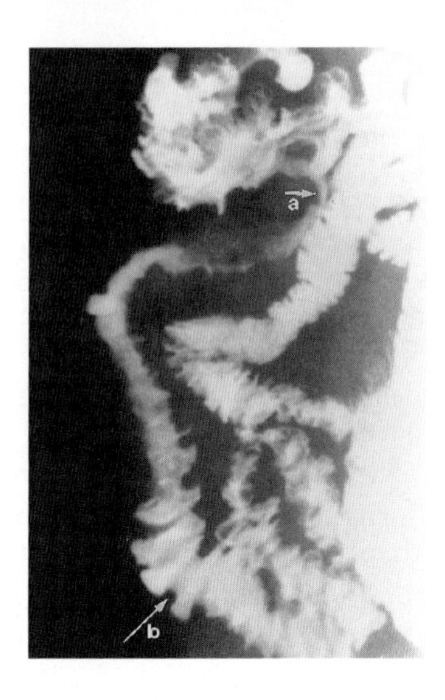

Figure 6.2
Barium follow-through showing stricturing of the small intestine (a) and edematous small bowel with thickening of the valvulae conniventes (b). (From Axford JS. Medicine. Oxford: Blackwell Science, 1998.)

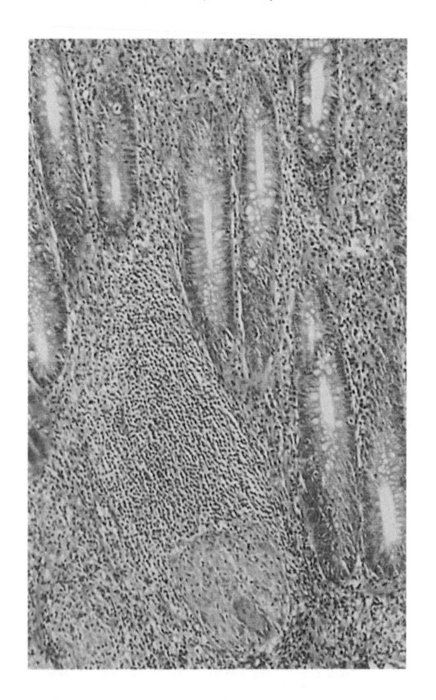

Figure 6.3
Histopathology of Crohn's colitis showing intense mucosal inflammatory cell infiltration and an epithelioid granuloma containing a giant cell (center, bottom). (From Axford JS. Medicine. Oxford: Blackwell Science, 1998.)

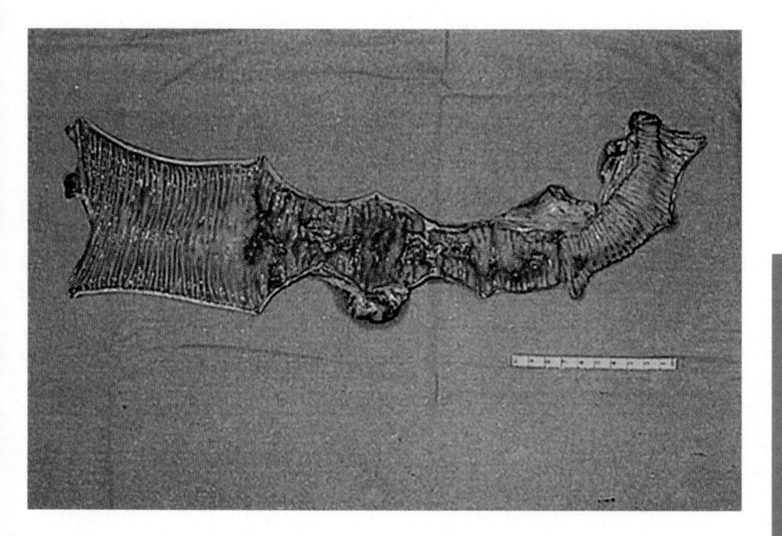

Figure 6.4
Resected small bowel showing segmental stricture with patchy deep ulcers and proximal intestinal dilation (left). The patient presented with subacute bowel obstruction. (From Axford JS. Medicine. Oxford: Blackwell Science, 1998.)

E. Malabsorption
   1. Malabsorption diarrhea characterized by high fat content
   2. Lose fat-soluble vitamins, iron, calcium, & B vitamins
   3. Can cause iron deficiency, megaloblastic anemia (vitamin B_{12} loss), & hypocalcemia
   4. Etiologies
      a. Celiac disease
         (1) Diarrhea 2° to gluten (gliadin fraction) sensitivity
            (a) Wheat, barley, rye, oats contain gluten
            (b) Rice & corn are gluten-free
         (2) Genetic & autoimmune components
         (3) **Dx: pathognomonic biopsy of small bowel shows blunting of intestinal villi, anti-gliadin, anti-endomysial, and anti-tissue trans-glutaminase antibodies also suggest the dz**
         (4) 10%–15% of pts develop cancer (usually lymphoma)
         (5) Sx/Si = ↓ weight, weakness, diarrhea with pale, frothy, foul-smelling stool, failure to thrive, growth retardation

(6) Classic rash = **dermatitis herpetiformis** = pruritic, red papulovesicular lesions on shoulders, elbows & knees that disappear after gluten withdrawal

b. Tropical sprue
   (1) Diarrhea probably caused by a tropical infection, responds to antibiotics (tetracycline + folate)
   (2) Si/Sx = glossitis, diarrhea, weight loss, steatorrhea

c. Whipple's disease
   (1) An inflammatory disorder of the GI tract due to infection by *Tropheryma whippelii*
   (2) Dx by periodic acid-Schiff (PAS)+ macrophages in intestinal mucosa
   (3) Note that PAS+ macrophages may also appear in *Mycobacterium avium intracellulare* in AIDS
   (4) Classic Si/Sx = diarrhea, arthritis, rash, anemia, malabsorption

d. Lactase deficiency
   (1) Most of world is lactase deficient as adults; people lose as they emerge from adolescence
   (2) Lactate ingestion → osmotic diarrhea as sugar draws water into bowel
   (3) Also, presence of carbohydrate in the colon allows for bacterial fermentation

e. Abetalipoproteinemia
   (1) Hereditary deficiency of apoprotein B → fat malabsorption
   (2) **Look for spur cells (acanthocytes) on blood smear**

f. Intestinal lymphangiectasia
   (1) Dilation of intestinal lymphatics leads to marked GI protein loss, hypoproteinemia, edema
   (2) Dx by jejunal biopsy, can be congenital or acquired

g. **Pancreatitis & cystic fibrosis frequently cause malabsorption**

h. A variety of infectious agents can cause malabsorption, including worms, bacteria & protozoa

F. Cancer

1. Very rare in small bowel
2. Most common are adenocarcinoma, also see lymphoma & carcinoid

3. Carcinoid = APUDoma (**a**mine **p**recursor **u**ptake & **d**ecarboxylate), occurs most frequently in the appendix
   a. Neoplasm of the neuroendocrine Kulchitsky cells (K-cells)
   b. Slow growing, low grade but is malignant, appendiceal tumors rarely metastasize, ileal tumors commonly do
   c. Carcinoid syndrome results from metastases to liver by tumors that secrete serotonin (5-HT)
   d. Liver normally degrades 5-HT, but metastases in liver secrete 5-HT into posthepatic circulation
   e. Causes flushing, watery diarrhea & abdominal cramps, bronchospasm, right-sided heart valve lesions
   f. Dx = High levels of urine 5HIAA (false-positives seen in patients who eat lots of bananas)
   g. Tx = somatostatin & methysergide

IV. Large Intestine

A. Hirschsprung's disease ("aganglionic megacolon")
   1. Congenital lack of myenteric plexus leads to static colon, with compensatory dilation proximal to the denervated bowel
   2. Due to loss of function mutation in *ret* oncogene
   3. Tx = excision of the denervated segment of the bowel

B. Diverticula
   1. Herniation of colonic mucosa through the muscle wall, common in older people, usually involves the sigmoid colon—considered a muscle defect, associated with low-fiber diet
   2. Diverticulosis = multiple diverticula without inflammation, causes bleeding that is bright red & can be massive
   3. Diverticulitis = inflammation of diverticula, complicated by bleeding, perforation, peritonitis, & fistula formation, **presents as acute abdomen but pain is localized to left lower quadrant**

C. Ischemic bowel disease
   1. Can be caused by atherosclerotic occlusion of AT LEAST 2 major mesenteric vessels
      a. Usually occurs at splenic flexure & rectosigmoid junction
      b. These are watershed areas, between superior mesenteric & inferior mesenteric supply zones
   2. Emboli can lead to rapid ischemia of entire gut segment
   3. Vasculitis causes local ischemic necrosis
   4. Venous thrombosis can cause ischemia

5. Low cardiac output can cause nonocclusive bowel ischemia
6. Mucosal layer is the most sensitive, **ischemia → necrosis & bleeding but no pain since the mucosa is not innervated**
7. **Ischemia of the deeper layers → severe pain, metabolic acidosis, shock, perforation, death**
8. 3 outcomes of bowel ischemia
   a. If only mucosa involved, reperfusion → complete restitution
   b. If deeper layers involved, healing → fibrosis & stricture
   c. Transmural infarction → perforation, peritonitis, death

D. Inflammatory disorders
1. Ulcerative colitis (UC) (inflammatory bowel disease)
   a. An idiopathic autoinflammatory disorder of the colon (see Figures 6.5 and 6.6)
   b. Always starts in rectum & spreads proximal
   c. If confined to rectum = ulcerative proctitis, a benign subtype
   d. Most characteristic feature is crypt abscess with numerous polymorphonuclear neutrophils (PMNs) in crypt of Lieberkuhn (see Figure 6.7)
   e. Also see bloody, distended capillaries in submucosa, UC lesions bleed very easily
   f. Watch for toxic megacolon!
2. Comparison of inflammatory bowel disease (IBD) (see Table 6.1)
3. Pseudomembranous colitis
   a. A prolific diarrhea caused by *Clostridium difficile* after a patient has received broad-spectrum antibiotics
   b. Classic endoscopy finding = gray, necrotic pseudo-membrane
   c. Tx = metronidazole or oral vancomycin

E. Colonic tumors
1. Pedunculated (stem) & sessile (broad base) polyps are most common benign tumors
2. Hyperplastic polyps occur anywhere in the colon, have no clinical significance besides misdiagnosis
3. Polyps 2° to chronic inflammation can bleed or perforate
4. Lymphoid polyps occur in rectum, small intestine, or colon
5. Hamartomatous polyps = juvenile polyps, rarely occur in adults
6. Hamartomatous polyps also seen in Peutz-Jeghers (see Section F.8)

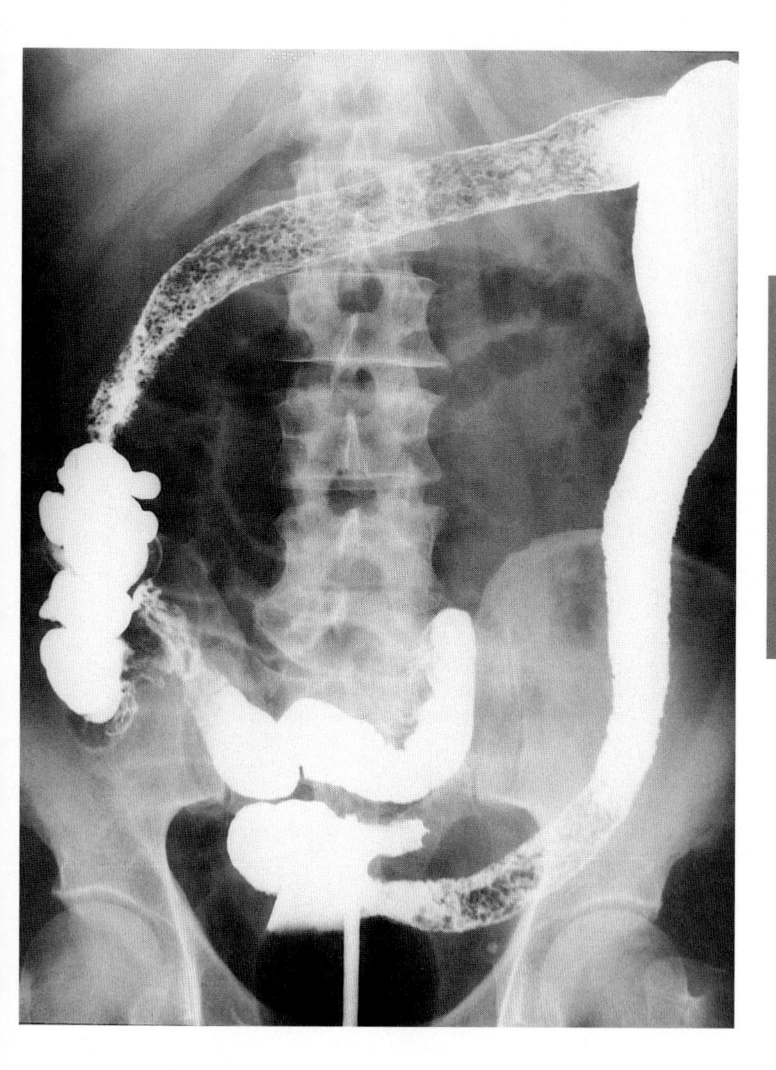

Figure 6.5 Barium Enema
Extensive diffuse mucosal ulceration in the large bowel, with loss of the normal haustral pattern in ulcerative colitis. (From Patel PR. Lecture Notes on Radiology. Oxford: Blackwell Science, 1996.)

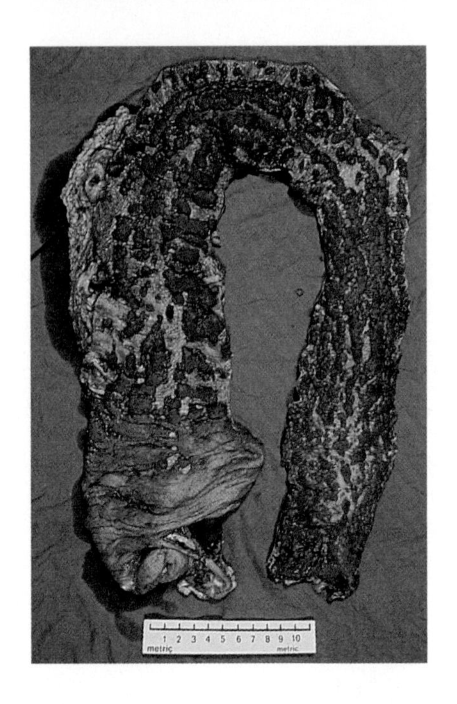

Figure 6.6
Colonic resection specimen from patient with UC. Note subtotal involvement with areas of ulceration and pseudopolyps. (From Axford JS, Callaghan CA. Medicine. 2nd ed. Oxford: Blackwell Science, 2004.)

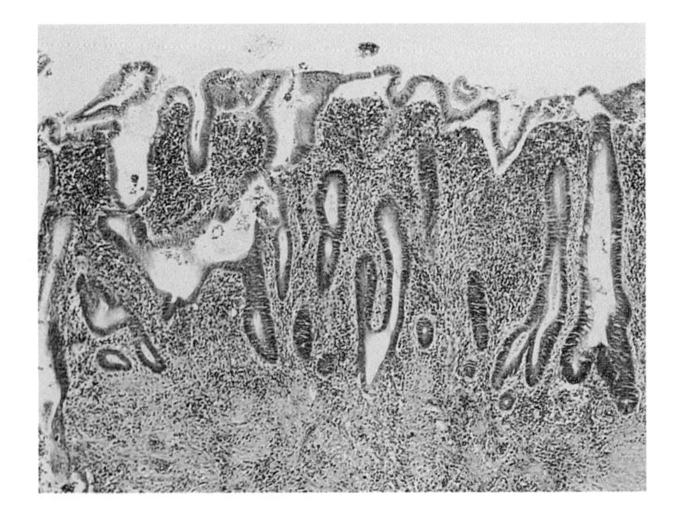

Figure 6.7
Histopathology of UC showing epithelial cell loss, inflammatory cell infiltrate in the lamina propria, separation and distortion of crypt architecture, and goblet cell depletion. (From Axford JS. Medicine. Oxford: Blackwell Science, 1998.)

Table 6.1 Ulcerative Colitis versus Crohn's Disease

	Ulcerative Colitis	Crohn's Disease
Location	Isolated to colon	Anywhere in GI tract
Lesions	Contiguously proximal from colon	Skip lesions, disseminated
Inflammation	Limited to mucosa/ submucosa	Transmural
Neoplasms	Very high risk for development	Lower risk for development
Fissures	None	Extend through submucosa
Fistula	None	Frequent: can be enterocutaneous
Granulomas	None	Noncaseating are characteristic
Extraintestinal manifestations	Seen in both: • Arthritis, iritis, erythema nodosum, pyoderma gangrenosum • Sclerosing cholangitis = chronic, fibrosing, inflammation of biliary system leading to cholestasis & portal hypertension	

F. Colonic cancers
1. Adenomatous polyps are usually aSx, but may bleed
2. Tubular adenomas are most common (75%), contain malignant foci, larger the polyp = ↑ odds malignant
3. Tubulovillous adenomas are a bridge between tubular & villous, middle morphology & median malignant
4. Villous adenomas are most rare (10%), large, sessile, 30% become malignant
5. Familial adenomatous polyposis (FAP) = autosomal dominant, hundreds of polyps with 100% chance of developing colon CA
6. Gardener's syndrome = FAP + triad of osteomas, desmoid tumors & sebaceous cysts

7. Turcot's syndrome = adenomatous polyps + CNS tumors
8. Peutz-Jeghers syndrome = autosomal dominant, melanin pigment of lips, oral mucosa, hands, genitals, **benign hamartomas**, ↑ risk of CA of stomach, breast & ovaries
9. Adenocarcinoma produce carcinoembryonic antigen (CEA), used to follow course of dz, but not Dx due to low specificity
10. CA may occur in the rectosigmoid, typically ulcerative, leading to stenosis & obstruction

V. Appendix

A. Acute appendicitis

1. Occurs most frequently in the second to third decades, usually due to obstruction by a fecalith
2. Histologic appearance: acute inflammatory infiltrate extending from mucosa through the full thickness of the wall
3. Si/Sx: diffuse periumbilical pain migrating to right lower quadrant (McBurney's point), ⊕ rebound tenderness, nausea/vomit, ↑ white cells (WBCs) with left shift, urinalysis → ⊕WBC, ⊕RBC
4. Psoas sign = pain on flexion of hip &/or extension of thigh
5. Obturator sign = pain on external rotation of hip

B. Tumor

1. Most common tumor is carcinoid

VI. Liver

A. Jaundice—visible when serum bilirubin exceeds 2 mg/dL

1. Physiologic jaundice of the newborn
   a. Clinically benign jaundice in first week of life
   b. Characterized by unconjugated hyperbilirubinemia
   c. Results from increased bilirubin production & relative deficiency in glucuronyl transferase in the immature liver (see Figure 6.8)
   d. **Physiologic jaundice develops 24–48hr after birth!, jaundice present AT birth is ALWAYS pathologic**
   e. Tx = UV light that breaks down bilirubin pigments
2. Congenital hyperbilirubinemia
   a. Gilbert's syndrome
      (1) Extremely common, occurring in 5% of population
      (2) ↑ serum unconjugated bilirubin, caused by ↓ bilirubin uptake by cells & ↓ activity of glucuronyl transferase

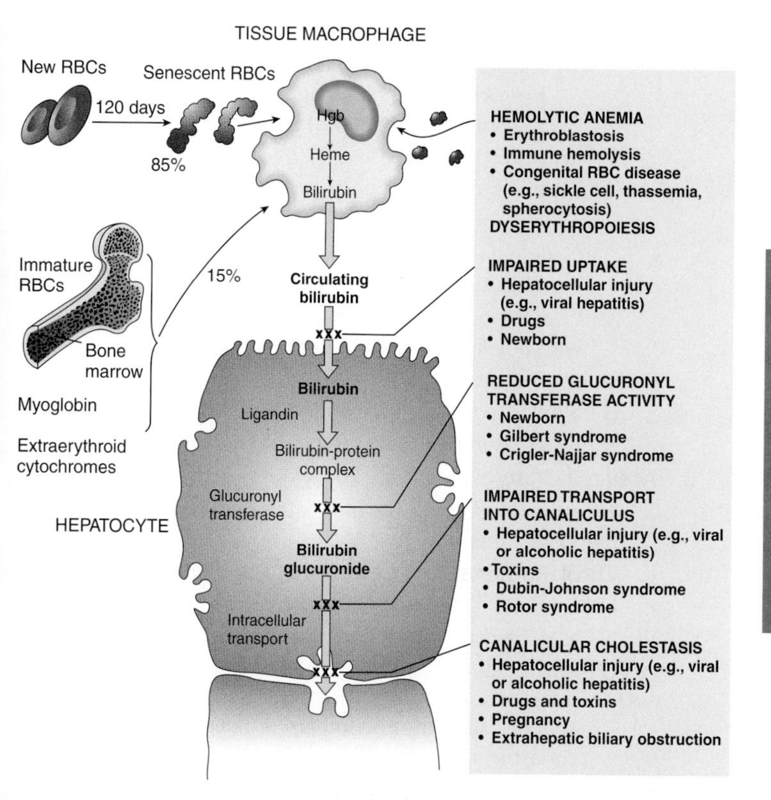

Figure 6.8 Mechanisms of Jaundice at the Level of the Hepatocyte Bilirubin is derived principally from the senescence of circulating red blood cells, with a smaller contribution from the degradation of erythropoietic elements in the bone marrow, myoglobin, and extraerythroid cytochromes. Jaundice results from overproduction of bilirubin (hemolytic anemia), dyserythropoiesis, or defects in its hepatic metabolism. The locations of specific blocks in the metabolic pathway of bilirubin in the hepatocyte are illustrated. (From Rubin E, Gorstein F, Rubin R, et al. Rubin's Pathology: Clinicopathologic Foundations of Medicine. 4th ed. Baltimore: Lippincott Williams & Wilkins, 2005.)

(3) Jaundice presents during stressful situations, clinically completely benign

b. Crigler-Najjar syndrome

(1) Severe familial disorder with ↑ unconjugated bilirubin caused by a deficiency of glucuronyl transferase

(2) Type 1 = total absence of glucuronyl transferase
(a) Causes markedly ↑ bilirubin levels & early death from kernicterus (damage to basal ganglia by unconjugated bilirubin)
(b) Autosomal recessive
(3) Type 2 = mild deficiency (autosomal dominant).

c. Dubin-Johnson syndrome
(1) Conjugated hyperbilirubinemia due to defective bilirubin excretion
(2) Characterized by black liver jaundice & not associated with any liver failure

d. Rotor syndrome
(1) Similar to Dubin-Johnson but no black liver
(2) Defect is in bilirubin storage, not excretion

3. Acquired causes
a. Excess production: ↑ unconjugated bilirubin seen in hemolytic anemias
b. Cholestasis: impaired excretion of conjugated bilirubin
c. Intrahepatic = hepatocellular cholestasis
(1) May be due to viral hepatitis or cirrhosis
(2) May be due to drug-induced hepatitis (carbon tetrachloride, acetaminophen, methotrexate, oral contraceptives, anabolic steroids, phenothiazines, halothane, INH, fluconazole, methyldopa)
d. Extrahepatic causes = choledocholithiasis (but not cholelithiasis), bile duct CA, CA at ampulla of Vater/head of pancreas, cholangitis, biliary cirrhosis
(1) Primary biliary cirrhosis
(a) An autoimmune disorder found in women
(b) Si/Sx = obstructive jaundice, pruritus, hypercholesterolemia
(c) **Antimitochondrial antibody test is 90% sensitive**
(2) Secondary biliary cirrhosis results from long-standing biliary obstruction due to any cause (e.g., cholangitis)
e. Clinical features of acquired jaundice = acholic stools (pale), fat malabsorption, pruritus, elevated serum cholesterol, xanthomas, urinary bilirubin

B. Hepatitis
1. Transaminases = ALT (SGPT) & AST (SGOT)
a. Alcoholics: AST higher than ALT (AST:ALT ratio ≥ 2:1)
b. Viral infection: often ALT = AST, but ALT may be higher

   c. **Mnemonic: toAST = alcohol, virALT = viral, so AST is higher in alcohol & ALT in viral**
2. Acute hepatitis can be due to virus, alcohol/drugs, vascular insufficiency, other infectious agents, trauma
3. Fulminant hepatitis
   a. Hepatic failure characterized by falling prothrombin levels & development of hepatic encephalopathy
   b. Complication of acute hepatitis, can occur over a period of less than 4wk
   c. Can be caused by viral agents (Hep A-E), drugs (INH), toxins & some metabolic disorders like Wilson's disease [see Neurology, Section VIII.E]
4. Viral hepatitis
   a. HBV & HCV can lead to macronodular cirrhosis
   b. Histologic appearance: large nodules with intact hepatic lobules
   c. **Viral cirrhosis develops into hepatocellular CA more often than other types**
   d. **Pearl: pts infected with HBV classically have anorexia & a distaste for cigarettes, can also see urticaria & arthralgias**
5. Granulomatous hepatitis
   a. Often not associated with symptoms, but can have pruritus, fever &/or jaundice
   b. Causes = tuberculosis (TB), *Coccidioides*, brucellosis, *Rickettsia*, spirochetes, sarcoidosis, Wegener's granulomatosis, Hodgkin's disease
6. Other inflammatory liver disorders
   a. Epstein-Barr virus: seen in infectious mononucleosis
   b. **HSV-1: histologically characteristic nuclear inclusion surrounded by a halo (OWL'S EYE)**
   c. Yellow fever characterized by mid-zonal hepatic necrosis
      (1) Dying hepatocytes condense into **eosinophilic contracted forms called "Councilman bodies"**
      (2) Similar bodies seen in all viral hepatitides
   d. Leptospirosis
      (1) Known as Weil's disease or icterohemorrhagic fever
      (2) Severe infection characterized by jaundice, renal failure & hemorrhagic phenomena
   e. *Echinococcus granulosa*
      (1) Ingestion of dog tapeworm (*Taenia*) results in hydatid cyst diseases

(2) Large parasitic cysts invade the liver, if rupture can lead to anaphylaxis

(3) Tx = careful surgical excystation without spillage of cyst contents

f. Schistosomiasis: *S. mansoni* or *S. japonicum*

(1) Adult worms lodge in portal vein & its branches

(2) Eggs stimulate granuloma formation, tissue destruction & portal hypertension

7. Microvesicular fatty liver

a. A group of serious disorders associated with the presence of small fatty vacuoles in hepatocytes

b. Reye's syndrome

(1) Encephalopathy, coma & microvesicular fatty liver

(2) Associated with aspirin administration to children with acute viral infections

c. Fatty liver of pregnancy = acute hepatic failure during the third trimester of pregnancy

d. Tetracycline toxicity is due to unpredictable hypersensitivity-like reaction

8. Alcoholic liver disease

a. Most common form of liver disease in United States

b. Early on reversible fatty changes seen, followed by development of hepatitis, with focal liver necrosis, PMN infiltrate, & **Mallory bodies**

c. Can lead to alcoholic cirrhosis (Laennec's cirrhosis)

d. Clinical manifestations

(1) Jaundice due to ↑ conjugated/unconjugated bilirubin

(2) ↓ liver synthesis leads to ↑ **PT, PTT (most sensitive laboratory sign of liver failure)**, ascites 2° to ↓ serum albumin (as well as portal hypertension, see below)—note, all coagulation factor levels are diminished except for von Willebrand factor, which is not synthesized in liver (synthesized in endothelial cells)

(3) ↑ estrogen leads to palmar erythema, **Dupuytren's contractures** (fibrous contraction of palmar fascia causing finger flexion at rest; see Figure 6.9), spider angioma (arteriole telangiectasia) of face, arms & chest, ↓ body & pubic hair, testicular atrophy, gynecomastia

(4) Peripheral edema, ascites, or hydrothorax caused by

(a) ↑ portal venous pressure leading to increased production of hepatic lymph

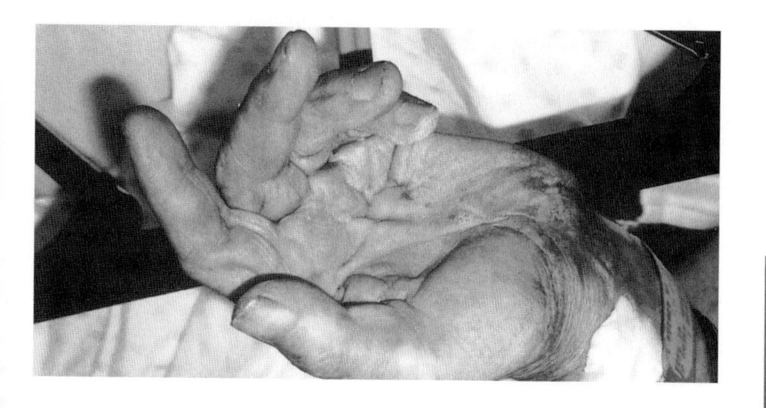

Figure 6.9
Dupuytren's contracture. (From Berg D. Advanced Clinical Skills and Physical Diagnosis. Oxford: Blackwell Science, 1999.)

(b) ↓ plasma oncotic pressure 2° to ↓ albumin
(c) Retention of sodium & water as a result of decreased hepatic degradation of aldosterone & activation of renin-angiotensin system
(d) Spontaneous bacterial peritonitis
   (i) Usually low protein ascites with no Sx of infection (see Table 6.2)
   (ii) Dx = ascitic fluid with absolute neutrophil count of >250 or ⊕ Gram stain/culture of ascitic fluid

Table 6.2 Ascites Differentials

	Portal Hypertension	No Portal Hypertension
Serum/ascites albumin gradient	>1.1g/dL	<1.1g/dL
Causes	Cirrhosis, alcoholic hepatitis, Budd-Chiari, liver metastases, CHF	Pancreatic dz, nephrosis, TB, peritoneal metastases, idiopathic
Other Labs	Ascites total protein >2.5 → heart dz Ascites total protein ≤2.5 → liver dz	Amylase ↑ in pancreatic dz

(iii) Common organisms include *Escherichia coli*, *Klebsiella*, *Enterococcus*, & *Streptococcus pneumonia*

(iv) Tx = third-generation cephalosporins

(5) Encephalopathy probably due to ↑ ammonia levels, characterized by asterixis (flapping tremor of the wrist upon flexion) & altered mental status

(6) Tx of encephalopathy is to lower NH_3 levels

(a) Lactulose metabolized by bacteria, acidifies the bowel, $NH_3 \rightarrow NH_4^+$, which cannot be absorbed

(b) Neomycin kills bacteria making NH_3 in gut

(c) Sodium benzoate binds NH_3 in blood & causes it to be excreted as hippurate via kidney

e. Delirium tremens (DTs)

(1) Alcohol (EtOH) withdrawal time course—**time from last drink**

(a) Within 12 hours, pt has headache, malaise, irritable

(b) **24–48 hours, seizures develop,** ⊕ resting tremor

(c) **72 hours autonomic instability (↑↑ BP/HR), delirium**

(2) DTs → agitation, delirium, confusion, **auditory & tactile hallucinations** (bugs crawling on skin), **generalized seizures that can be lethal, hypertension/tachycardia**

f. Treatment of inpatient alcoholics

(1) IV thiamine & B_{12} supplements to correct deficiency (very common), also **must give thiamine before IV glucose or will precipitate Wernicke's encephalopathy**

(2) Give IV glucose, fluids & electrolytes

(3) Correct any underlying coagulopathy

(4) Benzodiazepine for prevention & Tx of delirium tremens

9. Autoimmune hepatitis

a. Variable presentation, several types of disease

b. Clinically similar to any other hepatitis, can lead to cirrhosis with 40% resultant mortality

c. Type I occurs in young women, ⊕ antinuclear antigen, ⊕ anti-smooth muscle antibody

d. Type II occurs mostly in children, linked to Mediterranean ancestry, ⊕ anti–liver-kidney-muscle (anti-LKM) antibody

e. Tx = prednisone +/− azathioprine

10. Can also see cirrhosis 2° to hemochromatosis [see Dermatology, Section III.D.9], galactosemia [see Appendix B], glycogen storage diseases [see Musculoskeletal, Section V.C] & biliary cirrhosis

C. Vascular disorders
   1. Portal hypertension can be presinusoidal, intrahepatic, or postsinusoidal in nature
   2. Presinusoidal is due to thrombosis & obstruction of portal or splenic veins
   3. Intrahepatic is due to obstruction of intrahepatic vessels by tumor, schistosomes, or cirrhosis
   4. Postsinusoidal is due to hepatic venous or vena caval occlusion
      a. **Budd-Chiari syndrome**
         (1) Rarely congenital, usually acquired thrombosis occluding hepatic vein or hepatic stretch of inferior vena cava
         (2) Associated with hypercoagulability (e.g., polycythemia vera, hepatocellular or other CA, pregnancy, etc.)
         (3) Sx = acute onset of abdominal pain, jaundice, ascites
         (4) Hepatitis quickly develops, leading to cirrhosis & portal hypertension
         (5) Px poor, less than 1/3 pts survive at 1yr
         (6) Dx = right upper quadrant ultrasound
         (7) Tx = clot lysis or hepatic transplant
      b. Veno-occlusive disease (VOD)
         (1) Occlusion of hepatic venules (not large veins)
         (2) Associated with graft vs. host disease, chemotherapy, & radiation therapy
         (3) Px = 50% mortality at 1yr
         (4) Tx = hepatic transplant, sometimes is self-limiting

D. Hepatic tumors
   1. Benign tumors
      a. Hemangioma is most common benign tumor of the liver
      b. Hepatic adenoma incidence related to oral contraceptives
      c. Adenomas may rupture → severe intraperitoneal bleed
   2. Malignant tumors
      a. Metastases are the most common malignant hepatic tumors
      b. Hepatocellular CA is the most common 1° hepatic malignancy
         (1) Associated with cirrhosis, HBV & HCV infection, aflatoxin B (nuts & grains)

(2) Frequently associated with increased α-fetoprotein
(3) **Note:** also called "hepatoma," incorrectly implying benign tumor (historical misnomer)

c. Cholangiocarcinoma = bile duct CA
(1) Frequently seen in Far East, associated with *Clonorchis sinensis* (liver fluke) infestation
(2) Can also occur as a late side effect of thorium dioxide (Thorotrast) administration
(3) Almost always an adenocarcinoma, carries very poor Px
(4) When the tumor occurs at the confluence of the hepatic ducts forming the common duct, the tumor is called "Klatskin's tumor" (mean survival = 9–12 months, no Tx, invariably lethal)

d. Hemangiosarcoma is associated with toxic exposure to polyvinyl chloride, thorotrast, & arsenic

VII. Gallbladder

A. Cholelithiasis 5 gallstones

1. Higher incidence in women, multiple pregnancies, obesity **(the 4 Fs: female, forty, fertile, fat)**
2. Stones may be cholesterol, pigmented, or mixed
   a. Cholesterol stones are often solitary LARGE stones that cannot enter the cystic/common bile duct
   b. Pigment stones seen in hemolytic anemia
      (1) Results from excess unconjugated bilirubin
      (2) **Gallstones in nulliparous child/very young adult is a clue to congenital hemolytic process (think sickle cell or thalassemia, rarely spherocytosis)**
   c. Mixed stones comprise 80% of stones, mix of cholesterol & calcium salts, can be seen on x-ray
3. Cholelithiasis is asymptomatic by definition, detected by ultrasound, often incidental finding that does not require therapy—10% of US population has gallstones
4. Complications of the disorder are what necessitate intervention
5. Biliary colic is due to gallstone impaction in cystic or common bile duct
   a. Sx = sharp, colicky pain made worse by eating, particularly fats

b. May have multiple episodes that resolve, but eventually this condition will lead to further complications so surgical resection of the gallbladder is required
c. **The vast majority of people who have asymptomatic gallstones WILL NEVER progress to biliary colic** (2%–3% progress per year, lifelong risk = 20%)

B. Cholecystitis
1. Cholecystitis is due to 2° infection of obstructed gallbladder
   a. The EEEK! bugs: *E. coli, Enterobacter cloacae, Enterococcus, Klebsiella* spp.
   b. First line Tx = second- & third-generation cephalosporins
2. Passage of stone through the cystic duct can obstruct common bile duct (CBD)
   a. Si/Sx = obstructive jaundice, ↑ conjugated bilirubin, hypercholesterolemia, ↑ alkaline phosphatase, **Murphy's sign** (sharp pain causing cessation of inspiration upon palpation of right upper quadrant)
   b. Utz → CBD > 9-mm diameter (Utz first line for Dx)
   c. **Passage of stone to CBD can cause acute pancreatitis if the ampulla of Vater is obstructed by the stone**
3. Ascending cholangitis
   a. Results from secondary bacterial infection of obstructed CBD, facilitated by obstructed bile flow
   b. **Charcot's triad = jaundice, RUQ pain, fever (85% sensitive for cholangitis)—for Reynold's pentad add altered mental status & hypotension**
4. Gallstone ileus
   a. Very rare disease due to intestinal obstruction caused by passage of a large gallstone through the eroded gallbladder wall into adjacent small bowel
   b. **Pathognomonic plain abdominal x-ray sign is free air in the biliary system (one of the few pathognomonic findings on plain x-rays)**
5. Cancer
   a. Gallstones are risk factors for developing cancer
   b. Most common 1° tumor of gallbladder is adenocarcinoma
   c. **Courvoisier's law** = non-tender gallbladder enlarges when CBD is obstructed by pancreatic CA but not enlarged when CBD is obstructed by stone
   d. CA of bile ducts is caused by liver flukes & ulcerative colitis, & is not associated with gallstones

VIII. Exocrine Pancreas

A. Congenital anomalies
   1. Ectopic pancreatic tissue
      a. Most commonly in stomach, small bowel, or Meckel's diverticulum
      b. Can be asymptomatic or cause bleeding & obstruction
   2. Annular pancreas = ring of pancreatic tissue encircling & obstructing duodenum
   3. Cystic fibrosis
      a. Meconium ileus results from ↑ viscosity of mucous secretions of intestinal tract
      b. *S. aureus* & *Pseudomonas* often infect these patients
      c. Dx = sweat test, except infants, for whom test not reliable
      d. Pathology shows mucous plugging of alveolar ducts with cystic dilation, fibrous proliferation, & atrophy
B. Acquired anomalies
   1. Acute pancreatitis (see Figure 6.10)
      a. Pancreatic enzymes autodigest pancreas → hemorrhagic fat necrosis, calcium deposition, & sometimes formation of pseudocysts (cysts not lined with ductal epithelium)

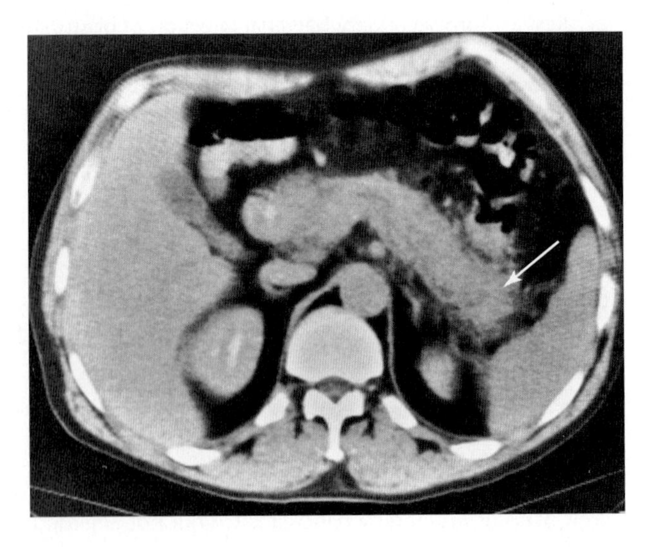

Figure 6.10 Acute Pancreatitis.
CT scan showing diffuse enlargement of the pancreas with ill-defined edges. (From Axford JS. Medicine. Oxford: Blackwell Science, 1998.)

b. Most common causes in United States = gallstones & alcohol
c. Other causes include infection, trauma, radiation, drug (thiazides, AZT, protease inhibitors), hyperlipidemia, hypercalcemia, vascular events, tumors, scorpion sting
d. Si/Sx = severe abdominal pain, prostration (fetal position opens up retroperitoneal space & allows more room for swollen pancreas), hypotension (due to retroperitoneal fluid sequestration), tachycardia, fever, ↑ serum amylase (90% sensitive)/lipase, hyperglycemia, hypocalcemia
e. **Classic x-ray finding = sentinel loop, or colon cut off sign** (loop of distended bowel adjacent to pancreas)
f. **Classic physical findings = Grey Turner's sign (discoloration of flank) & Cullen's sign (periumbilical discoloration)**
g. Complications = abscess, pseudocysts, duodenal obstruction, shock lung & acute renal failure

2. Pancreatic pseudocyst
   a. Collection of fluid in pancreas surrounded by a fibrous capsule, no communication with fibrous ducts
   b. **Suspect anytime a patient is readmitted with pancreatitis complaints within several weeks of being discharged after a bout of pancreatitis**
   c. Occurs from pancreatitis or trauma as in steering wheel injury
   d. New cysts contains blood, necrotic debris, leukocytes
   e. Old cysts contain straw-colored fluid
   f. Can become infected with purulent contents, causing peritonitis after rupture
3. Chronic pancreatitis due to recurrent episodes of inflammation, resulting in fibrosis & atrophy of the organ with early exocrine & later endocrine insufficiency (see Figure 6.11)
4. Pancreatic cancer
   a. 60% of adenocarcinomas are in head of pancreas (see Figure 6.12)
   b. Frequently invade duodenum, ampulla of Vater, common bile duct & can also cause biliary obstruction
   c. **Classic sign is Trousseau's syndrome = migratory thrombophlebitis, occurs in 10% of patients**
   d. Px very poor, 5-year survival rate after resection is 5%

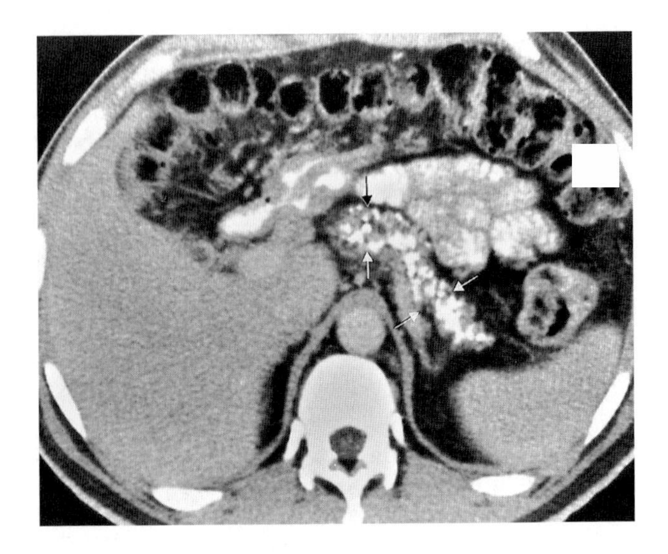

Figure 6.11 Chronic Pancreatitis
CT scan showing numerous small areas of calcification within the pancreas (arrows). (From Axford JS. Medicine. Oxford: Blackwell Science, 1998.)

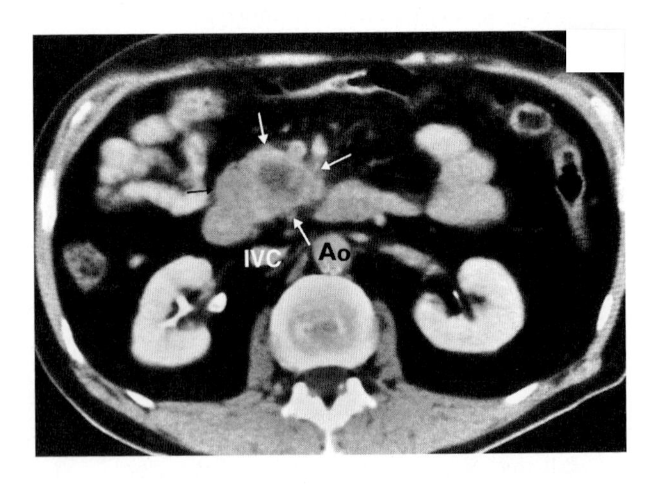

Figure 6.12 CT Scan Showing Focal Mass in Head of Pancreas (arrows)
Ao = aorta; IVC = inferior vena cava. (From Armstrong P, Wastie M. Diagnostic Imaging. 4th ed. Oxford: Blackwell Science, 1998.)

5. Endocrine pancreatic neoplasm
   a. Insulinoma due to hyperplasia of insulin producing β-cells
   b. Hyperglucagonemia = α cell tumor → hyperglycemia & exfoliative dermatitis
6. Zollinger-Ellison syndrome (see Section III.B.10 above)

7. NEPHROLOGY

I. Congenital Anomalies

A. Bilateral renal agenesis (Potter's Syndrome)
   1. Incompatible with fetal life
   2. Mother will have oligohydramnios (decreased amniotic fluid)
      a. Fetus normally swallows large quantities of amniotic fluid & then urinates it out
      b. Because fetus has no kidneys, cannot excrete swallowed fluid, results in oligohydramnios
   3. Seen in conjunction with multiple fetal anomalies, including hypoplastic lung & defects in extremities

B. Unilateral renal agenesis
   1. Unilateral renal agenesis is more common than bilateral, & is compatible with life
   2. Patient may develop progressive glomerular sclerosis

C. Renal ectopia
   1. Kidney may be in pelvis or other abnormal location
   2. Resulting tortuosity of ureters may predispose to pyelonephritis

D. Horseshoe kidney
   1. May cause urinary tract obstruction because of impingement on ureters
   2. Also may predispose to renal calculi

II. Urinary Tract Infection

A. Characteristics
   1. Infections much more common in women, possibly due to shorter female urethra
   2. ↑ incidence during pregnancy, possibly due to urinary stasis
   3. Most infections caused by gram-negative rods, & of these *Escherichia coli* causes 80% of all urinary tract infections (UTIs)
   4. *Staphylococcus saprophyticus* is second most common cause of UTI in young, healthy women
   5. Others include *Pseudomonas*, *Enterococcus*, & *Candida* (↑ risk with catheterization, nursing home, nosocomial)
   6. If ⊕ urethritis, look for *Neisseria*, herpes, *Chlamydia trachomatis*

7. Obstruction, surgery, catheters, anatomic abnormalities all predispose to infection
8. Signs/symptoms (Si/Sx) = ↑ frequency urination, dysuria, pyuria (↑↑ polymorphonuclear neutrophils [PMNs] in urine), hematuria, bacteriuria (minimum of 10^5 colonies/mL)

B. Acute bacterial pyelonephritis
   1. Often bilateral, occurs by ascension from perineum via urethra/ureters
   2. Gram negative rods the most common cause, rarely *Enterococcus*
   3. Causes inflammatory destruction of cortex, while glomeruli & vessels often spared
   4. PMNs infiltrate interstitium & tubules, **patchy appearance to involvement**
   5. Diagnosis (Dx) = fever, ↑ WBC, **costovertebral angle (CVA) tenderness & white cell casts in the urine—the latter is pathognomonic of renal inflammation** (also seen in glomerulonephritis, or noninfectious tubular/interstitial disease [dz])
   6. Complications: papillary necrosis, pyonephrosis, perinephric abscess
   7. Papillary necrosis also occurs in diabetics, pale gray necrosis of renal pyramids
   8. Perinephric abscess = penetration of the inflammation through the renal capsule
   9. Pyonephrosis is due to almost complete obstruction of renal pelvis, so pus cannot drain out of kidney
   10. The pyelonephritic scar causes fibrosis of the underlying renal calyx & pelvis, so **the calyces become dilated & blunted, & covered by a thick, contractile scar**

C. Chronic bacterial pyelonephritis
   1. Difference is long-time course causes renal atrophy, calyceal deformity & parenchymal scarring
   2. Histologic appearance: parenchymal scar causing retraction of adjacent papilla
   3. Clinical Si/Sx are vague & often not helpful as in acute infection
   4. **Urogram showing dilated calyces with overlying scar is the most accurate tool for diagnosis**
   5. Atrophic tubules with eosinophilic casts resemble thyroid follicles—**classic histologic description is thyroidization of the kidney**

6. Patients can have normal renal function for > 20 years after onset of infection

III. Renal Tubular and Interstitial Disorders

A. Acute interstitial nephritis (AIN)
   1. This is a form of acute renal failure
      a. Penicillin, sulfonamides, diuretics, & nonsteroidal anti-inflammatory drugs (NSAIDs) cause hypersensitivity reactions
      b. Variable presentation, but Sx may include fever, dysuria, pyuria, flank pain, maculopapular rash, eosinophilia suggesting hypersensitive etiology, & oliguria
   2. Earliest finding is interstitial edema (swollen kidneys), followed by mononuclear & eosinophilic infiltrate, with few PMNs
   3. Often nephrotic range proteinuria, hematuria, & marked pyuria with eosinophils in urine—**eosinophiluria is rare, but is pathognomonic for hypersensitivity acute interstitial nephritis or atheroembolic dz**
   4. Other signs due to failure of tubules to concentrate urine include polyuria, volume depletion, hyperkalemia, metabolic acidosis
   5. Withdrawal of offending drug often restores renal function, some can be irreversible
   6. Treatment (Tx) = corticosteroids, may accelerate recovery of renal function
   7. Some agents cause characteristic histology in early stage, prior to complete necrosis
      a. Mercuric chloride causes acidophilic inclusions in tubular cells
      b. Carbon tetrachloride causes lipid accumulation in injured cells
      c. Ethylene glycol causes calcium oxalate crystals with vacuolar ballooning of proximal tubules

B. Chronic tubular interstitial nephritis
   1. This is a grab-bag term that encompasses all chronic kidney disorders where tubulointerstitial areas are more affected than glomerular or vascular lesions
   2. Kidneys are small & atrophic, tubular lumens show marked dilation
   3. Infiltrate is mononuclear & there is prominent interstitial fibrosis with tubular atrophy, but nonscarred areas are normal

4. Edema is usually not present, minimal proteinuria, BP normal or mildly ↑
5. Many etiologies: pyelonephritis, transplant rejection, toxic intake, metabolic diseases including nephrocalcinosis/lithiasis, cystinosis, gout, polycystic disease, sickle cell, Sjögren's, sarcoid, multiple myeloma, radiation nephritis, idiopathic

C. Renal papillary necrosis = necrotizing papillitis
   1. Defined as ischemic necrosis of tip of renal papillae
   2. Usually associated with diabetes mellitus, infection, sickle cell disease, &/or renal vascular disease
   3. Occasionally a catastrophic consequence of acute pyelonephritis
   4. Chronic phenacetin, aspirin & other NSAID use can cause chronic analgesic nephritis = loss of tubules & interstitial fibrosis & inflammation

D. Acute renal failure (ARF) (see Table 7.1)
   1. Syndrome defined as rapidly ↑ azotemia (↑ serum creatinine &/or urea), with or without oliguria ($\equiv < 500$ mL/day urine)
   2. Categories of ARF: 1) prerenal (hypoperfusion), 2) postrenal (obstruction), 3) renal
   3. Prerenal failure
      a. Caused by volume depletion, heart failure, liver failure, sepsis, heatstroke (myoglobinuria), burns & bilateral renal artery stenosis
      b. ↓ glomerular filtration rate (GFR) leads to oliguria, ↑ resorption of Na & water, & very concentrated urine
      c. GFR = $(140 - \text{age}) \times (\text{weight (kg)}) \times (0.85 \text{ for females}) / (72 \times \text{creatinine})$
   4. Postrenal ARF caused by obstruction 2° to BPH, bladder/pelvic tumors & calculi
   5. Intrinsic renal causes
      a. Acute tubular necrosis [see below, Section III.E] is most common type of intrinsic renal disease
      b. Others include vasculitis and glomerulonephritis
   6. Edema, nephrotic syndrome & arteritis in skin & retina suggest glomerulonephritis
   7. **Hemoptysis suggests Wegener's granulomatosis or Goodpasture's syndrome**
   8. Skin rash suggests polyarteritis or SLE
   9. History of drug ingestion, maculopapular or purpuric rash, suggest allergic nephritis

10. Urinary sediment may give valuable etiologic clues
    a. Sediment is usually unremarkable in prerenal azotemia
    b. Renal injury leads to tubular cells & casts in sediment
11. Urinary eosinophils suggests allergic nephritis or atheroembolic disease
12. **RBC casts virtually pathognomonic for glomerulonephritis (can be vasculitis)**
13. **Progressive, daily rise in serum creatinine is Dx for ARF**
14. Laboratory characteristics of renal failure (Table 7.1)
15. BUN/creatinine ratio < 10 can also be due to extrarenal causes
    a. Anything that increases serum creatinine levels, or decreases BUN causes a low BUN/creatinine ratio
    b. Rhabdomyolysis causes spillage of excess creatinine from muscle into blood, lowering ratio
    c. Cimetidine & trimethoprim/sulfamethoxazole (Bactrim) inhibit renal secretion of creatinine, elevating levels, lowering ratio
    d. Malnutrition leads to negative nitrogen balance, lowering BUN, lowering ratio
16. Ratio can also be > 15 for metabolic reasons
    a. ↑ protein intake puts into positive nitrogen balance, elevating ratio
    b. Steroids cause a breakdown of proteins, leading to increase in circulating BUN, elevating ratio
    c. Infection, uncontrolled diabetes, & cachexia (neoplastic) can also increase protein catabolism

E. Acute tubular necrosis (ATN)
   1. Most common cause of acute renal failure, falls into the intrinsic renal category

Table 7.1 Laboratory Characteristics of Renal Failure

Test/Index	Prerenal	Postrenal	Renal
Urine osmolality	>**500**	<350	<350
Urine Na	<**20**	>40	>20
FE_{Na}	<1%	>4%	>2%
BUN/creatinine	>20	>15	<**15**

FE_{Na} = (urine sodium × serum creatinine) / (urine creatinine × serum sodium)

2. Most common etiology of ATN is renal ischemia caused by prolonged hypotension secondary (2°) to gram-negative sepsis, trauma, hemorrhage, heart failure, etc.
3. Crush injury or rhabdomyolysis leading to myoglobinuria also cause ATN
4. Can also be caused by direct toxins, including mercuric chloride
5. If not treated it is invariably fatal, but it is usually reversible if treated properly
6. 3 phases of injury: 1) prodromal, 2) oliguric, 3) postoliguric
7. Prodromal phase is variable depending upon etiology (e.g., amount of toxin, duration of hypotension)
8. Oliguric phase, urine output is 50–400mL/day, most lethal time period
   a. Note some patients may NEVER be oliguric
   b. Avg. oliguric phase lasts 10–14 days, creatinine increases by 1–2/day, BUN by 10–20/day
9. Postoliguric phase is gradual return to normal levels, tubular dysfunction may persist
   a. Can see Na wasting, polyuria unresponsive to antidiuretic hormone (ADH), & hyperchloremic metabolic acidosis
   b. Creatinine & BUN levels may remain elevated for several days into the convalescent phase

F. Renal tubule functional disorders
1. Renal tubular acidosis (RTA)
   a. A group of intrinsic renal defects → metabolic acidosis
   b. Type I = **distal tubular defect** in establishment of urinary H^+ gradient → **metabolic acidosis with urine pH > 5.5**
   c. Type II = **proximal tubule failure** to resorb HCO_3^-, urine pH > 5.5 early but then < 5.5 as acidosis worsens
   d. RTA IV = ↓ **aldosterone** → hyperkalemia & hyperchloremia
      (1) Usually due to ↓ aldosterone secretion (**hyporeninemic hypoaldosteronism**), seen in diabetes, interstitial nephritis, NSAID use, angiotensin converting enzyme (ACE) inhibitors & heparin
      (2) Also due to aldosterone resistance, seen in urinary obstruction & sickle cell dz
      (3) **Urine pH < 5.5**
   e. There is no RTA III for historical reasons
2. Fanconi's syndrome is a generalized dysfunction of proximal renal tubules, congenital or acquired
   a. Characterized by impaired reabsorption of glucose, amino acids, phosphate, & bicarbonate

   b. Associated with RTA Type II
   c. Clinically see glycosuria, hyperphosphaturia, hypophosphatemia (vitamin D resistant rickets), aminoaciduria (generalized, not cystine specific), systemic acidosis, polyuria, polydipsia
   d. Often congenital Fanconi's presents with cystinosis
   e. This is a totally distinct disorder from Fanconi's anemia
   f. Acquired Fanconi's syndrome caused by 6-mercaptopurine, tetracycline, renal transplantation, multiple myeloma, amyloidosis, heavy metal toxins & vitamin D deficiency
3. Cystinuria is congenital failure of tubular reabsorption of cystine
   a. Autosomal recessive, also see impaired reabsorption of dibasic amino acids (lysine, ornithine, arginine)
   b. Clinically see cystine stones
   c. Sx appear between 10 and 30 years, renal colic is most common presenting complaint, may see UTI
   d. Tx = hydration to ↑ urine volume, alkalinization of urine with bicarbonate & acetazolamide
4. Hartnup's disease
   a. Autosomal recessive defect in tryptophan absorption at renal tubule
   b. **Sx mimic pellagra, the 3 Ds—dermatitis, dementia, diarrhea** (tryptophan is niacin precursor)
   c. Rash is on sun-exposed areas
   d. Can see cerebellar ataxia, mental retardation, psychosis
   e. Tx = niacin supplements
5. Diabetes insipidus (DI)
   a. Caused by ↓ ADH secretion (central) or failure of renal tubule response to ADH (nephrogenic)
   b. Causes massive loss of free water in urine
   c. Si/Sx = polyuria, polydipsia, nocturia, urine specific gravity < 1.010, urine osmolality (U_{osm}) ≤ 200, serum osmolality (S_{osm}) ≥ 300
   d. Central DI
      (1) 1° (idiopathic) or 2°(acquired)
      (2) 2° due to trauma (basilar skull fractures), posterior pituitary infarct, or granulomatous infection (e.g., sarcoidosis, histiocytosis, tuberculosis, *Coccidioides immitis*, etc.)
      (3) Tx = DDAVP (ADH analogue) nasal spray
   e. Nephrogenic DI
      (1) 1° disease is X-linked, seen in infants, may regress with time

(2) 2° disease seen in sickle cell anemia, pyelonephritis, nephrotic syndrome, amyloidosis, multiple myeloma, iatrogenic (aminoglycoside, lithium, demeclocycline)
(3) Tx = ↑ water intake, sodium restriction

f. **Dx = water deprivation test**
(1) Hold all water, check hourly U_{osm}
(2) When U_{osm} stable for 3 hours, check S_{osm}, give vasopressin
(3) Normal people: U_{osm} after deprivation > S_{osm}, vasopressin causes ↑ U_{osm} of less than 10%
(4) Central DI: U_{osm} after deprivation no greater than S_{osm}, but ↑ ≥ 10% after vasopressin given
(5) Nephrogenic DI: U_{osm} after deprivation no greater than S_{osm} & vasopressin does not ↑ U_{osm}

6. Syndrome of inappropriate antidiuretic hormone (SIADH)
a. ↑ ADH secretion → hypotonic hyponatremia
b. SIADH is most common cause of inpatient hyponatremia
c. Etiologies
(1) CNS dz: trauma, tumor, Guillain-Barré syndrome, subarachnoid hemorrhage, hydrocephalus
(2) Pulmonary dz: pneumonia, tumor, abscess, COPD
(3) Endocrine dz: hypothyroidism, Conn's syndrome
(4) Drugs: NSAIDs, antidepressants, chemotherapy, diuretics, phenothiazine, oral hypoglycemics

d. Dx = hyponatremia with U_{osm} > 300 mmol/liter
e. Tx = usually resolves with time, otherwise correct hyponatremia with normal saline, demeclocycline for resistant cases—**beware:** too rapid correction of sodium can cause central pontine myelinolysis

G. Chronic renal failure
1. Always associated with azotemia of renal origin
2. Can be due to any cause, not just tubular or interstitial dz
3. 3 Stages: 1) diminished renal reserve, 2) renal insufficiency (azotemia), 3) uremia
4. Uremia = biochemical & clinical syndrome of the following characteristics
a. Azotemia
b. Acidosis due to accumulation of sulfates, phosphates, organic acids
c. Hyperkalemia due to inability to excrete K^+ in urine

d. Fluid volume dysregulation (early can't concentrate urine, late can't dilute urine)
e. Hypocalcemia due to lack of vitamin D production
f. Anemia due to lack of erythropoietin production
g. Hypertension 2° to activated renin-angiotensin axis
h. Clinical presentation of uremia
   (1) Anorexia, nausea, vomit
   (2) Neurologic Sx = dementia, convulsions, eventually coma
   (3) Bleeding due to platelet dysfunction
   (4) Fibrinous pericarditis

5. Chronic renal failure (CRF) differentiated from ARF by multiple tests
   a. Renal ultrasound → small kidneys in chronic dz
   b. Hematocrit to check for anemia from chronic lack of EPO
   c. Metabolic bone survey → diffuse osteopenia to establish long-term lack of vitamin D production
6. Organ manifestations
   a. Neuromuscular → twitching, peripheral neuropathy, muscle cramp, convulsions
   b. GI → anorexia, nausea/vomit, stomatitis, unpleasant taste in mouth, GI ulcers/bleeding
   c. Cardiovascular → hypertension, hypervolemia, CHF, edema, pericarditis
   d. Skin → yellow-brown macules, uremic frost (urea crystals from sweat), pruritus
7. Laboratory findings = ↑ BUN, ↑ creatinine,↑ urea, acidosis, anemia

IV. Glomerular Diseases

A. Nephrotic syndrome (see Tables 7.2 and 7.3)
   1. Characterized by proteinuria > 3.5 g/day, generalized edema (anasarca), lipiduria with hyperlipidemia, marked ↓ albumin, hypercoagulation (loss of antithrombin III in urine, ↑ platelets)
   2. Proteinuria due to ↓ charge selectivity (minimal change disease), ↓ size selectivity (membranous glomerulonephritis), or ↑ permeability due to factors released by lymphocytes (focal segmental glomerulosclerosis)

Table 7.2 Nephrotic Glomerulonephropathies

Disease	Characteristics
Minimal change disease (MCD) (See Figure 7.1)	• Classically seen in young children • Light microscope (LM) → lipid laden renal cortices, Nml glomerulus • Electron microscopy (EM) → epithelial foot process process fusion • Most often responds to corticosteroid therapy
Focal segmental glomerulosclerosis	• Clinically similar to MCD, but occurs in adults with refractory HTN • LM → glomerular sclerosis with focal (some glomeruli affected) & segmental (only part of a glomerulus affected) distribution • Usually idiopathic, but heroin, HIV, diabetes, sickle cell are associated • Idiopathic typically presents in young, hypertensive African American males

Membranous glomerulonephritis (See Figure 7.2)	• Most common primary cause of nephrotic syndrome in adults
	• Idiopathic immune complex dz, ↑ incidence in teens & young adults
	• LM → markedly thickened capillary walls
	• EM → classic findings
	  • 5–10-fold thickening of the basement membrane
	  • Subepithelial (epimembranous) immune complexes
	  • Resulting pattern is the classic "spike & dome" appearance
	  • Spikes = basement membrane, domes = immune omplexes
	• Slowly progressive disorder with ↓ response to steroid treatment seen
	• Causes of this disease are numerous
	  • Infections include HBV, HCV, syphilis, malaria
	  • Drugs include gold salts, penicillamine (note, both used in RA)
	  • Malignancy
	  • SLE (10% of patients develop)

(continued)

Table 7.2 *Continued*

Disease	Characteristics

Membranoproliferative glomerulonephritis	• Characterized clinically by a slow progression to chronic renal disease
	• LM → basement membrane thickening & cellular proliferation
	• **Classic LM → "tram track appearance,"** which is a double-layered basement membrane best seen with silver stain
	• Disease has 2 forms
	  • Type I = subendothelial immune complex (IgG) deposition—tram track appearance is striking
	  • Type II (dense deposit disease) = complement abnormalities
	    • Very electron dense C3 subendothelial deposits due to activation of alternate complement pathway
	    • Most of these patients have an autoantibody against C3 convertase called **"C3 nephritic factor"**
	    • **Characterized clinically by decreased serum levels of C3**

Systemic diseases	See Table 7.3

3. Hyperlipidemia (↑ cholesterol, ↑ low-density lipoproteins) due to ↑ production & ↓ catabolism of apolipoprotein B-containing lipoproteins
4. Classic physical finding → Muehrcke's nails = paired narrow horizontal white bands on all fingernails, seen most often in hypoalbuminemia associated with nephrotic syndrome

B. Nephritic syndrome (see Table 7.4)
   1. Results from diffuse glomerular inflammation
   2. Characterized by sudden onset of gross or microscopic hematuria (smokey brown urine), ↓ GFR resulting in azotemia (↑ BUN & creatinine), oliguria, hypertension & edema

C. Urinalysis evaluation of primary glomerular disease (see Table 7.5)

D. Secondary vs. tertiary hyperparathyroidism
   1. The natural physiological response to elevated serum phosphorous is stimulation of parathyroid hormone (PTH) secretion by the parathyroid glands
   2. Renal failure prevents excretion of phosphorous → ↑ serum phosphorous levels → ↑ PTH secretion—this is secondary

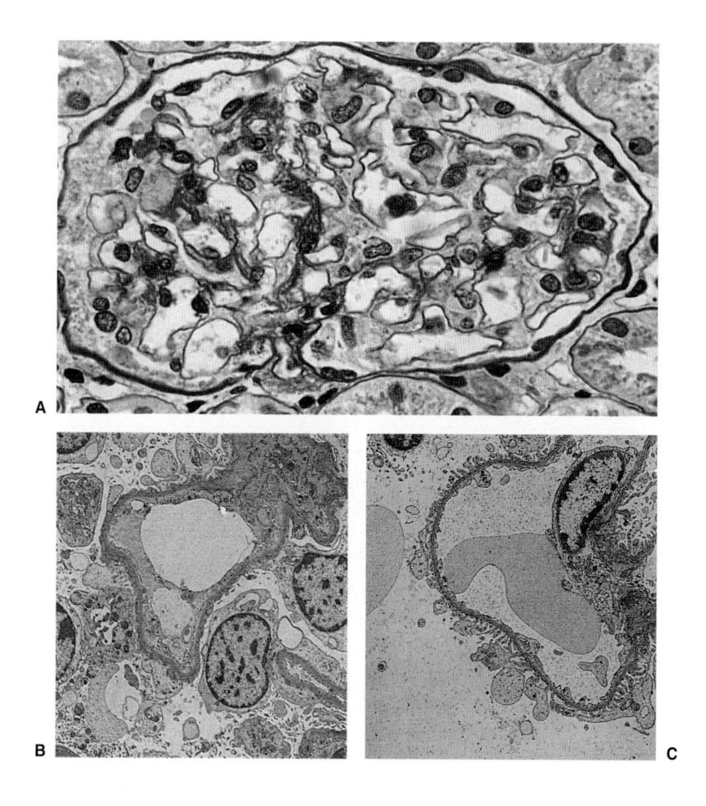

Figure 7.1 Minimal Change Nephropathy.
A. Appearance on electron microscopy is normal. **B.** Appearance on electron microscopy shows characteristic fusion of the foot processes. Compare with **C.**, an electron micrograph of a normal kidney. (From Axford JS, Callaghan CA. Medicine. 2nd ed. Oxford: Blackwell Science, 2004.)

hyperparathyroidism (primary hyperparathyroidism is when the gland develops hyperplasia or adenoma and oversecretes PTH without any antecedent elevations in phosphorous levels)

3. Because PTH normally acts via stimulation of renal secretion of phosphorous, and because this mechanism does not work in renal failure, PTH levels keep increasing in patients with renal failure as the body keeps trying to excrete the phosphorous—eventually the chronic stimulation of the parathyroid gland leads to glandular hypertrophy and resulting autonomous hypersecretion of PTH, so that even if calcium-phosphorous levels are later corrected, hyperparathyroidism continues, this is tertiary hyperparathyroidism

Table 7.3 Systemic Glomerulonephropathies

Disease	Characteristic Nephropathy
Diabetes	• ↑ glomerular basement membrane thickness • ↑ mesangial matrix either diffusely or in nodular accumulations called **"Kimmelstiel-Wilson nodules" (pathognomonic)**
Renal amyloidosis	• Subendothelial & mesangial amyloid deposits visible by special stains (e.g., Congo Red), birefringent under polarized light • EM shows criss-cross fibrillary pattern of amyloid • Amyloid comprised of β_2 microglobulin (from hemodialysis)
Lupus	
Type I	No renal involvement
Type II	Mesangial disease with focal segmental glomerular pattern
Type III	Focal segmental proliferative disease
Type IV	• Diffuse proliferative disease, the most severe form of lupus nephropathy • Presents with a combination of nephrotic/nephritic disease • Extensive scarring & thrombosis involves almost all glomeruli • **Classic LM → wire-loop abnormality**
Type V	Membranous form, indistinguishable from other 1° membranous GNs

4. Osteitis fibrosa cystica
   a. PTH also stimulates calcium resorption from bone, and this mechanism is intact in patients with renal failure
   b. Bony demineralization and cystic bone lesions develop in patients with renal failure as a result of the secondary hyperparathyroidism
   c. However, if phosphorous levels are exogenously lowered (by dialysis or oral phosphate binders), the feed-forward stimulation of PTH levels is lost, PTH levels fall to normal, and bone resorption ceases

V. Renal Artery Stenosis (RAS)

A. Presentation
   1. **Classic dyad = sudden hypertension with low K^+** (pt not on diuretic)

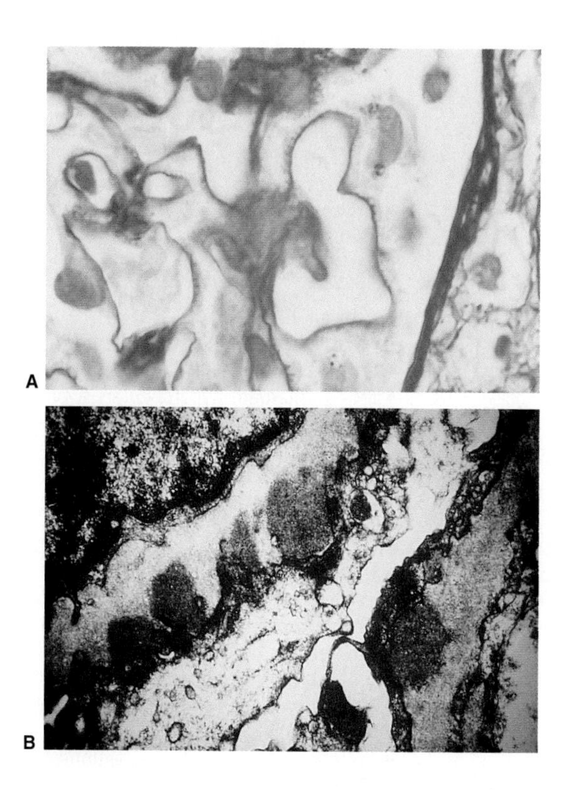

Figure 7.2
A. Silver stain of membranous GN. Note the appearance of "spikes" on the outside of the capillary loop. The immune deposits between the "spikes" of basement membrane do not stain with silver. **B.** The immune deposits are electron dense and appear as black lumps in the basement membrane. (From Axford JS. Medicine. Oxford: Blackwell Science, 1998.)

2. Caused by ↓ blood flow to juxtaglomerular apparatus of involved kidney, leading to renin-angiotensin activation, culminating in ↑ aldosterone levels
3. 2 most common causes are atherosclerotic plaques & fibromuscular dysplasia (see below, Section C)
4. Screening Dx = oral captopril induces ↑ renin, which is more marked in RAS than in essential hypertension
5. Dx confirmed with angiography
6. Tx = surgery vs. angioplasty

B. Atherosclerotic plaque
   1. This is the most common cause of RAS
   2. Seen in males over 50yr, due to hypercholesterolemia

Table 7.4 Nephritic Glomerulonephropathies

Disease	Characteristics
Poststreptococcal (postinfectious) glomerulonephritis (PSGN/PIGN)	• Prototype of nephritic syndrome (acute glomerulonephritis) • Classically due to immune complex deposition following infection with group A β-hemolytic *Streptococcus* (*S. pyogenes*) • Can follow infection by virtually ANY organism, viral or bacterial • Patient typically completely recovers • Laboratory → urine red cells & casts, azotemia, ↓ serum C3, ↑ **ASO titer** • Grossly see many punctate hemorrhages on both kidneys • LM → enlarged, hypercellular, swollen, bloodless glomeruli with proliferation of mesangial cells, endothelial cells & neutrophils • **EM → characteristic subepithelial "humps"** • **Immunofluorescence → coarse granular IgG or C3 deposits**

Crescentic (rapidly progressive) glomerulonephritis	• Nephritis progresses to renal failure within wk or mo
	• **Crescents seen between Bowman's capsule & glomerular tuft** due to deposition of fibrin & proliferation of epithelial cells & monocytes
	• May be part of PIGN or other systemic diseases
	• Goodpasture's disease
	• Crescentic GN caused by antiglomerular basement antibodies
	  • **Disease causes glomerulonephritis with pneumonitis**
	  • **90% pts present with hemoptysis**, only later get glomerulonephritis
	  • Peak incidence in men in mid-20s
	  • **Classic immunofluorescence → smooth, linear deposition of IgG** (antibody deposited, not antigen/antibody complexes)

Alport's syndrome	• Hereditary nephritis due to genetic abnormality of collagen • **Results in renal disease, deafness, ocular abnormalities** (dislocated lens, corneal dystrophy cataracts) • Usually X-linked • Classic EM → glomerular basement membrane splitting

(Continued)

Table 7.4 *Continued*

Disease	Characteristics
Berger's disease (IgA nephropathy)	• **Most common worldwide nephropathy** • Due to IgA deposition in the mesangium • Presents with recurrent hematuria with low-grade proteinuria • Whereas PIGN presents weeks after infection, **Berger's presents concurrently or within several days of infection** • 25% of pts slowly progress to renal failure, otherwise harmless
Henoch-Schönlein purpura (HSP)	• Also an IgA nephropathy, but almost always presents in children • Presents with abdominal pain, vomiting, hematuria & GI bleeding • **Classic physical finding = "palpable purpura" on buttocks & legs in children, & on shins adults** • Often follows respiratory infection
Multiple myeloma	• ↑ production of light chains → tubular plugging by Bence-Jones proteins • 2° hypercalcemia also contributes to development of "myeloma kidney" • Myeloma cells can directly invade kidney parenchyma • Defect in normal antibody production leaves pt susceptible to chronic infections by encapsulated bacteria (e.g., *E. coli*) → chronic renal failure

Table 7.5 Urinalysis of Glomerulonephropathies

	Nephrotic Syndrome	Nephritic Syndrome	Chronic Disease
Proteinuria	↑↑↑↑	+/−	+/−
Hematuria	+/−	↑↑↑↑	+/−
Cells	−	**⊕RBCs ⊕ WBCs**	+/−
Casts	**Fatty casts**	**RBC casts, granular casts**	**Broad waxy casts, pigmented granular casts**
Lipids	Free fat droplets, oval fat bodies	−	−

C. Fibromuscular dysplasia
   1. An idiopathic disorder that presents most commonly in young women
   2. Angiography showing "string of beads" sign due to luminal narrowing at various points along the vessel

VI. Diffuse Cortical Necrosis

A. General characteristics
   1. Rare form of arterial infarction, causes necrosis & calcification of renal cortex, with sparing of medulla
   2. Usually occurs in infancy or childhood, can occur at any age
   3. In neonates, 50% caused by abruptio placentae, next most common cause is sepsis
   4. In children infections, volume depletion, shock, hemolytic-uremic syndrome cause it
   5. In adults, pregnancy accidents (abruptio placentae, eclampsia, placenta previa, puerperal sepsis, etc.) cause > 50% of all cases, bacterial sepsis causes another 30%
   6. Difficult to distinguish from acute renal failure, Dx depends upon biopsy, although clinical Hx is suggestive
   7. May be caused by a combination of end organ vasospasm & DIC

VII. Urinary Tract Obstruction

A. General characteristics
   1. Most common causes in children are congenital
   2. Most common causes in adults are benign prostatic hyperplasia (BPH) & stones
   3. Obstruction leads to urinary stasis proximal to the block, predisposes to infxn that can spread to renal parenchyma

B. Nephrolithiasis (see Figure 7.3)
   1. Calcium pyrophosphate stones
      a. Cause 80–85% of all stones in urinary tract, are **radiopaque**, associated with hypercalciuria
      b. Hypercalciuria can be idiopathic or caused by ↑ intestinal calcium absorption, ↑ 1° renal calcium excretion, or hypercalcemia (1° hyperparathyroidism or malignancy induced, sarcoid, milk-alkali, & vitamin D intoxication)
      c. 50% associated with idiopathic hypercalciuria

2. Ammonium magnesium phosphate stones ("struvite stones")
   a. Second most common form of stones, are **radiopaque**
   b. Facilitated by alkaline urine, most often due to urease ⊕ *Proteus* or *S. saprophyticus*
   c. Can form large staghorn or struvite calculi (casts of renal pelvis & calyces) (see Figure 7.3)
3. Uric acid stones
   a. 50% of pts with stones have hyperuricemia
   b. Can be 2° to gout or ↑ cell turnover (leukemia, myeloproliferative disorders)
   c. Stones are **radiolucent**
4. Cystine stones caused by cystinuria or congenital aminoaciduria
5. Urinary colic is sharp, 10/10 pain, often described as the worst pain in the patient's life, which may radiate from the back through to the anterior portion of the pelvis—classic finding for urinary stones
6. Hydronephrosis
   a. Defined as progressive dilation of the renal pelvis & calyces with blunting of renal pyramids
   b. Caused by stones, BPH, pregnancy, neurogenic bladder, tumor, or congenital
   c. Causes high pressure in the collecting system resulting in renal atrophy & ischemia

VIII. Cystic Diseases of the Kidney

A. Adult polycystic kidney disease
   1. Autosomal dominant inheritance, slowly progressive over many years, ALWAYS bilateral
   2. Clinical onset usually in early or middle adult life, may rarely escape clinical detection until autopsy
   3. Sx = lumbar pain, hematuria, infection, nephrolithiasis, uremia
   4. 33% of cases have cysts in liver as well, but they have no functional or pathologic significance
   5. 10–20% cases have intracranial aneurysms, hypertension is present in 50% of patients at time of Dx
   6. Ultrasound & computed tomography (CT) show classic "moth-eaten" appearance due to cysts (see Figure 7.4)
   7. Differential diagnosis is chronic renal failure, differentiated by ultrasound finding of small kidneys in CRF & large kidneys in polycystic disease

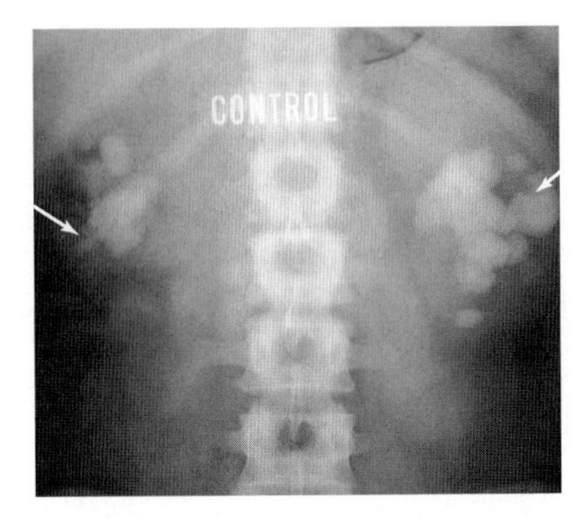

Figure 7.3
Bilateral staghorn (i.e., filling renal pelvis and calyces) renal calculi. (From Axford JS. Medicine. Oxford: Blackwell Science, 1998.)

8. **External surface shows multiple cysts** (see Figure 7.5)
9. This is the most common inherited disorder of the kidney

B. Juvenile onset polycystic disease
   1. Autosomal recessive, much rarer than adult type, but most common childhood congenital kidney lesion
   2. Almost all cases have cysts in liver & portal bile duct proliferation = "congenital hepatic fibrosis"
   3. Variable age of onset, those presenting early in childhood → mainly renal symptoms, poor prognosis (Px)
   4. Those presenting later in adolescence → mainly hepatic related symptoms, better Px
   5. Affected neonates have pulmonary involvement & typically die very quickly
   6. Cysts are closed & not connected to collecting system, **external surface is smooth, no cysts visible**

C. Solitary renal cyst
   1. Common, often aSx lesion in adults

D. Medullary cystic disease
   1. Congenital or acquired disease, family history is common
   2. Presents with insidious onset of uremia
   3. ADH resistant polyuria, Na wasting, retarded growth, bone disease, small kidneys on ultrasound
   4. Variable disease progression, slow but inexorable, patients do well with transplants

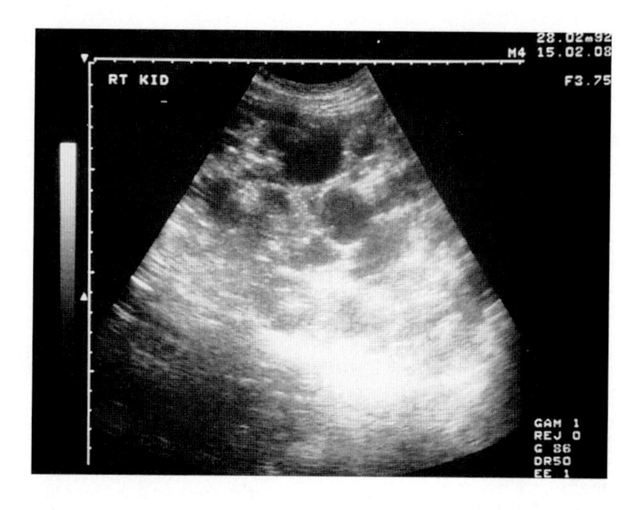

Figure 7.4
Ultrasound of polycystic kidney (cysts of different sizes are scattered throughout kidney substance). (From Axford JS. Medicine. Oxford: Blackwell Science, 1998.)

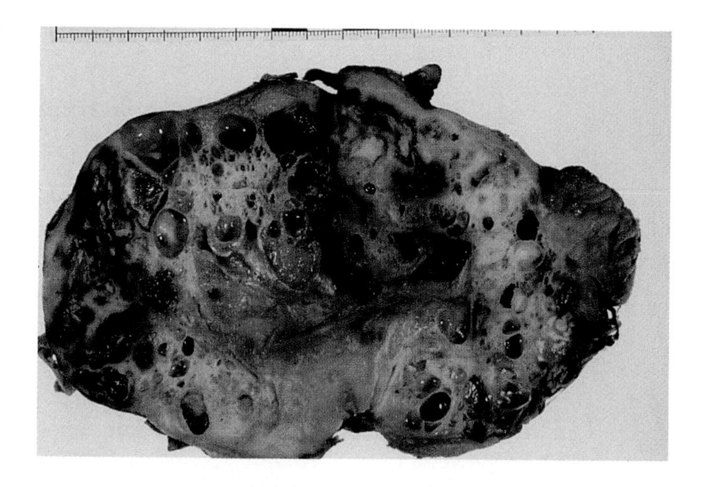

Figure 7.5 A polycystic kidney
There are multiple cysts of different sizes, some filled with blood. (From Axford JS. Medicine. Oxford: Blackwell Science, 1998.)

5. Pathology = medullary cysts with significant tubular atrophy & interstitial fibrosis
6. Grossly kidneys are small, with contractile granular surfaces

E. Medullary sponge kidney
1. Tubular ectasia or dysplasia causing congenital dilation of collecting tubules only
2. Unrelated to medullary cystic disease
3. Sx = urinary stasis & calcinosis
4. Usually aSx, most common complaint is colic, can see infection or hematuria
5. Excellent Px (contrast to medullary cystic disease), renal failure rarely develops

IX. Tumors of the Kidney

A. Benign renal tumors
1. Adenomas are small & aSx, always present in the cortex, are derived from tubules
2. They may be a precursor to adenoCA
3. Angiomyolipoma is a hamartoma, often associated with tuberous sclerosis syndrome
   a. Tuberous sclerosis syndrome = cerebral cortical glial nodules/distorted neurons
   b. Sx/Si = epileptic seizures, mental retardation, adenoma sebaceum (facial skin lesion with malformed blood vessels & connective tissue), cardiac rhabdomyomas, & renal angiomyolipomas

B. Malignant renal tumors
1. Renal cell CA is most common renal malignancy
   a. Occurs most often in men ages 50–70, often in smokers
   b. Associated with chromosome 3 deletions & von Hippel-Lindau disease
   c. Originates in renal tubules, often in the upper renal pole
   d. **Can hematogenously disseminate by invading renal veins or the vena cava**
   e. Histologically looks like **polygonal clear cells**, reminiscent of adrenal cortex
   f. Also called "hypernephroma" due to gross yellow color & histologic resemblance of clear cells to adrenal cortex
   g. Clinically presents with hematuria (most common), palpable mass, flank pain, fever, 2° polycythemia (EPO),

ectopic hormone production (adrenocorticotropic hormone, prolactin, follicle-stimulating hormone/ leuteinizing hormone, PTHrp, renin)

2. Wilms' tumor = nephroblastoma
   a. Most common renal malignancy of childhood, incidence peaks at 2–4 years
   b. Presents with palpable flank mass (often huge)
   c. Histologically looks like immature stroma, primitive tubules & glomeruli, can have striated muscle
   d. Associated with deletions of chromosome 11, the WT-1 tumor suppressor gene
   e. Can be part of WAGR complex = **W**ilms' tumor, **A**niridia, **G**enitourinary malformations, mental motor **R**etardation
   f. **Also associated with hemihypertrophy of the body**

X. Acid-Base Disorders. See Figure 7.6 and the Accompanying Algorithms 7.1 to 7.8.

Disorder	pH	PCO_2	HCO_3^-
Respiratory acidosis			
Acute	↓	↑	↑
Chronic	N	↑	↑
Respiratory alkalosis			
Acute	↑	↓	↓
Chronic	N	↓	↓
Metabolic acidosis			
Acute	↓	N	↓
Chronic	N	↓	↓
Metabolic alkalosis	↑	↑	↑

Figure 7.6
Acid/base disorders. (Adapted from Axford JS. Medicine. Oxford: Blackwell Science, 1998.)

Algorithm 7.1

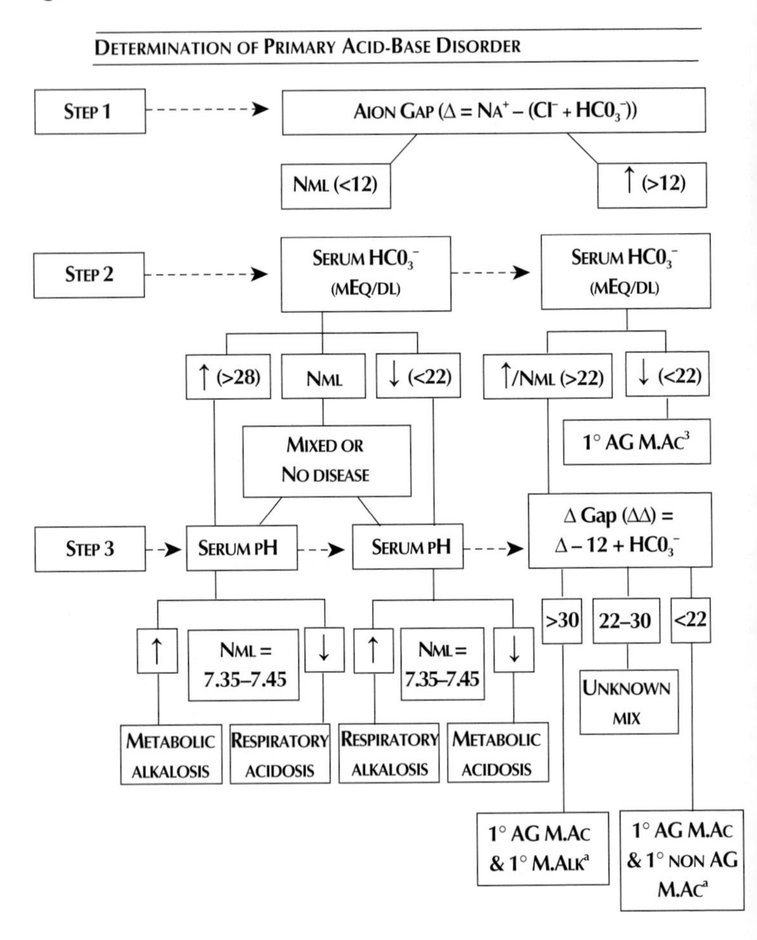

[a] AG = anion gap. M.Alk = metabolic alkalosis. M.Ac = metabolic acidosis.

Algorithm 7.2

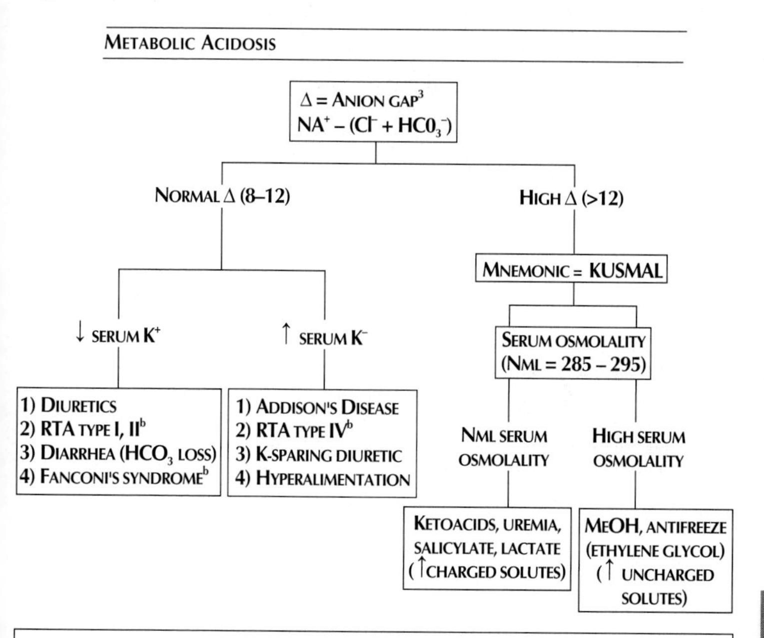

Check for compensation or the presence of a mixed disorder. Winter's formula predicts the CO_2 if there is compensation: $CO_2 = 1.5 * HCO_3^- + 8 \pm 2$. If the CO_2 is higher than expected, there is an additional acidotic process occurring. If the CO_2 is lower than expected, there is an additional alkalotic process occurring.

[a] Calculate Δ in *all* patients, regardless of pH or HCO_3^-. Mixed acidosis and alkalosis can cancel each other out, causing neutral pH. Perform the following steps to search for a mixed disorder.
1) Calculate Δ: if $\Delta \geq 12$, the disorder is a 1° anion gap acidosis
2) Calculate $\Delta\Delta = [\Delta - 12 + HCO_3^-]$: if $\Delta\Delta \geq 31$, there is also a 1° metabolic alkalosis
if $\Delta\Delta \leq 21$, there is also a 1° nonanion gap acidosis
Example: A diabetic in ketoacidosis who is vomiting can have a 1° anion gap acidosis from the ketoacidosis and a 1° metabolic alkalosis from the the vomiting. In this case, the $\Delta > 12$, the $\Delta\Delta \geq 31$. A diabetic with renal failure who presents with ketoacidosis can have a 1° anion gap and a nonanion gap acidosis, with a $\Delta > 12$ and a $\Delta\Delta \leq 21$. Note that this patient may also be vomiting and either tachypneic or bradypneic from obtundation. Thus the patient may have three 1° metabolic acid-base disorders (1° AG acidosis, 1° nonAG acidosis, 1° metabolic alkalosis) and a respiratory disorder. in this case, the disorders must be discriminated clinically or by changes in status in response to therapy.

Our thanks to Dr. Arian Torbati for his assistance with the ΔΔ algorithm.

[b] See Nephrology, Section III.F for description of RTA and Fanconi's syndrome.

NEPHROLOGY

Algorithm 7.3

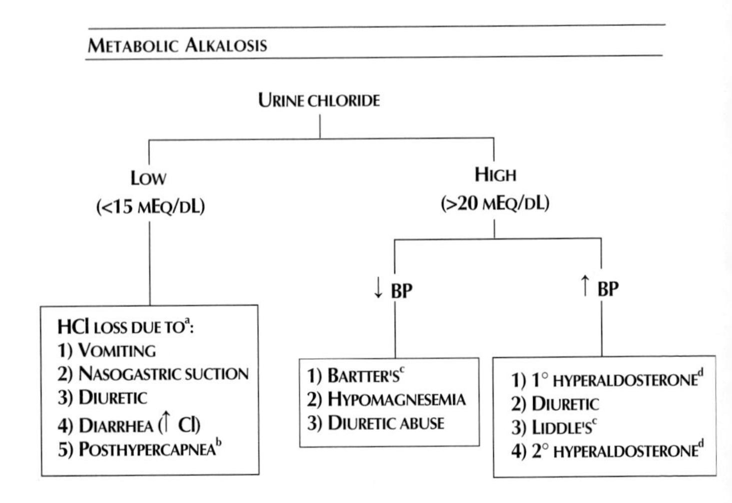

[a] These conditions are all known as " contraction alkaloses," or "chloride-responsive alkaloses." The concentration in extracellular volume creates a hypochloremic state. The kidney resorbs extra bicarbonate from the tubules due to the loss of chloride anion (tubules need a different anion to maintain electrical neutrality). Administration of chloride anion in the form of normal saline will correct the alkalosis.

[b] Patients who are hypercapnic undergo renal compensation, with resorption of extra bicarb from the tubules to offset the respiratory acidosis. When the hypercapnia is corrected (e.g., via intubation) the kidneys must adjust and resorb less bicarb. Until they adjust, the patient will have a posthypercapnic metabolic alkalosis.

[c] See Appendix B for Bartter's & Liddle's.

[d] 1° hyperaldosterone is known as Conn's syndrome. See Endocrinology, Section III.D.1. 2° hyperaldosteronism can be caused by renal artery stenosis (see Nephrology, Section V), Cushing's syndrome (see Endocrinology, Section III.B), congestive heart failure, and hepatic cirrhosis.

Algorithm 7.4

RESPIRATORY ACID-BASE DIFFERENTIAL

RESPIRATORY ALKALOSIS	RESPIRATORY ACIDOSIS
• CNS LESION	• MORPHINE/SEDATIVES
• PREGNANCY	• STROKE IN BULBAR AREA OF BRAIN STEM
• HIGH ALTITUDE	• ONDINE'S CURSE (CENTRAL SLEEP APNEA)
• SEPSIS/INFECTION	• COPD (EMPHYSEMA, ASTHMA, BRONCHITIS)
• SALICYLATE TOXICITY	• ADULT RESPIRATORY DISTRESS SYNDROME
• LIVER FAILURE	• CHEST WALL DISEASE (POLIO, KYPHOSCOLIOSIS, MYASTHENIA GRAVIS, MUSCULAR DYSTROPHY)
• ANXIETY (HYPERVENTILATION)	• OBESITY
• PAIN/FEAR (HYPERVENTILATION)	• HYPOPHOSPHATEMIA (DIAPHRAGM REQUIRES LOTS OF ATP DUE TO HIGH ENERGY DEMAND) SUCCINYLCHOLINE (PARALYSIS FOR INTUBATION)
• CONGESTIVE HEART FAILURE	• PLEURAL EFFUSION
• PULMONARY EMBOLUS	• PNEUMOTHORAX
• PNEUMONIA	
• HYPERTHYROIDISM	
• COMPENSATION FOR A 1° ACIDOSIS	

Check for the presence of a mixed disorder by comparing the change in CO_2, and HCO_3^- from normal (normal $CO_2 = 40$, normal $HCO_3^- = 24$).

Acute respiratory acidosis: HCO_3^- increases by 1 for every 10 the CO_2 increases.
Acute respiratory alkalosis: HCO_3^- decreases by 2 for every 10 the CO_2 decreases.
Chronic respiratory acidosis: HCO_3^- increases by 3.5 for every 10 the CO_2 increases.
Chronic respiratory alkalosis: HCO_3^- decreases by 5 for every 10 the CO_2 decreases.

It's easy to remember the compensations by organizing them into the following table.

	ACIDOSIS	ALKALOSIS
Acute	1	2
Chronic	3–4 (3.5)	5
Change in HCO_3^- per 10 change in CO_2. Just remember = 1:2:3–4:5!		

As usual, if the CO_2 is higher than predicted, there is a mixed acidotic process. If the CO_2 is lower than predicted, there is a mixed alkalotic process.

Algorithm 7.5

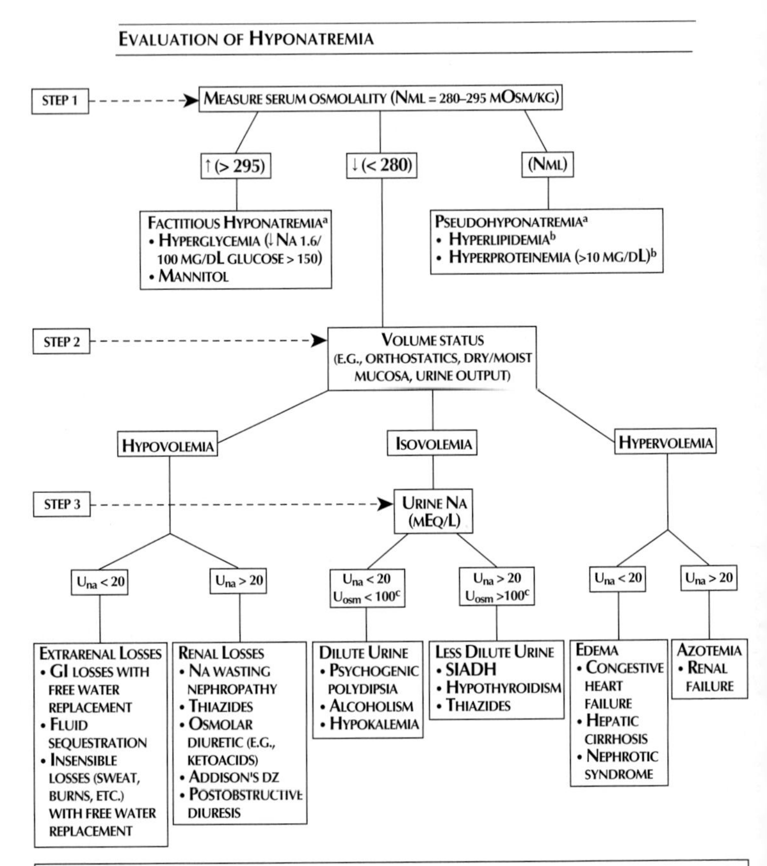

[a] Pseudohyponatremia is a lab artifact due to serum volume occupation by lipid or protein, resulting in an apparent decrease in the amount of Na per given volume of serum. Factitious hyponatremia is a true decrease in serum Na concentration (but normal total body Na) caused by glucose or mannitol osmotically drawing water into the serum.

[b] These disorders are characterized by ≥ 10mOsm/kg gap between the calculated and the measured serum osmolarity. Serum osmolarity is calculated by (2*Na) + (BUN/2.8) + (glucose/18). The gap is due to the presence of solutes detected by the lab but not accounted for in the osmolality calculation.

[c] U_{osm} = urine osmolality.

Algorithm 7.6

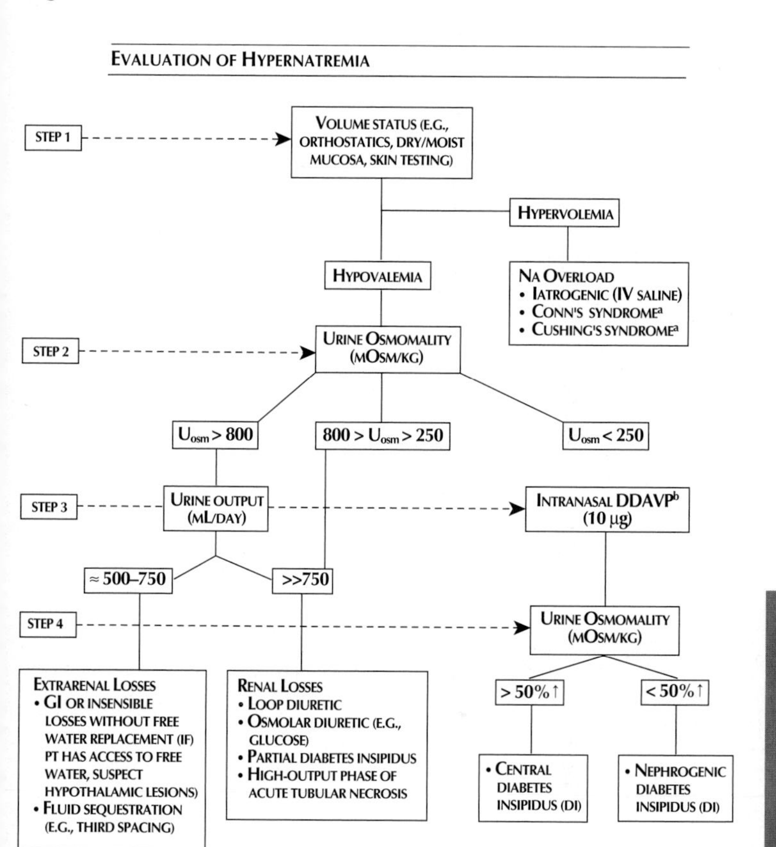

[a] See Endocrinology, Section III.B1 and III.D.1 for Cushing's syndrome and Conn's syndrome.
[b] DDAVP = long-acting antidiuretic hormone analogue. Patients with central DI respond by successfully increasing the concentration of their urine by 50%. Patients with nephrogenic DI are unable to concentrate their urine in the presence of DDAVP. Patients with DI tend to be only mildly hypernatremic.

Algorithm 7.7

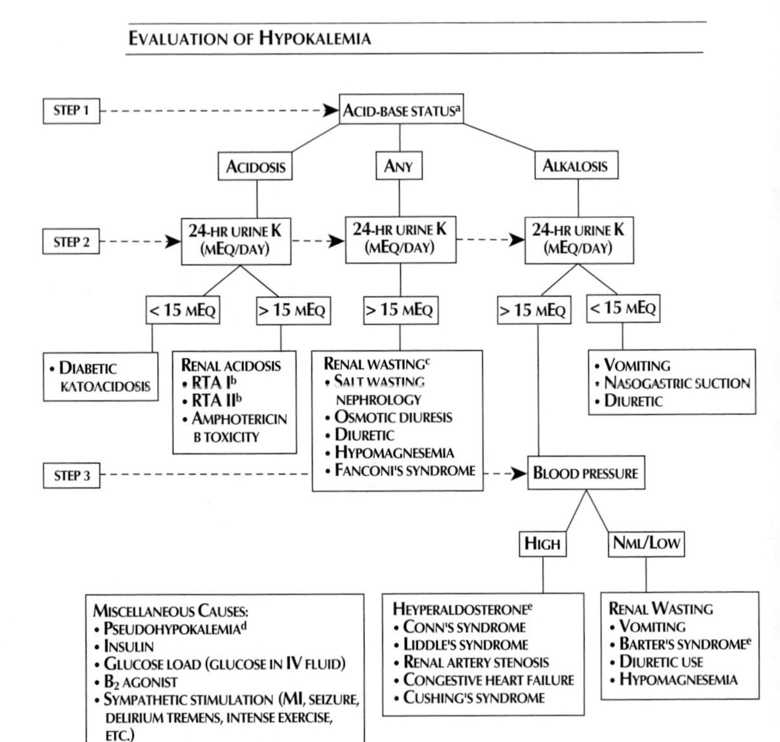

[a] Metabolic acidosis or alkalosis. Please see Acid-Base algorithms to determine acid-base status.
[b] RTA = renal tubular acidosis. See Nephrology, Section III.F.1 for full description.
[c] Salt wasting nephropathies are tubulointerstitial disorders (e.g., pyelonephritis, renal medullary dz, acute tubular necrosis and allergic interstitial nephritis). For Fanconi's syndrome, see Nephrology, Section III.F.2.
[d] Pseudohypokalemia is seen in conditions with very high white blood cell counts (e.g., leukemia). The white cells take up potassium while they are sitting in the blood draw tube, creating spurious results.
[e] See Endocrinology, Sections III.B & D for Cushing's and Conn's syndromes, IV.C.1 for congenital adrenal hyperplasia, Nephrology, Section V for renal artery stenosis, and Appendix B for Liddle's disease and Bartter's syndromes.

Algorithm 7.8

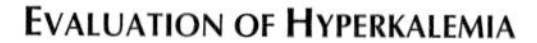

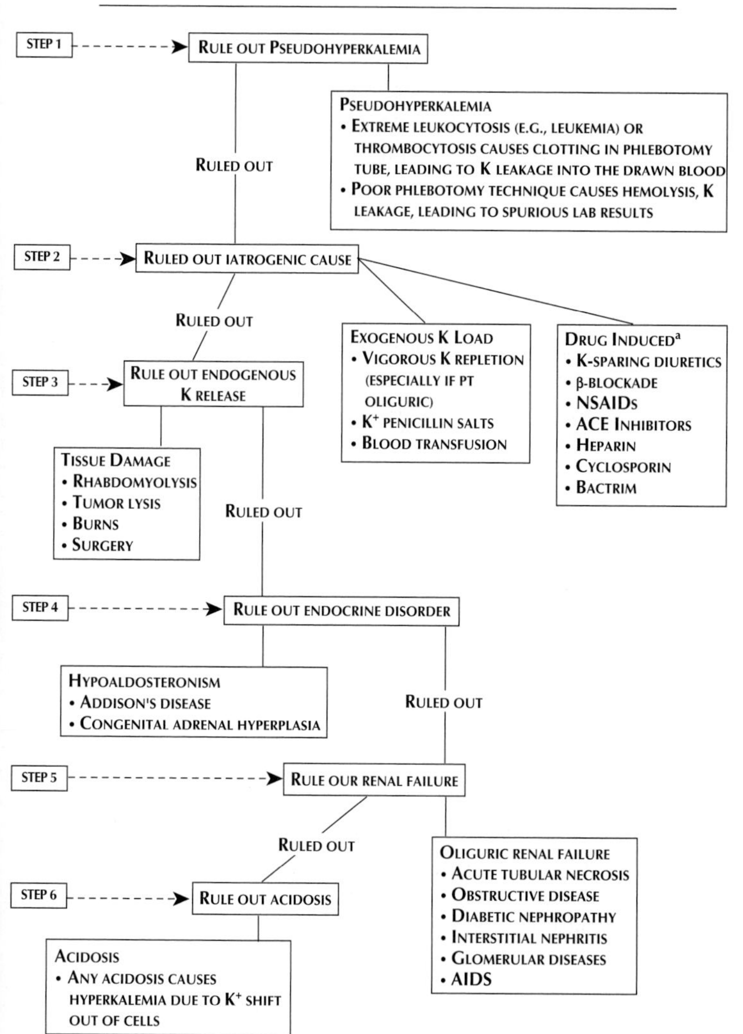

[a] **NSAIDs** = nonsteriodal anti-inflammatories, inhibit prostaglandins →↓ renal perfusion →↓ K delivery to nephron. **ACE inhibitors** block efferent arteriole constriction →↓ GFR →↓ K delivery to the nephron. Heparin blocks aldosterone production, while **cyclosporine** blocks aldosterone activity. **Bactrim** (trimethoprim) has K-sparing diuretic effect on tubules.

NEPHROLOGY

8. GENITOURINARY

I. Male Genitourinary Tract

A. Cryptorchidism
   1. Testes develop embryologically in abdomen, descend into scrotum during development
   2. Cryptorchidism ≡ retention of testis at any point along line of descent prior to reaching the scrotum
   3. Imparts 40-fold ↑ risk of developing testis cancer later in life

B. Scrotal masses
   1. Hydrocele is fluid filling tunica vaginalis, usually idiopathic
      a. May be congenital due to persistent processus vaginalis connecting to abdominal peritoneum
      b. Diagnosis (Dx) by transillumination of scrotum
   2. Masses in epididymis almost always benign, commonest benign neoplasm is adenomatoid tumor
   3. Masses in testis nearly always malignant, 95% germ cell tumor

C. Carcinoma in situ
   1. Often a history of cryptorchidism
   2. 70% of patients develop invasive testis cancer
   3. Histology: enlarged cells in basal layer with nuclei about 2 times the size of spermatogonia

D. Germ cell tumors (90% of all Testes Tumors)
   1. Seminoma
      a. Peak incidence in 40s
      b. Monotonous cellular appearance, arranged in lobules or nests with associated lymphoid or granuloma reaction
      c. **Never cause ↑ α-fetoprotein (αFP) levels but can rarely cause ↑ human chorionic gonadotropin (HCG)**
      d. Radiosensitive, often curable
   2. Spermatocytic seminoma
      a. Peak incidence in 50s
      b. Histologically see cells of various sizes
      c. Excellent prognosis
      d. **Never cause ↑ HCG levels, but can cause ↑ αFP levels**
   3. Embryonal carcinoma
      a. Peak incidence in 20s
      b. Variable sizes, form structures with many patterns

c. Often combined with teratoma
d. Much worse prognosis than seminoma

4. Teratomas
   a. **Almost always malignant (ovarian teratomas almost always benign)**
5. Yolk sac tumor (endodermal sinus tumor)
   a. Peak incidence in infancy & childhood
   b. Open pattern with anastomosing cords of cells
   c. **These tumors cause elevations in αFP**
6. Choriocarcinoma
   a. Peak incidence in teens & 20s
   b. Its villous structures resemble mature human placenta
   c. Most hemorrhagic of the germ cell tumors
   d. **HCG is always elevated**

E. Interstitial cell tumors
   1. Leydig cell tumor
      a. Cells contain intracytoplasmic Reinke crystals
      b. Can produce testosterone, estrogen, or corticosteroids
      c. Kids present with precocious puberty, adults with galactorrhea
   2. Sertoli cell tumor
      a. Usually benign
      b. Do not see endocrine abnormalities
   3. Lymphoma
      a. Seen in patients older than 60 years
      b. Despite local testicular presentation, lymphoma usually spreads or is already present in other sites in the body
      c. Poor prognosis

F. Bladder
   1. Congenital diseases
      a. Diverticula = evaginations of bladder wall
         (1) Leads to urinary stasis & infection
         (2) Can be congenital due to abnormal muscle development
         (3) Can be acquired due to obstruction of urethra or bladder neck

b. Exstrophy of bladder wall is complete absence of anterior musculature of bladder & abdominal wall
    (1) Due to failure of mesoderm growth over anterior bladder
    (2) Site of severe chronic infections & increased incidence of adenocarcinoma
c. Patent urachus is a fistula connecting bladder with umbilicus
d. Urachal cyst is persistence of central urachus along line from umbilicus to bladder, CAs may develop in cysts

2. Cancer
    a. Carcinoma more common in males than females
    b. Risks = smoking, cyclophosphamide, phenacetin (old analgesic), aniline dyes (used in paints), β-naphthylamine (found in rubber), chronic *Schistosoma hematobium* infection
    c. Signs/symptoms (Si/Sx) = hematuria, dysuria, frequency, urgency
    d. Transitional carcinoma
        (1) Comprises 90% plus of invasive bladder cancers, remainder are squamous CAs & adenocarcinomas
        (2) Usually flat & ulcerated
        (3) Common in males older than 60 years
        (4) Prognosis (Px) depends on depth of invasion & whether it reaches muscularis propria
    e. Papillary neoplasm (papilloma)
        (1) Always exophytic, are multifocal & recur
        (2) If multiple tumors exist, may progress to higher grades
        (3) Less than 10% invade or metastasize

3. Cystitis
    a. Hemorrhagic cystitis due to viral infection, radiation, or chemotherapy (cyclophosphamide)
    b. Emphysematous cystitis occurs in diabetics, see submucosal gas bubbles
    c. Encrusted cystitis due to precipitation of urinary salts (especially phosphates) on bladder wall

4. Malakoplakia
    a. Soft, broad yellow plaques in bladder mucosa
    b. Composed of foamy macrophages & multinucleated giant cells with concretions (Michaelis-Gutman bodies)

5. Ulcerated interstitial cystitis
   a. Idiopathic, seen in young females
   b. Presents with pain, inflammation, fibrosis throughout bladder wall

G. Prostate
   1. Anteromedial portion is estrogen sensitive, most common area of hyperplasia
   2. Posterolateral portion is androgen sensitive, most common area of adenocarcinoma (only 60% are actually palpable rectally)
   3. Benign prostatic hyperplasia (BPH)
      a. Narrows urethral canal, pt present with difficulty urinating
      b. Common after age 45 (at autopsy 90% of men over 70 have BPH)
      c. Does not predispose to prostate cancer
      d. Prostate-specific antigen (PSA) elevated in up to 50% of patients, not specific—not useful marker for BPH
      e. Treatment (Tx) = α-blockers & finasteride, both ↓ retention Sx
   4. Prostatitis
      a. Chronic or acute inflammation of prostate
      b. Chronic form usually nonbacterial, but can be due to chronic *Chlamydia* infection
      c. Acute form usually caused by gram-negative bacteria (e.g., *Escherichia coli*)
      d. No biopsy is needed, urine culture can be diagnostic
      e. Tx = antibiotics if bacterial
   5. Prostate cancer
      a. Most common cancer in males, second most common cause of cancer death (first = lung)
      b. It is adenocarcinoma histologically
      c. More common in African Americans, rare in Asians
      d. PSA ↑ in 90% of adenocarcinoma patients, but not specific, **controversy over use as a screening tool**, used to follow therapy by watching for dropping PSA levels
      e. Gleeson score (pathological grading) (see Figure 8.1)
         (1) Add scores of 2 of most common patterns (scored from 1 to 5)
         (2) If only one pattern multiply by 2
         (3) Scores range from 2 to 10, higher score → worse Px

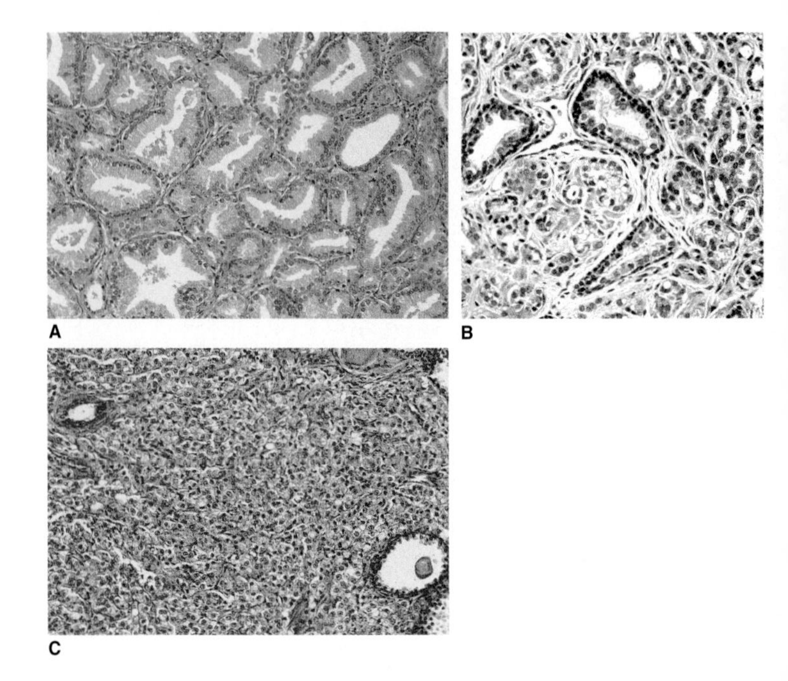

Figure 8.1 Gleason Grading System
A. Gleason grade 1. **B.** Gleason grade 3. **C.** Gleason grade 5. (From Rubin E, Gorstein F, Rubin R, et al. Rubin's Pathology: Clinicopathologic Foundations of Medicine. 4th ed. Baltimore: Lippincott Williams & Wilkins, 2005.)

f. Metastasis occurs via lymph or blood, commonly causes **osteoblastic** lesions in bone (see Figure 8.2)

II. Female Genitourinary Tract

A. Neoplastic diseases

1. Vaginal neoplasms

a. Condyloma acuminata

(1) Genital warts caused by the STD human papilloma virus (HPV)

(2) Virus infects keratinocytes in the stratum germinativum, causing aberrant growth of epidermis

(3) Histologic appearance: koilocytes & large epithelial cells with clear cytoplasmic halo around atypical nucleus

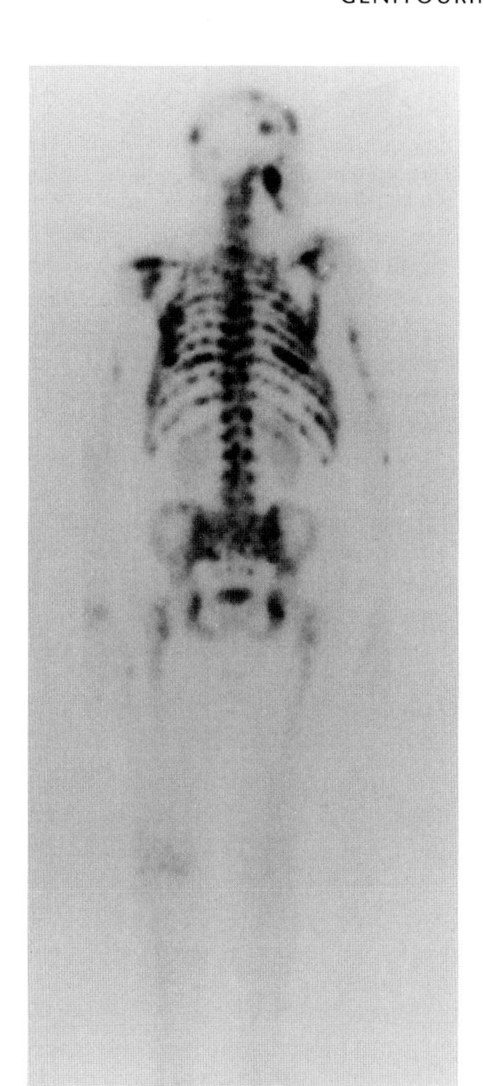

Figure 8.2
Bone scan showing multiple metastases secondary to prostatic cancer.

b. Squamous cell carcinoma
    (1) Caused by HPV serotypes 16, 18, 31, 33, 35
    (2) Proceeds through orderly continuum of neoplastic development, from dysplasia to carcinoma in situ to frankly invasive cancer
    (3) **Pap smear has been very successful at reducing mortality due to early detection (screening)**
    (4) Can occur at any site on external genitalia or cervix
c. Clear cell CA of the vulva is a rare cancer that develops at a markedly **increased frequency in the daughters of women exposed to diethylstilbestrol** (DES)
d. Endometriosis
    (1) Ectopic growth of endometrial tissue (occurs anywhere in pelvis)
    (2) Tissue is responsive to hormonal cycles, can cause ectopic bleeding
    (3) Most common symptom is severe cyclical pain, but can also cause infertility
    (4) **3 Ds = dyspareunia** (painful intercourse), **dyschezia** (painful defecation), **dysmenorrhea** (painful menses)

2. Uterine neoplasms
    a. Fibroid (leiomyoma)
        (1) **This is the most common tumor in women**
        (2) Benign tumor that is responsive to estrogen
        (3) ↑ in size by pregnancy & shrinks during menopause
        (4) Major symptom is vaginal bleeding
    b. Endometrial hyperplasia (see Figure 8.3)
        (1) Caused by ↑ estrogen, major Sx = excess vaginal bleeding
        (2) Is considered premalignant
        (3) Note that while it typically occurs in the uterus, ectopic endometrial tissue (endometriosis) can develop hyperplasia
    c. Endometrial CA (see Figure 8.4)
        (1) The most common urogenital malignancy in females
        (2) May be proceeded by endometrial hyperplasia, most common Sx = bleeding
        (3) Exogenous estrogen intake is a major risk factor
        (4) Incidence markedly ↑ in older women, is associated with nulliparity & delayed onset menopause

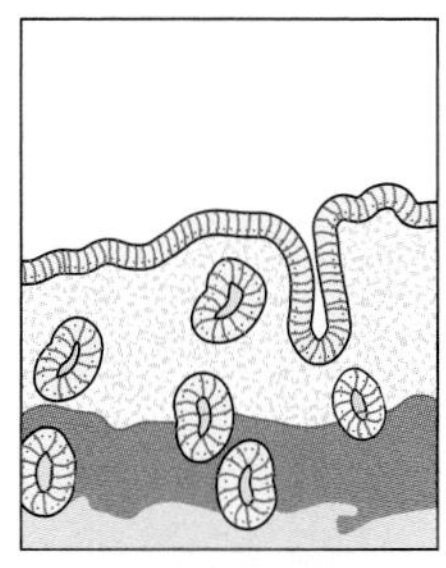

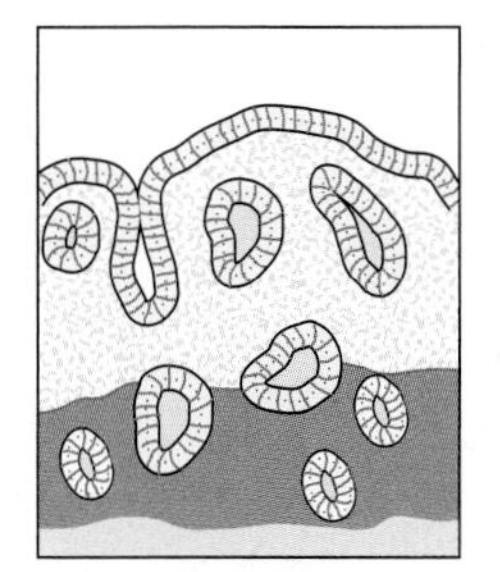

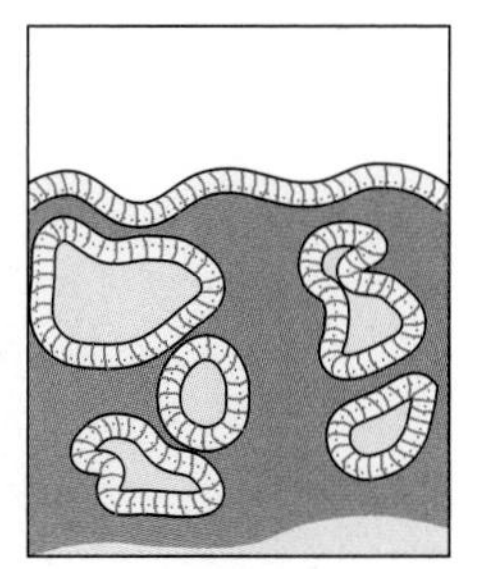

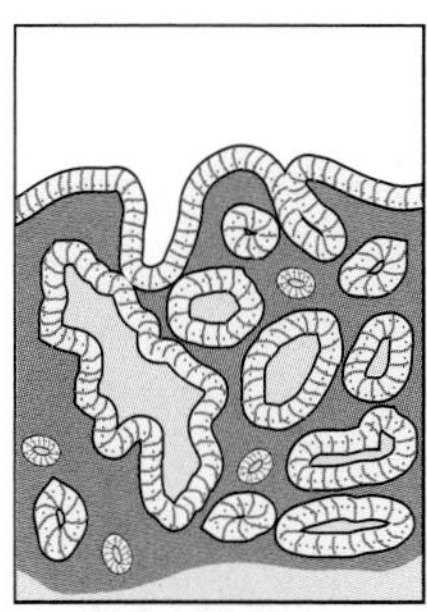

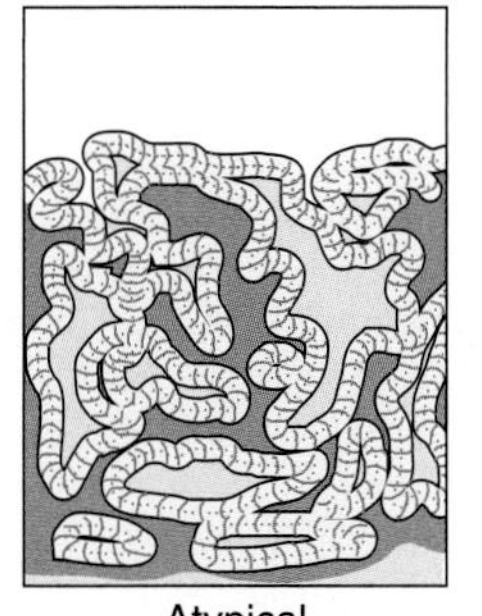

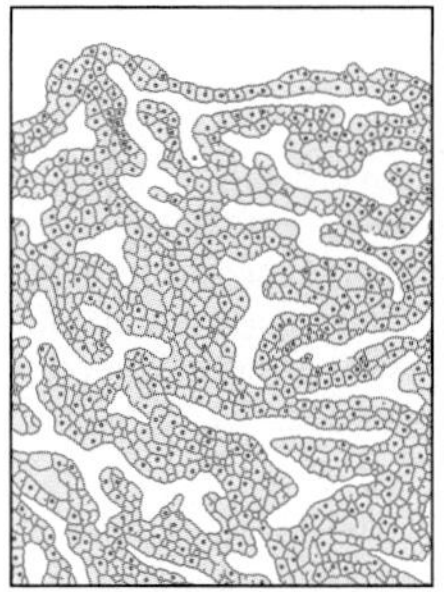

Figure 8.3
Endometrial histology from hyperplasia to carcinoma. (Reproduced with permission by Beckman CC, Ling F. Obstetrics and Gynecology for Medical Students. Baltimore: Williams & Wilkins, 1992: 407.)

(5) Obesity is also a risk factor due to ↑ circulating estrogen levels

3. Ovarian neoplasms
   a. Epithelial tumors comprise 75% of all ovarian tumors
      (1) Cystadenomas are benign cysts of 2 types
         (a) Serous cystadenomas are frequently bilateral & cause 20% of all ovarian tumors
         (b) Mucinous are less common, lined by mucus-secreting columnar cells
      (2) Serous cystadenocarcinoma is frequently bilateral—causes 50% of all ovarian malignant neoplasms

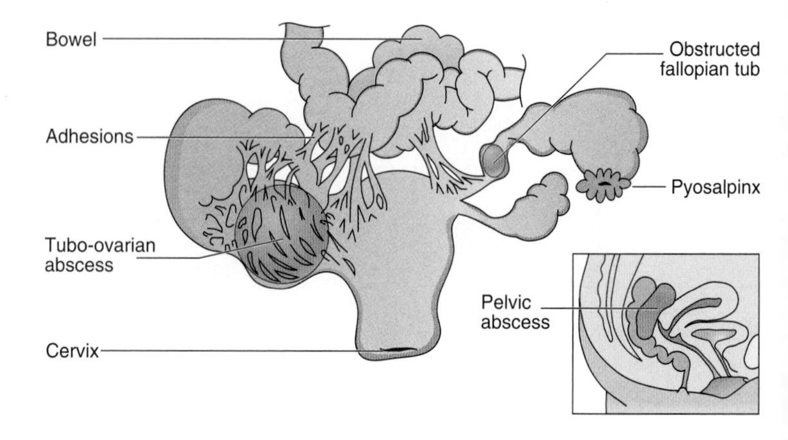

Figure 8.4
Findings associated with chronic pelvic inflammatory disease, including tubo-ovarian abscess, adhesions, pyosalpinx, and an abscess located in the posterior cul-de-sac. (Reproduced with permission by DeCherney A, Pernow M. Current Obstetrics and Gynecologic Diagnosis and Treatment. Norwalk, CT: Appleton & Lang, 1994: 755.)

(3) Mucinous cystadenocarcinoma is less common, can lead to **pseudomyxoma peritonei**
  (a) Pseudomyxoma peritonei is due to peritoneal seeding of the cancer
  (b) Peritoneum engorged with mucinous material secreted by the cancer
(4) Clear cell tumor is rare, in the ovaries it is also associated with DES exposure
(5) Brenner tumor is also rare, characterized by cells resembling bladder transitional epithelium

b. Germ cell tumors comprise 25% of all ovarian tumors, but account for majority of tumors in women younger than 20 years
  (1) Dysgerminoma is homologous to male seminoma, malignant
  (2) Endodermal sinus tumor (yolk sac tumor) is homologous to tumor of same name in males & **is also associated with elevated αFP**
  (3) Teratomas
    (a) Unlike in males, mature teratomas in females are benign tumors, occurring either within the ovaries

or at any midline structure in the body (e.g., thyroid, pituitary, etc.)
(b) Immature teratomas are very rare but aggressive cancers
(4) Choriocarcinoma
(a) An aggressive cancer that **produces HCG**
(b) As in males, this tumor is very bloody
(c) This cancer frequently occurs during pregnancy & then is even more malignant
(d) Can often be preceded by hydatidiform mole
c. Stromal neoplasms
(1) Fibroma is comprised of fibroblastic tissue, can cause **Meigs' syndrome**
(a) **Meigs' triad = fibroma + ascites + hydrothorax**
(b) Tumor seeds pleural & peritoneal cavities, secretes fluid
(2) Thecoma consists of fibroblasts plus lipid containing cells, can sometimes produce estrogen
(3) Granulosa cell tumor
(a) **Produce estrogen, in adults this leads to endometrial hyperplasia or CA, while in adolescents it causes precocious puberty**
(b) **Classic histologic finding = Call-Exner bodies, which are follicles filled with eosinophilic secretions**
(4) Sertoli-Leydig tumors are androgen producers, cause virilization

B. Polycystic ovaries (Stein-Leventhal Syndrome)
1. Excess excretion of leuteinizing hormone in young women leads to infertility
2. Classic Sx = amenorrhea, infertility, obesity, hirsutism
3. Tx = surgery, steroids, hormone replacement, depending upon patient preference

C. Inflammatory conditions
1. Toxic shock syndrome
a. Caused by enterotoxins of *S. aureus*
(1) Enterotoxins bind to nonpolymorphic regions of T-cell receptors & thereby activate such cells in an indiscriminate manner
(2) ↑ cellular activation & cytokine secretion lead to septic-like shock

(3) Clinically seen in the past due to use of certain tampons that had been seeded with *Staphylococcus*

2. Salpingitis/Pelvic inflammatory disease (PID)
   a. Salpingitis = infection/inflammation of fallopian tubes
   b. PID refers to salpingitis or any STD spreading to cause peritonitis
   c. #1 cause is *Chlamydia trachomatis* (*Neisseria gonorrhea* is second)
   d. Generally onset follows menses, can present with acute abdomen (PID is major appendicitis differential diagnosis [DDx] in young women)
   e. Chronically → pelvic adhesions, menstrual changes & infertility
   f. Si/Sx = rigid abdomen, ⊕ rebound tenderness, nausea/vomiting, ileus, fever, ↑ WBC, vaginal discharge
   g. Dx is by history and physical
      (1) **Bimanual examination elicits cervical motion tenderness**
      (2) **The infected tube is on the same side as the motion of the cervix, i.e., if stretching the cervix to the patient's left hurts, then the patient's left tube is infected**
3. Tubo-ovarian abscess (TOA) (See Figure 8.4)
   a. PID can lead to development of TOAs, which are also in the differential for acute abdomen in young women
   b. TOA perforation is a surgical emergency; antibiotics are ineffective
   c. Can quickly lead to septic shock
   d. Infertility is a common sequela if the abscess is not treated quickly
4. Vulvovaginitis (see Table 8.1)
   a. 50% of cases due to *Gardnerella* ("bacterial vaginosis"), 25% due to *Trichomonas* (for both, see Section III below)
   b. *Candida* (yeast infection) causes 25% of cases, increased frequency in diabetics, in pregnancy & in HIV
   c. Presents with milky-white, watery, or mucinous discharge from cervix
   d. Pain, burning sensation, itching may be present
   e. Dx by pelvic examination with microscopic examination of discharge

	Candida	Trichomonas	Gardnerella
Vaginal pH	4–5	>6	>5
Odor	None	Rancid	"Fishy" on KOH prep
Discharge	Cheesy white	Green, frothy	Variable
Si/Sx	Itchy, burning erythema	Severe itching	Variable to none
Microscopy	Pseudohyphae, more pronounced on 10% KOH prep	Motile organisms	Clue cells (large epithelial cells covered by dozens of small dots)
Treatment	Fluconazole	Metronidazole	Metronidazole

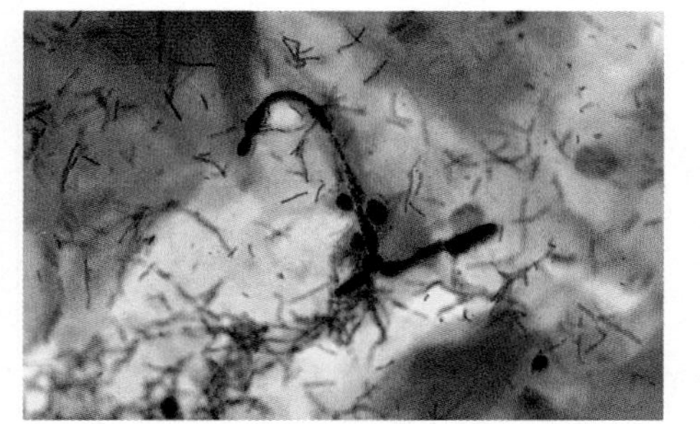

Gram's stain appearance of candidal pseudo-hyphae and cells.

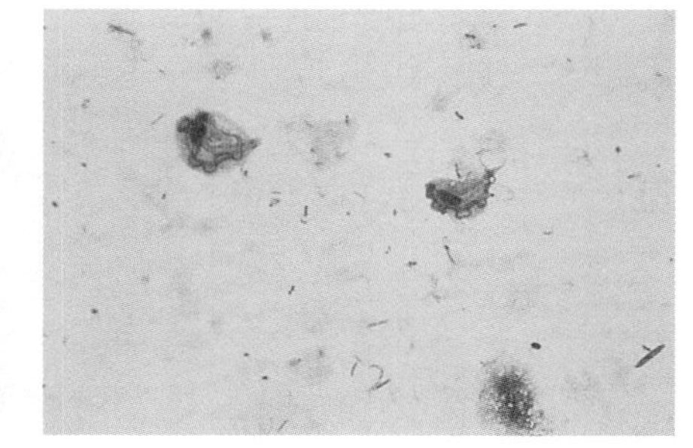

Scanning electron micrograph of *Trichomonas vaginalis*. The undulating membrane and flagellae of *Trichomonas* are its characteristic features.

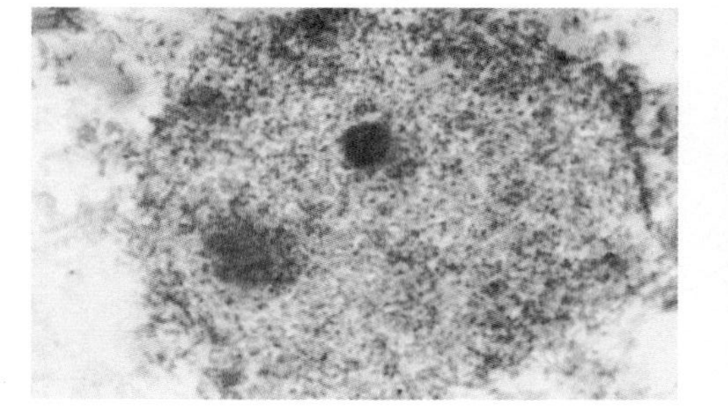

Gram's stain appearance of a "clue cell"—a vaginal epithelial cell covered with bacteria. No lactobacilli are present.

(A and C from Axford JS. Medicine. Oxford: Blackwell Science, 1998; Figure B adapted from Axford JS, Callaghan CA. Medicine. 2nd ed. Oxford: Blackwell Science, 2004.)

D. Pregnancy
  1. Normal physiology of pregnancy
    a. Dating pregnancy (Nägele's rule)
      (1) Dated from beginning of last menstrual period (LMP)
      (2) Formula = LMP − 3 months + 7 days + 1 yr
      (3) If LMP began 5/20/99, delivery due 2/27/2000
    b. Diagnosis
      (1) Si/Sx = missed periods, swollen breasts, fatigue, nausea
      (2) Urine/blood HCG test can Dx within 2–3 weeks of fertilization
      (3) **Common sign is melasma (chloasma), "the mask of pregnancy," a brownish discoloration of brow & both cheeks**—can also see ↑ pigmentation of areolae
    c. Cardiovascular circulation
      (1) Cardiac output rises 50%, heart rate rises to 80–90 bpm
      (2) BP drops (pulse pressure widens), but often returns to normal by third trimester
      (3) Both blood & plasma volumes ↑; however, plasma volume ↑ is greater, so hematocrit falls
      (4) White count often rises above 10,000, probably due to demargination of leukocytes
      (5) Due to pressure of expanding uterus on great veins, lower extremity dependent edema is common
      (6) Iron supplements should be given to mother to prevent anemia (↑ iron demand)
    d. Pulmonary physiology
      (1) Tidal volume & respiratory rate rise at expense of reserve volumes; therefore, vital capacity is not changed
      (2) ↑ in respiration blows off CO_2 so that mother's CO_2 levels run below 40—this allows the fetal circulation to remain near 40 & still be able to give off CO_2 to maternal blood (sets up a CO_2 concentration gradient across maternal–fetal circulation)
    e. Renal physiology
      (1) GFR ↑ (up to 50%) to match the cardiac output ↑
      (2) BUN typically falls to less than 10, creatinine falls as well
    f. GI physiology
      (1) Constipation common due to uterus pressing against colon

(2) Elevations in systemic progesterone cause systemic smooth muscle relaxation, which interferes with motility & can exacerbate constipation
(3) Relaxation of cardiac sphincter along with slower gastric emptying cause dyspepsia/heartburn

g. Endocrine
(1) Pregnant women often have ↑ thyroid-binding globulin & a goiter, so they can appear as hyperthyroid although functionally they are euthyroid
(2) Corticoid levels increase, probably responsible for striae that accompanies pregnancy
(3) Placenta produces HPL factor, which causes insulin resistance
(4) Gestational diabetes affects up to 5% of pregnancies (up to 40% in Hispanics)
(5) **The cure for gestational diabetes is delivery of the placenta!!!**

2. Abruptio placentae
   a. **Painful uterine bleeding** caused by premature separation of the placenta from the uterine wall, usually in third trimester
   b. Leads to fetal death & can cause disseminated intravascular coagulation (DIC) in mother due to seepage of fetal thromboplastin into maternal circulation
3. Placenta accreta
   a. Defective decidual layer allows direct connection of placenta to myometrium
   b. Prior C-section or endometrial inflammation predisposes
   c. Placenta does not separate properly during delivery, leading to massive maternal hemorrhage
4. Placenta previa
   a. Implantation of embryo at the bottom of the uterus, possibly even obstructing the cervical os
   b. Causes sudden, **painless vaginal bleeding** in any trimester
5. Ectopic pregnancy
   a. Most common location is fallopian tubes
   b. Predisposed by prior PID & endometriosis
   c. Can lead to tubal rupture that can kill the mother due to hemorrhage
6. Erythroblastosis fetalis (EF)
   a. Rh incompatibility leads to maternal IgG translocation across placenta, causing fetal hemolytic anemia

b. Develops in Rh^- mothers who have PREVIOUSLY given birth to Rh^+ children & are now pregnant with another Rh^+ child

c. **Aside from anemia, kernicterus is often fatal to the fetus**
   (1) Kernicterus is due to precipitation of bilirubin in brain
   (2) Caused by hemolytic liberation of excess intravascular bilirubin in the fetus
   (3) Clinically kernicterus presents with poor feeding, flaccidity, opisthotonus, seizures, apnea & death in the newborn
   (4) Those babies that survive untreated kernicterus often suffer long-term sequelae including mental retardation & deafness
   (5) Tx = placement of infant under UV lamp to degrade bilirubin

d. EF rare today due to Tx of mother with RhoGAM at 28 weeks gestation & after delivery of an Rh-incompatible child
   (1) Immunoglobulin binds to Rh^+ cells in maternal circulation & masks the Rh from the mother's immune system
   (2) Because mother's immune system is not sensitized during the first delivery, subsequent Rh^+ fetuses will not be recognized by the maternal immune system

7. Eclampsia

a. Progresses from preeclampsia, which is more common & much less severe
   (1) Preeclampsia presents after twentieth week of pregnancy with hypertension, proteinuria, edema
   (2) Preeclampsia occurs in 5% of pregnancies, often in women with preexisting hypertension
   (3) Preeclampsia can progress spontaneously to eclampsia
   (4) Tx is $MgSO_4$, which can improve some of the symptoms, but only cure is delivery of the child

b. Eclampsia includes preeclampsia symptoms & adds seizures &/or coma, & sometimes DIC

c. Classic eclampsia Sx = **HELLP**: **H**emolytic anemia, **E**levated **L**iver enzymes (transaminases), **L**ow **P**latelets

d. Untreated eclampsia is usually fatal

e. Tx = IV $MgSO_4$ to control seizures (if not, add diazepam)—delivery must be induced as soon as possible

8. Hydatidiform mole
   a. Occurs early in pregnancy, presents with vaginal bleeding, rapid swelling of uterine size
   b. Placenta appears like a large, bloody bunch of grapes
   c. Usual cause of preeclampsia prior to twentieth week of gestation
   d. 2 varieties, complete & partial, depending upon if fetal tissue is present or not
   e. 90% of complete moles are 46 XX
   f. 90% of partial moles are triploid = 69, XXY
   g. **HCG levels ↑↑↑ (>100,000)**, mimicking pregnancy
   h. Ultrasound → **classic "snowstorm" pattern**
   i. Can precede choriocarcinoma (premalignant)
   j. Tx = methotrexate &/or surgical evacuation

III. Sexually Transmitted Diseases

A. Gonorrhea
   1. Usually symptomatic in men; however, in women it is often aSx
   2. Characterized by purulent discharge from urethra
   3. Extragenitourinary manifestations are numerous
      a. In women is a common cause of PID
      b. The most common cause of septic arthritis in sexually active adults, **classically a monarthritis (one joint)**
      c. Can also cause anorectal infections & pharyngitis
      d. Ophthalmic neonatorum
         (1) Formerly a common eye infection in babies delivered by women infected with gonorrhea
         (2) Now is prophylaxed for with silver nitrate or erythromycin eye drops given to the infant after birth
   4. Dx = **gram-negative diplococci in PMNs is pathognomonic in discharge from males, in women cultures are necessary to diagnose**
   5. Culture media = **Thayer-Martin media** = chocolate agar + a cocktail of antibiotics to suppress endogenous flora
   6. Tx = cephalosporin (or ciprofloxacin in penicillin-allergic patients)

B. Lymphogranuloma venereum (*Chlamydia trachomatis*)
   1. **Chlamydia is the most common STD in the world**
   2. Causes nongonococcal urethritis that may progress to epididymitis or PID in women

3. Lymphogranuloma venereum characterized by small papule that ulcerates & lymph node swelling in inguinal region
4. **Classic physical finding = "the groove sign,"** a groove-like skin fold over the inguinal ligament created by profuse inguinal lymphadenopathy
5. Dx by culture or now have PCR-based methods
6. Tx = doxycycline or azithromycin
7. Neonates born to mothers infected with *C. trachomatis* can develop conjunctivitis or pneumonia characterized by eosinophilia & a very classic **"staccato" cough**

C. Syphilis (*Treponema pallidum*)

1. **Chancre = pathognomonic nontender ulcer occurring at the site of initial infection within 2–10 weeks (1° disease)**
2. 1–3 months later, secondary (2°) disease begins with **disseminated maculopapular rash that involves palms & soles**
3. Condyloma lata occur in genital areas, are very infectious by contact
4. 2/3 of patients never progress to tertiary (3°) disease, although people who are not treated can have repeated bouts of 2° disease
5. 3° disease occurs years later, presents with gummas of skin & bone, tabes dorsalis & dementia, ascending aortic aneurysms, and Argyll Robertson pupil (see Head and Neck chapter)
6. **Syphilis transplacental transmission is almost always AFTER the first trimester**
7. Syphilis CANNOT be cultured
8. Dx is by serology
   a. RPR & VDRL tests measure antibodies that cross-react to syphilitic antigens, but are not direct measurements of syphilis—frequently false-positive in collagen-vascular disease (dz) (e.g., lupus)
   b. Fluorescent treponemal antibody absorption test (FTA-ABS) is specific for the treponeme, but is more expensive & less sensitive
   c. Rapid plasma reagin test (RPR) & Venereal Disease Research Laboratory test (VDRL) are used for screening, FTA-ABS is used for subsequent specificity
   d. RPR & VDRL disappear in convalescence, but FTA-ABS usually ⊕ forever, despite resolution with treatment
9. Tx = penicillin G

10. Jarisch-Herxheimer reaction
    a. A septic-like condition that occurs after penicillin administration possibly due to release of endotoxin-like substances from the dead treponemes
    b. Can pretreat patients with antihistamines & NSAIDs before giving penicillin to avoid

D. Chancroid (*Hemophilus ducreyi*)
1. Presents with painful ulcers + local lymphadenitis
2. Dx by culture or Gram's stain of pus
3. Tx = azithromycin, cephalosporin, ciprofloxacin

E. Granuloma inguinale (*Calymmatobacterium granulomatis*)
1. Presents with genital ulceration & soft tissue/bone destruction that can be very disfiguring
2. Dx made by Gram's stain visualization, will show **classic Donovan bodies** = stained organisms within large macrophages
3. Tx = tetracycline

F. Genital herpes
1. Usually caused by HSV-2
2. Presents with perigenital/perianal painful vesicular rash, in 1° disease will see fever & lymphadenopathy
3. Both males & females can be aSx carriers
4. **Sexual transmission CAN occur in pts with latent dz!**
5. Dx by H&P, culture, or **Tzanck smear** = Giemsa stain of vesicular biopsy, ⊕ stain shows multinucleated giant cells at base of vesicle
6. Tx = acyclovir, shortens duration of lesions but will NOT eradicate dz

G. *Trichomonas vaginalis*
1. 25–50% of women in United States carry this organism, symptomatic dz is far rarer
2. Infected men are usually asymptomatic
3. See Table 8.1 for Dx & Tx

9. ENDOCRINOLOGY

I. The Hypothalamic Pituitary Axis

A. Anatomy

1. Pituitary lies in sella turcica atop the roof of the sphenoid sinus
2. Cavernous sinus with carotids & cranial nerves (CN) 3, 4, 6 bound the pituitary laterally, optic chiasm lies superiorly
3. Dural roof of pituitary = diaphragma sella, lies between gland & the chiasm
4. Blood → anterior pituitary via internal carotid & superior hypophyseal arteries
5. Hypothalamus-pituitary portal circulation supplies blood to anterior lobe (See Figure 9.1)
6. Inferior hypophyseal artery supplies blood to posterior pituitary
7. Cell types
   a. Somatotrophs are acidophilic, secrete growth hormone
   b. Corticotrophs are basophilic, secrete pro-opiomelanocortin, which then splits into: corticotropin (ACTH) & β-lipotropin, which is further split into β-melanocyte stimulating hormone (β-MSH), endorphins, & enkephalins
   c. Thyrotrophs stain basophilic to chromophobic & secrete thyrotropin (TSH)
   d. Gonadotrophs also stain basophilic to chromophobic & secrete follicle stimulating hormone (FSH) & luteinizing hormone (LH)
   e. Lactotrophs stain acidophilic to chromophobic, secrete prolactin
   f. Nonsecretory cells are resting forms of secretory cells
8. Anterior pituitary glycoprotein hormones are TSH, LH, & FSH
9. Posterior pituitary (neurohypophysis) hormones are synthesized by hypothalamus & transported down axons to posterior pituitary (see Figure 9.1)
10. Oxytocin induces uterine contraction & ejection of milk
11. Vasopressin = ADH, promotes water retention via action on renal collecting ducts

B. Hypopituitary syndrome

1. **First lose growth hormone (GH)**, then FSH/LH, then TSH, then ACTH

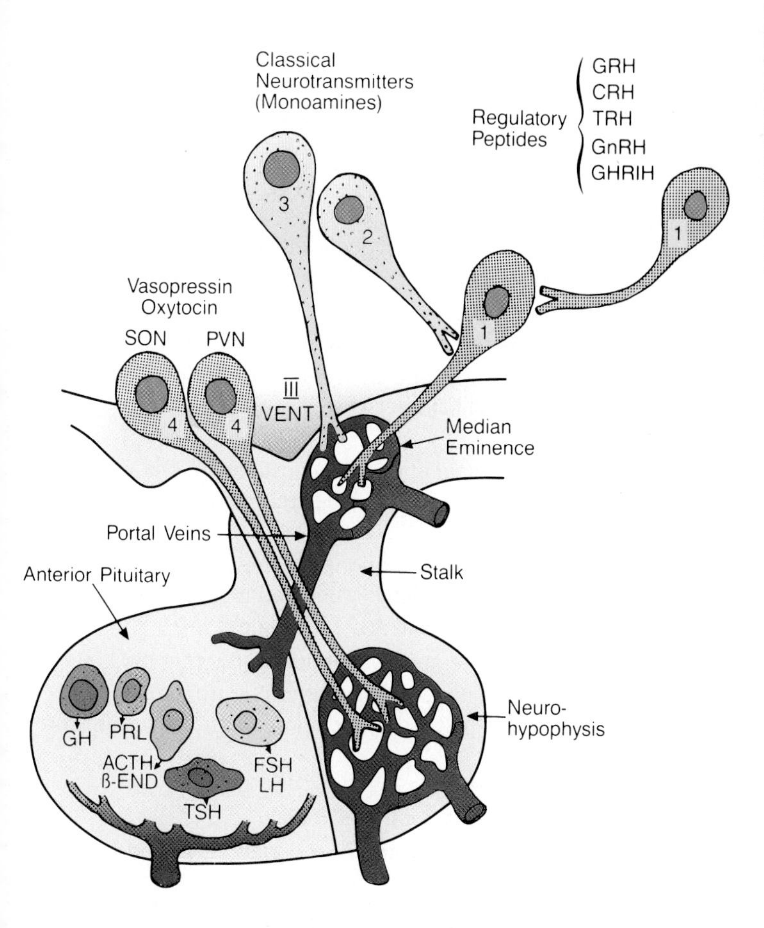

Figure 9.1 Diagram Representing the Hypothalamic-Pituitary Axis
Neuron 4 represents the magnocellular peptidergic neurons at the hypothalamoneurohypophyseal tract with cell bodies in the supraoptic nuclei (SON) and paraventricular nuclei (PVN) and terminals in the neurohypophysis. Neurons 2 and 3 are monoaminergic neurons. Neuron 2 represents a neuron contacting the cell body of a peptidergic neuron whereas neuron 3 represents a dopaminergic neuron projecting to the median eminence where release of dopamine occurs. The neurons 1 are the peptidergic neurons that secrete the regulatory peptides into the pituitary portal lexus. The regulatory peptides as well as dopamine are involved in the control of the secretion of the different anterior pituitary hormones. β-END = beta-endorphin; GHRIH = growth hormone release inhibiting hormone; VENT = ventricle.

2. Causes: congenital, trauma, radiation, sarcoidosis, histiocytosis, infection, infarction, tumor (craniopharyngioma or prolactinoma), amyloidosis, hemochromatosis, empty sella syndrome, idiopathic
3. Si/Sx:
   a. GH loss
      (1) ↓ growth, fasting hypoglycemia, delayed puberty
      (2) Children have round face & are chubby
   b. FSH/LH loss
      (1) No puberty, amenorrhea, delayed long bone closure
      (2) If occurs postpuberty, see gonadal atrophy, decreased body/facial hair, decreased libido
   c. TSH loss
      (1) Lethargy, cold intolerant, constipation, bradycardia, delayed deep tendon reflex relaxation
   d. ACTH loss
      (1) Orthostatic hypotension, weakness, hypothermia, nausea, vomit, dehydration, lethargy, coma, death
4. Pituitary apoplexy (Simmonds' syndrome)
   a. Defined as acute, massive pituitary infarct
   b. Risks = pregnancy, tumor, clotting disorder, trauma, diabetes, atherosclerosis, radiation, ↑ intracranial pressure (ICP)
   c. Sheehan's syndrome
      (1) Postpartum pituitary infarction
      (2) Caused by hypotension secondary (2°) to postpartum hemorrhage
      (3) Can be insidious, **first symptom (Sx) = can't lactate after birth**
   d. Sx = headache, diplopia, photophobia, visual blurring, vomiting, fever, other neurologic Sx
5. Tumors
   a. Prolactinomas are most common, 33% of pituitary tumors
      (1) Sx = impotence, amenorrhea, gynecomastia, galactorrhea, ↓ estrogen causing osteopenia or osteomalacia, ↑ androgens in females → virilization
      (2) **50% of prolactinoma patients have hypopituitarism, caused by mass effect of the tumor, coexistent with hyperprolactinemia**
      (3) TRH test will not cause a prolactin (PRL) surge when a tumor is present

b. GH secretors cause gigantism or acromegaly
   (1) Can be acromegaloid, which means that GH levels are not ↑, may be due to undiscovered hormone
   (2) Differential diagnosis (DDx) = 2° ↑ GH, occurs in anorexia, malnutrition, diabetes, renal failure, porphyria, cirrhosis, stress, lung adenocarcinoma & breast cancer
   (3) To screen for acromegaly, measure insulin growth factor (IGF), normals NEVER have acromegalic levels

II. Diabetes/Hypoglycemia

A. Type I diabetes
   1. Treatment (Tx) = insulin, insulin levels near 0, ketosis prone, early onset, minimal FHx
   2. Monozygotic concordance = 30–50%, HLA-linked autoimmune disease (dz)
   3. Diabetic ketoacidosis (DKA) due to lack of insulin ⇒ ↑ hormone-sensitive lipase ⇒ ↑ free fatty acid to liver, where ketogenesis occurs due to lack of insulin & ↑ glucagon as body attempts to get sugar inside cells
   4. Symptoms/signs (Sx/Si) of DKA = **Kussmaul hyperpnea** (Rapid, DEEP, respirations w/o dyspnea), psychoses/dementia, hyperthermia, nausea/vomit, **abdominal pain** (may resemble acute abdomen), **dehydration**
   5. **Mucormycosis**
      a. Uncommon but rapidly fatal fungal infection that classically presents in diabetics in DKA
      b. Any patient in DKA with facial pain MUST be worked up for *Mucor* sinusitis/facial infections
      c. Dx by immediate CT of sinuses
      d. Tx = urgent surgical débridement with adjunctive amphotericin B
      e. If Tx is not begun quickly, mortality >50% despite antifungal Tx
   6. **DKA labs = acidemia & "anion gap"** = Na − (Cl^- + HCO_3^-)
      a. Normal anion gap should be 12 ± 4
      b. LOOKS increased in DKA due to ketoacids occupying negative charge, causing ↓ in the Cl & HCO_3^- levels
   7. Labs also show ↑ urine/blood ketones, ↑ blood sugar, ↑ K^+
   8. ↑ K^+ due to 1) ↓ insulin, 2) ↑ H^+ ⇒ shifting of K^+ from intracellular pool to extracellular

9. If serum K^+ is NOT ↑, BEWARE of massive underlying hypokalemia
10. DKA Tx: **(1°) Tx = FLUIDS!!!, (2°) = K+ & insulin, (3°) = add glucose to insulin drip if patient (pt) becomes normoglycemic to prevent hypoglycemia**—purpose of insulin is to shut down ketogenesis, NOT to ↓ glucose, so insulin must be given beyond normalization of glucose levels until ketones are gone!

B. Type II diabetes
1. Tx = insulin if severe, otherwise utilize diet, exercise, oral hypoglycemic agents
2. Insulin production can be ↑, normal, or ↓
3. Usually adult onset, not ketosis prone, often strong family history
4. Monozygotic concordance ≈ 100%, not HLA linked, no autoimmune etiology
5. Disease progresses sequentially through several stages of severity
6. Insulin physiology in different stages of diabetes—see Table 9.1

Table 9.1 Stages of Diabetes

Condition	OGTT*	Insulin Level	Insulin Sensitivity	Comments
Normal	Nml	Nml	Nml	
Obese	Nml	↑	↓	↑ insulin necessary to maintain Nml blood sugar
IFG†	↑ then Nml	↑↑↑	↓↓↓↓	↑ sugar postprandial, returns to Nml during fast
Early diabetes	↑↑	↑↑	↓↓↓↓	Still making insulin, but cannot overcome ↓ sensitivity
Late diabetes	↑↑↑	↓	↓↓↓↓	Final loss of insulin production worsens blood sugar

*OGTT = oral glucose tolerance test.
†IFG = impaired fasting glucose.

7. Diabetic Si/Sx
    a. Acute = dehydration, polydipsia/polyphagia/polyuria, fatigue, weight loss
    b. Subacute = infections (typically vaginitis, often yeast), mucor/zygomycoses, staphylococcal boils
    c. Chronic
        (1) Macrovascular = stroke, coronary artery disease
        (2) Microvascular = retinitis, nephritis
        (3) Neuropathy = ↓ sensation, paresthesias, glove-in-hand burning pain, autonomic insufficiency
    d. If catch nephropathy early (measuring microalbuminuria), can slow progression with ACE inhibitors
8. Hyperosmolar hyperglycemic nonketotic coma (HHNK)
    a. In Type II diabetes, residual insulin levels protect against DKA unless alternative stress (e.g., infection) is present, while HHNK is typically seen in type II patients but not type I diabetics
    b. HHNK caused by progressive hypovolemia, can be precipitated by acute infection, trauma, dehydration, etc.
    c. Blood sugar can rise above 1000 mg/dL, no acidosis but there is severe mental depression & acute renal failure
    d. Tx = rehydrate (may require 10L), mortality approaches 50%
    e. **Note: if DKA presents instead of HHNK, search carefully for an infection or other stressor!!!**
9. Maturity onset diabetes of youth (MODY)
    a. Autosomal dominant, nonobese young adolescents
    b. Defect in pancreatic/liver hexokinase isozyme = glucokinase
    c. Enzyme has ↓ affinity for glucose, blood sugar has to ↑↑ for the enzyme to work
    d. Result is higher blood sugar before insulin secretion begins & liver begins to utilize sugar
10. Gestational diabetes
    a. Affects 2–5% of pregnancies, 40% of mothers become diabetic postnatally
    b. Placenta causes gestational diabetes, anti-insulin peptides secreted (chiefly HPL)
    c. Si/Sx = macrosomia, neonatal hypoglycemia
    d. Often C-section required for successful delivery of large babies

11. Dx of any diabetes
    a. Random plasma glucose over 200 with symptoms or
    b. Fasting glucose over 125 twice or
    c. 2-hr oral glucose tolerance test (OGTT) glucose >200 with or without symptoms
12. Glycosylated hemoglobin A1c (HgA1c)
    a. Due to high blood glucose, intravascular hemoglobin becomes glycosylated in vivo (mechanism not known)
    b. HgA1c used to follow glucose control (marker of need to adjust regimen & also patient compliance to regimen!), ideal value of <8
    c. Because of serum half-life of hemoglobin, HgA1c is a marker of the prior 3 months of therapeutic regimen
    d. **Tight glucose control has been shown to reduce complications & mortality in IDDM & NIDDM, thus HgA1c is a key tool to follow diabetic Tx regimens**

C. Hypoglycemia
1. Gluconeogenesis is inhibited by insulin, stimulated by glucagon; GH & cortisol are permissive
2. Glucagon & epinephrine allow acute recovery of hypoglycemia, cortisol & GH act longer term
3. Whipple's triad of hypoglycemia (for Dx)
    a. Patient's Sx should be consistent with hypoglycemia
    b. Sx should occur while patient is hypoglycemic
    c. Sx should be relieved by sugar administration
4. Si/Sx due to adrenergic & neuroglycopenic responses
    a. Adrenergic Si/Sx = weak, diaphoretic, tachycardia, palpitations, tremor, nervous, irritable, perioral/peripheral paresthesias
    b. Neuroglycopenic responses = headache, hypothermia, visual disturbances, altered mentation, confusion, amnesia, seizure, coma
5. Causes of fasting hypoglycemia are myriad, include drugs (e.g., exogenous insulin, sulfonylureas, propranolol), EtOH, liver or kidney failure, enzyme defects (liver storage diseases), sepsis, adrenal insufficiency, GH deficiency, insulinomas **& EARLY type II diabetes**
6. Fasting hypoglycemia NOT Dx by looking at blood sugar, people can have low sugar & be normal
7. Dx by I/G ratio (insulin/glucose), should be below 0.3, will be above 0.3 in insulinomas

8. Factitious hypoglycemia 2° to insulin use is diagnosed by C-peptide level, will be low even though insulin levels are high
9. To detect factitious sulfonylurea use must test for urine metabolites, C-peptide levels will be normal

III. Adrenal Disorders

A. Adrenal physiology
   1. Synthesis of adrenal cortex hormones is regional
      a. Zona **g**lomerulosa makes **a**ldosterone
      b. Zona **f**asciculata makes **c**ortisol
      c. Zona **r**eticularis makes **t**estosterone (hormone)
      d. **Adrenal Mnemonic: GFR** (as in renal clearance) **makes ACT**(H)
   2. Conversion of cholesterol to pregnenolone is rate-limiting in cortisol formation
   3. Glucocorticoid secretion oscillates with 24-hr periodicity (levels highest at dawn, lowest in evening)
   4. Effects of cortisol on the body—see Table 9.2
   5. Anti-inflammatory effects of glucocorticoids due to:
      a. Induction of lipocortin, an inhibitor of phospholipase A2, which is the enzyme that liberates arachidonic acid
      b. Inhibition of the production of interleukin 2, thereby inhibiting T-cell activation & proliferation
      c. Induction of lymphocyte apoptosis
      d. Inhibition of release of histamine & serotonin from mast cells & platelets
      e. Other mechanisms not yet characterized
   6. Cortisol → cortisone by 11-β-hydroxysteroid dehydrogenase in kidneys & colon

Table 9.2 Effects of Cortisol on the Body

Glycogen/ Gluco-neogen-esis/ serum glucose	Lipol-ysis	Protein catabolism	Immune function	Bone density	Wound healing/ Fibrob-last activity	GI acid/ GI prosta-glandin
↑/↑/↑	↑	↑	↓↓	↓	↓	↑/↓

7. Cortisone has ↓ mineralocorticoid effect, enzyme protects mineralocorticoid reactive tissues from cortisol
8. Aldosterone → ↑ Na resorption/K+ secretion in distal tubules (Na/K pump)
9. ↑ renin ⇒ ↑ angiotensin ⇒ ↑ aldosterone production

B. Cushing's syndrome
   1. 5 causes
      a. Iatrogenic/exogenous cortisol (most common)
      b. Pituitary adenoma (Cushing's disease)
      c. Adrenal hyperplasia/cancer
      d. Ectopic ACTH producing tumor
         (1) Ectopic ACTH tumor can be small cell lung CA, thymoma, islet cell CA, carcinoid, pheochromocytoma, thyroid medullary CA
         (2) Frequently lack classic signs due to **RAPID** dz progression
      e. Ectopic CRH production
   2. Si/Sx = **buffalo hump, central obesity, moon facies, striae,** plethora, hyperglycemia, proximal weakness, hypertension, altered mentation, easy bruising, hirsutism, oligo/amenorrhea, impotence, acne, edema, backache, polydipsia/uria (see Figure 9.2, Figure 9.3, and Figure 9.4)
   3. Dx: 24-hr urine cortisol & dexamethasone (DEX) suppression
      a. If low dose DEX does NOT suppress cortisol, look for pituitary disease (Cushing's disease)

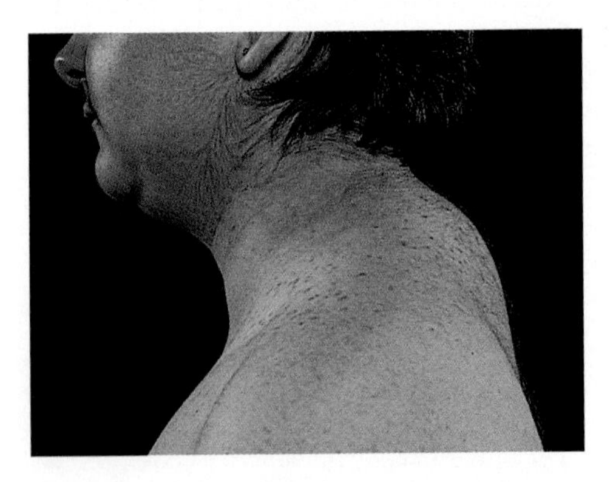

Figure 9.2
Buffalo hump. (From Axford JS. Callaghan CA. Medicine. 2nd ed. Oxford: Blackwell Science, 2004.)

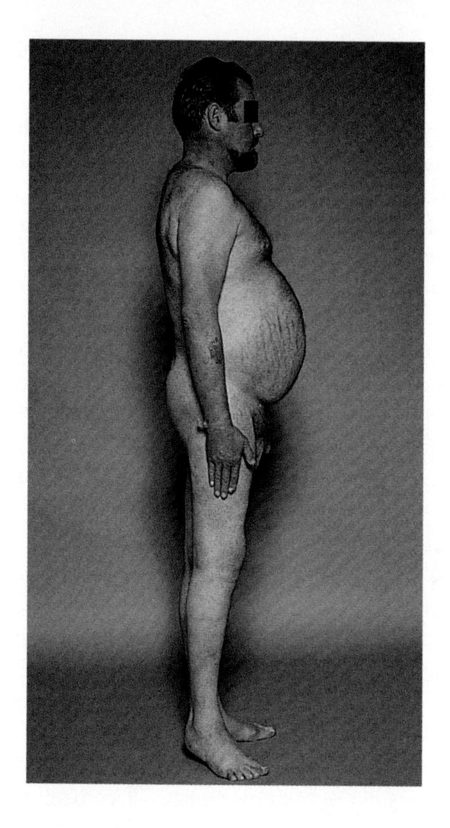

Figure 9.3
Truncal obesity with abdominal striae. (From Axford JS. Callaghan CA. Medicine. 2nd ed. Oxford: Blackwell Science, 2004.)

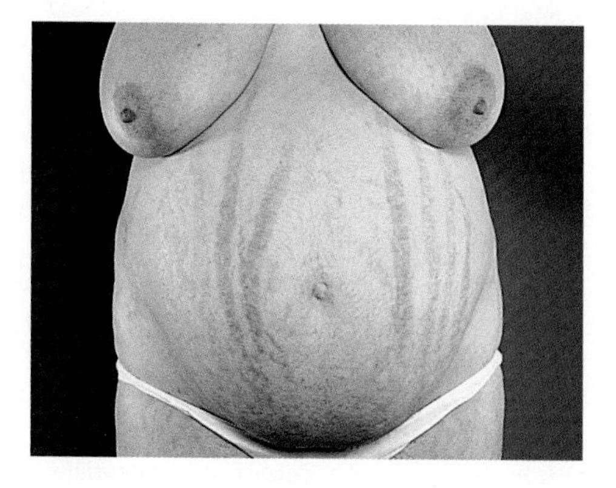

Figure 9.4
Abdominal striae. (From Axford JS. Callaghan CA. Medicine. 2nd ed. Oxford: Blackwell Science, 2004.)

   b. **High-dose DEX suppresses cortisol in Cushing's disease**
   c. **If high-dose DEX does not suppress cortisol & ACTH is low, look for adrenal disease**
   d. **If high-dose DEX does not suppress cortisol & ACTH is high, look for ectopic ACTH (small cell CA most common) or more rarely ectopic CRH production**
4. Pseudo-Cushing's = ↑ CRH ↑ ACTH ↑ cortisol 2° to alcohol, stress, renal failure, anorexia, obesity, depression
5. Tx: remove tumor, mitotane (adrenolytic), ketoconazole (inhibits P450), metyrapone (blocks adrenal enzyme synthesis), aminoglutethimide (inhibits P450)
6. Nelson's syndrome = postadrenalectomy, expansion of pituitary leading to hyperpigmentation

C. Adrenal insufficiency
1. Si/Sx of adrenal insufficiency due to any cause = fatigue, anorexia, nausea/vomit, constipation, diarrhea, salt craving (pica), postural hypotension, **hyponatremia**, **hyperkalemia, non-gap metabolic acidosis, eosinophilia**
2. Testing of hormonal axis can help differentiate between causes of insufficiency
   a. ACTH testing is DANGEROUS, only do in the hospital
   b. Give insulin ⇒ hypoglycemia ⇒ ↑ cortisol: contraindicated in adrenal failure, elderly, heart disease, seizures
   c. Metyrapone ⇒ inhibit cortisol synthesis, give at night, cortisol should be ↓ in morning, ACTH ↑
   d. Cortrosyn test = give ACTH, if cortisol does not ↑↑, = 1° adrenal failure
   e. Give CRH, if cortisol does not ↑↑ = 1° pituitary failure—in Cushing's see ↑↑↑↑ cortisol response
3. 1° Disease = Addison's disease
   a. 7 Causes = autoimmune (most common), granulomatous disease, CA, vascular, HIV, iatrogenic, DIC (Waterhouse-Friderichsen syndrome)
      (1) **Waterhouse-Friderichsen syndrome**: classic syndrome of hemorrhagic necrosis of adrenal medulla during the course of meningococcemia (see Figure 9.5)
      (2) Beware of this disease during meningococcal meningitis (look for truncal rash + meningitis)
      (3) Causes acute onset catastrophic adrenal insufficiency!!!
   b. **1° disease shows hyperpigmentation, ↑ ACTH, ↓ cortisol response to ACTH (Cortrosyn test)**

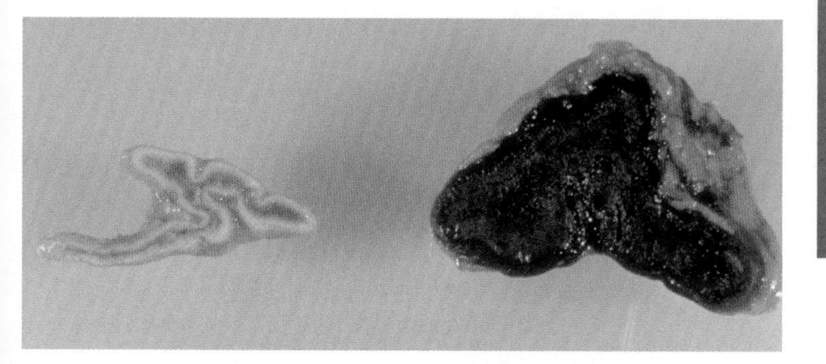

Figure 9.5 Waterhouse-Friderichsen Syndrome
A normal adrenal gland (left) in contrast to an adrenal gland enlarged by extensive hemorrhage (right), obtained from a patient who died of meningococcemic shock. (From Rubin E, Gorstein F, Rubin R, et al. Rubin's Pathology: Clinicopathologic Foundations of Medicine. 4th ed. Baltimore: Lippincott Williams & Wilkins, 2005.)

4. 2° Disease = ↓ ACTH secretion by pituitary, 3° Disease = ↓ CRH by hypothalamus
   a. Causes of either include tumor, vascular, trauma, idiopathic, radiation, granulomatous
   b. **2° shows NO hyperpigmentation, ↓ ACTH, ↑ cortisol response to ACTH**
5. Acute hypoadrenal crisis = marked hypotension, dehydration, shock, nausea, vomit, abdominal pain
6. Tx = cortisol replacement, ↑ replacement for times of illness or stress—**must taper replacement off slowly to allow HPA axis to restore itself**
7. Congenital adrenal hyperplasia [see below, Section IV.C.1]
   a. Shows ↓ cortisol, ↑/Nml androgens, ↑ ACTH
   b. Due to synthetic enzyme defects → steroids shunting away from glucocorticoids
   c. Causes virilization, hirsutism, edema due to ↑ androgens & mineralocorticoids

D. Adrenal cortical hyperfunction
1. 1° hyperaldosteronism = Conn's syndrome
   a. Adenoma or hyperplasia of zona glomerulosa → ↑ mineralocorticoid production
   b. Si = HTN, ↑ Na, ↑ Cl, ↓ renin (due to feedback inhibition), hypervolemia, ↓ K, alkalosis, weakness,

paresthesias, transient paralysis & tetany, polyuria/polydipsia

c. No edema seen due to ↑ excretion as body adapts to fluid overload

d. Dx: ↑ aldosterone ↓ renin

2. 2° hyperaldosteronism

a. Defect outside the adrenal → hypertension, edema, cirrhosis with ascites & cardiac failure

b. Due to increased renin production 2° to renal ischemia (e.g., congestive heart failure [CHF], shock, renal artery stenosis) or tumor

c. Can be due to defect in 11-β-hydroxysteroid dehydrogenase, allowing cortisol to stimulate the mineralocorticoid receptor in the kidney & colon

d. Dx = ↑ renin (renin levels differentiate 1° vs. 2° hyperaldosteronism)

E. Adrenal medulla

1. Pathologies are rare, most common is malignancy

a. Pheochromocytoma

(1) Derived from chromaffin cells of the adrenal medulla

(2) Usually benign, characterized by ↑ urinary excretion of catecholamines & their metabolites (VMA)

(3) Sx = hypertension (episodic or chronic), diaphoresis, palpitations, tachycardia, headache, nausea/vomit, flushing, dyspnea, paresthesias, blurry vision

(4) Rule of 10: 10% malignant, 10% bilateral, 10% extra-adrenal (tumor occurs in embryologic derivative cells that reactivate outside the adrenal gland)

(5) **Extra-adrenal pheochromocytoma**

(a) **May occur in the organs of Zuckerkandl** (para-aortic sympathetic chain), a rest of chromaffin cells

(b) Can occur within bladder wall, **presents with tachycardia, palpitations & syncope during urination**

b. Neuroblastomas are ↑ malignant catecholamine-producing tumors

(1) Usually seen in childhood, originates in the adrenal medulla

(2) Characterized by amplification of *N-myc* oncogene with thousands of gene copies per cell

IV. Gonadal Disorders

A. Male gonadal axis
   1. Normal physiology
      a. Puberty initiated by hypothalamic pulsatile GnRH release
      b. Testosterone synthesized & secreted by the Leydig cells
      c. LH ↑ testosterone synthesis by stimulating cholesterol desmolase
      d. FSH acts on Sertoli cells to maintain spermatogenesis
      e. Sertoli cells also secrete inhibin, which feedback-inhibits secretion of FSH from anterior pituitary
      f. Accessory sex organs contain 5-α-reductase, which converts testosterone to dihydrotestosterone (the most active form)
      g. Finasteride inhibits 5-α-reductase, used to Tx benign prostatic hypertrophy (BPH) & male pattern baldness
   2. Klinefelter's syndrome
      a. XXY chromosome inheritance, extremely variable expressivity
      b. Appear tall, eunuchoid, with small, firm testes & gynecomastia
      c. Most cases are undiagnosed until puberty, when diminished virilization is noted
      d. Some individuals go through puberty normally, others require testosterone supplements
      e. ↓ circulating testosterone leads to ↑ LH, FSH due to lack of feedback inhibition (useful laboratory markers for the disease)
      f. **Dx = buccal smear analysis for presence of Barr bodies**
      g. Individuals with ↑ X chromosomes (XXXY, XXXXY) have ↑ mental retardation & developmental abnormalities
   3. XYY Syndrome
      a. ↑ incidence of violence & antisocial behavior; HOWEVER, the vast majority of XYY individuals (98%) live completely normal lives NOT MARKED BY violence or antisocial behavior
      b. Therefore XYY may predispose to criminal/violent behavior, but it is NOT DIRECTLY CAUSAL
      c. Can see mild mental retardation, severe acne & tend to be tall

4. Testicular feminization syndrome
    a. Defect in the dihydrotestosterone receptor
    b. Leads to development of female external genitalia with sterile, undescended testes
    c. Patients appear as normal females, but are sterile & the vagina is blind-ended
    d. **Levels of testosterone, estrogen & LH are all high**
5. 5-α-reductase deficiency
    a. Patients have ambiguous genitalia until puberty
    b. At puberty, burst in testosterone synthesis overcomes the lack of dihydrotestosterone & external genitalia become masculinized
    c. **Levels of testosterone & estrogen are normal, LH is normal or increased**

B. Female gonadal axis
1. Normal physiology
    a. Day 1 of menstrual cycle = first day of menstrual bleeding
    b. Cycles can be 18–40 days in length, divided into 3 phases (see Figure 9.6 and Table 9.3)
    c. LH stimulates theca cells of ovum to produce androgens
    d. Androgens diffuse to granulosa cells, which contain aromatase stimulated by FSH to convert androgen to estrogen
2. Turner's syndrome (XO)
    a. **Most common cause of 1° amenorrhea**
    b. Newborns have ↑ skin at dorsum of neck (**neck webbing**)
    c. Also see short stature, ptosis, **coarctation of aorta, amenorrhea but uterus is present**, juvenile external genitalia, bleeding due to GI telangiectasias
    d. **No mental retardation is present**
    e. Classic finding is **ovaries replaced by fibrous streaks**

C. Hypogonadism of either sex
1. Congenital adrenal hyperplasia (CAH)
    a. Several types, each with defect in synthetic enzymes in the steroid pathway (see Figure 9.7)
    b. Block in normal synthetic pathways leads to shunting & altered production of sex hormones
    c. Causes either virilization of females or failure to virilize males
    d. Tx for all = replacement of necessary hormones

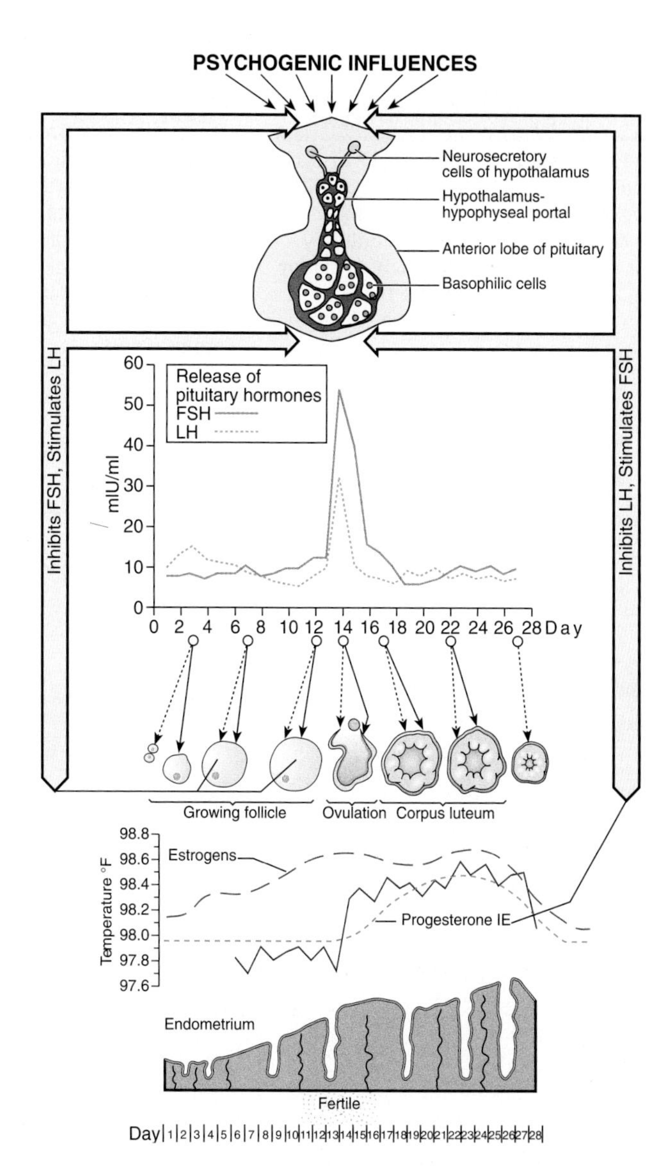

Figure 9.6 Normal Menstrual Cycle
Note the suprahypothalamic (cerebral, pineal), hypothalamic, pituitary, ovarian, and endometrial interrelations. (Adapted from Axford JS. Medicine. Oxford: Blackwell Science, 1998.)

Table 9.3 Phases of the Menstrual Cycle

Follicular Phase	Ovulatory Phase	Luteal Phase
Day 1–13 of cycle: estrogen-induced negative feedback on FSH & LH in anterior pituitary	**Day 13–17 of cycle:** estrogen-induced positive feedback to anterior pituitary FSH & LH, ovulation occurs 16–32 hr after the LH surge	**Day 15–first day of menses:** corpus luteal progesterone acts on hypothalamus, causing negative feedback on FSH & LH, resulting in ↓ to basal levels prior to next cycle

e. 21-α-hydroxylase deficiency causes 95% of all CAH
   (1) ↑↑↑ androgens leads to virilization of females
   (2) Severe disease presents in infancy with ambiguous genitalia & salt loss (2° to ↓↓ aldosterone)
   (3) Less severe variants → minimal virilization & salt loss, & can have Dx delayed for several years

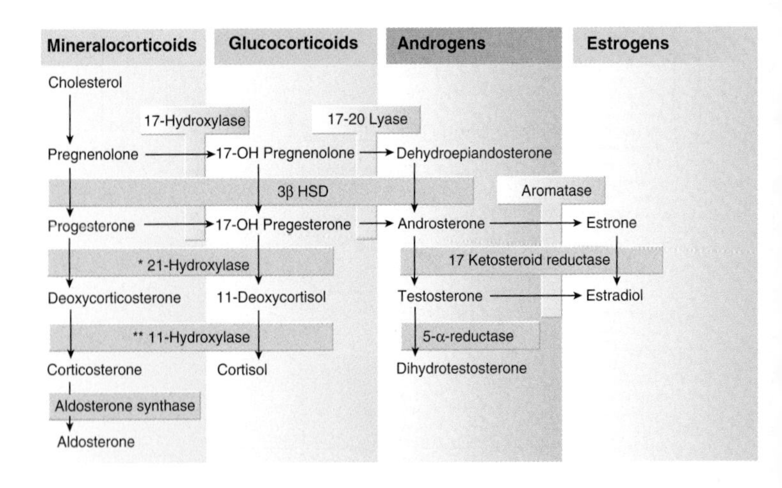

Figure 9.7 Pathways of Steroid Synthesis
The synthetic pathway of steroids and the enzymes facilitating each step. 17-Hydroxylase and 17–20 lyase activity are mediated by a single microsomal enzyme. The enzymes for sex steroids occur mainly outside of the adrenal gland: aromatase in granulosa cells and fat tissue, 5-α-reductase in skin and prostate glands, 17-ketosteroid reductase in gonads. *The most common defect in congenital adrenal hyperplasia is 21-hydroxylase deficiency. **Site of action of metyrapone is 11-hydroxylase. (From Axford JS. Callaghan CA. Medicine. 2nd ed. Oxford:Blackwell Science, 2004.)

(4) Complete virilizations can also be missed until puberty, as females will be thought to be males until that time

f. 11-β-hydroxylase deficiency
   (1) Hypertension (HTN) due to ↑ salt & water retention (hypertensive virilizing adrenal hyperplasia)
   (2) ↑↑↑ androgens leads to extreme virilization of females

g. 3-β-hydroxysteroid dehydrogenase & 17-α-hydroxylase
   (1) Both cause failure of virilization of males due to block in androgen secretion, does not virilize females
   (2) 17-α-hydroxylase deficiency is distinguished by simultaneous block in cortisol & sex hormones

2. Prader-Willi syndrome
   a. Autosomal with paternal imprinting (only gene from dad is expressed)
   b. Presents in infancy with floppy baby & obtundation
   c. Si/Sx = short limbs, obesity due to gross hyperphagia, nasal speech, retardation
   d. Classic craniofacies
      (1) Almond-shaped eyes with strabismus
      (2) High-arched palate, narrow skull
   e. **Mnemonic: H_3O: H**ypogonadism, **H**ypotonia, **H**ypomentation (i.e., retarded), **O**besity
3. Laurence-Moon-Biedl syndrome
   a. Autosomal recessive inheritance
   b. Contrast to Prader-Willi, patients are not usually short
   c. Children are obese, but have normal craniofacies, may be retarded
   d. Typical limb finding is polydactyly
   e. **Mnemonic: H_2O: H**ypogonadism, **H**ypomentation, **O**besity
4. Kallmann's syndrome
   a. Congenital hypogonadism with anosmia (can't smell)
   b. Autosomal dominant, variable penetrance
   c. Due to a lack of production/secretion of GnRH by hypothalamus
   d. Dx by lack of circulating LH & FSH
   e. Tx = pulsatile GnRH administration, which induces virilization

V. Thyroid

A. Physiology
   1. TRH secreted by hypothalamus, stimulates TSH secretion by anterior pituitary

2. The α-subunit of TSH is identical to that of FSH, LH, & HCG—the β-subunit gives specificity
3. Thyroid hormones = thyroxin (T4) & triiodothyronine (T3)
4. Synthesis depends upon sufficient quantities of iodine from diet
5. Iodine absorbed in upper GI tract, enters blood stream, is trapped by an active transport system in thyroid follicular cells
6. Iodine + thyroid peroxidase → iodide + hydrogen peroxide + tyrosine → MIT/DIT, MIT + DIT → T3, DIT + DIT → T4 (MIT = mono-iodinated thyroxine, DIT = di-iodinated thyroxine)
7. TSH binds to thyroid cell membrane receptors, activates adenylate cyclase, ↑ cAMP & ↑ thyroid hormone
8. Serum T3 & T4 are bound to thyroid-binding globulin (TBG)
9. In peripheral tissues T4 is converted to T3 or reverse T3 (rT3)
10. T3 is 4 times more biologically active than T4, rT3 is inactive
11. In the perinatal period maturation of CNS is absolutely dependent on thyroid hormone
    a. Deficiency causes irreversible mental retardation
    b. All neonates undergo mandatory screening for hypothyroidism

B. Congenital thyroid disease
1. Thyroid develops as outpouching of endoderm at base of tongue
2. Gland migrates caudally to its final resting position in the developed infant
3. During this migration, the gland remains connected to its starting point by the thyroglossal duct (site is marked in the developed organism by the foramen cecum)
4. Thyroglossal duct normally involutes during development, but cysts can present along tract of the duct during adolescence (or, rarely, adulthood) as thyroglossal cysts
5. Thyroglossal cysts are ALWAYS midline (main DDx = branchial cleft cysts, which lie laterally on the neck, & dermoid cysts)
6. **Thyroglossal cysts elevate with swallowing or sticking tongue out, whereas others do not**
7. Islets of ectopic thyroid tissue may lie anywhere along the tract of the resorbed thyroglossal duct

C. Goiter
1. Enlargement of the thyroid gland, implies NOTHING about thyroid function

2. Potential causes = normal physiologic enlargement (puberty/pregnancy), dietary iodine deficiency, inflammation, gland hyperfunction, goitrogens (compounds in food or drugs that suppress gland's hormone production)
3. The term *toxic* implies hyperthyroidism (↑ levels of serum thyroxine)

D. Hyperthyroidism
1. General
   a. Causes = Grave's disease, iatrogenic, Plummer's disease, adenoma, subacute thyroiditis, apathetic hyperthyroidism, struma ovarii, silent thyroiditis, 2° disease
   b. Si/Sx of hyperthyroidism = tachycardia, **isolated systolic hypertension**, tremor, a-fib, anxiety, diaphoresis, weight loss with increased appetite, insomnia/**fatigue**, diarrhea, **exophthalmus, heat intolerance**
   c. T4/3 levels fluctuate with changes in TBG levels, so serum levels are not strictly useful to measure
      (1) Pregnancy elevates TBG levels via estrogen, falsely elevating the lab value of the serum T4
      (2) Nephrotic syndrome & cirrhosis lower TBG levels, falsely lowering T4 levels
2. Graves' disease (diffuse toxic goiter) is the most common cause (90% of US hyperthyroid cases)
   a. Graves disease is seen in young adults & is 8x more common in females than males (see Figure 9.8)
   b. Caused by idiopathic autoimmune response to the TSH receptor, autoantibody stimulates the receptor
   c. **Graves' disease Si/Sx include 2 characteristic findings only seen in hyperthyroid due to Graves' disease: infiltrative ophthalmopathy & pretibial myxedema**
   d. **Infiltrative ophthalmopathy**
      (1) Similar to exophthalmus, but blurry/double vision is acquired due to weakness of ocular muscles
      (2) Whereas simple exophthalmus resolves when the thyrotoxicosis is cured, infiltrative ophthalmopathy may not be reversible (waxes & wanes, with no correlation to the pt's thyroid status)
      (3) Because of the above finding, it is clear that thyrotoxicosis is not responsible for infiltrative ophthalmopathy—instead it is hypothesized that autoantibodies damage retrobulbar tissues

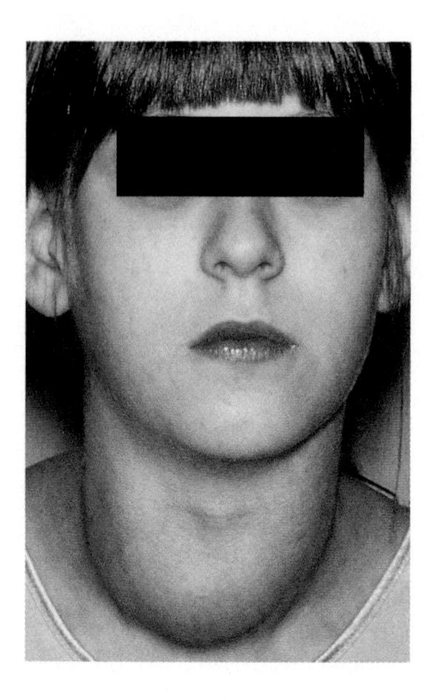

Figure 9.8
Patients with Grave's disease appear thin, nervous, hyperactive, and unable to sit still, often with a wide-eyed expression and symmetrical thyroid enlargement that moves on swallowing. (From Axford JS. Callaghan CA. Medicine. 2nd ed. Oxford: Blackwell Science, 2004)

   e. **Pretibial myxedema**
      (1) Dermopathy, usually on the shins, characterized by brawny, pruritic, nonpitting edema
      (2) Unlike infiltrative exophthalmus, pretibial myxedema often spontaneously remits after months to years
3. Plummer's disease (toxic multinodular goiter)
   a. Due to multiple foci of thyroid tissue that cease responding to T4 feedback inhibition
   b. More common in older people, as opposed to Grave's
   c. Dx
      (1) Physical examination → feel multiple nodules whereas Grave's is diffusely enlarged
      (2) Radioactive iodine uptake tests show hot nodules, with abnormally cold background gland due to suppression of normal tissue by overactive nodules
4. Thyroid adenoma due to overproduction of hormone by tumor in the gland

5. Subacute thyroiditis (granulomatous, giant cell, or de Quervain's thyroiditis)
   a. **BEWARE:** this disease presents with hyperthyroidism that then later turns into hypothyroidism
   b. Due to inflammation of the thyroid gland with early spilling of hormone from the damaged gland
   c. See below under Hypothyroid, Section V.E.3 for more
6. Apathetic hyperthyroidism is idiopathic condition seen in elderly where only Sx is often intractable CHF with atrial fibrillation
7. Silent thyroiditis
   a. Occurs mostly in women, often in postpartum period
   b. Characterized by mild, transient thyrotoxicosis with goiter
8. Struma ovarii
   a. An ovarian teratoma containing ectopic thyroid tissue
   b. Usually benign, 5% pts develop clinical hyperthyroidism
9. 2° hyperthyroidism very rare, due to hypersecretion of TSH from pituitary (3° even rarer, due to ↑ TRH)
10. Labs
    a. TBG sites are low in hyperthyroidism & T3RU (T3 resin uptake) is high in hyperthyroidism
    b. Radioiodine uptake ↑ in Grave's, Plummer's, toxic adenoma
    c. Radioiodine uptake ↓ in subacute thyroiditis, exogenous hormone, struma ovarii
11. Treat hyperthyroidism medically or surgically
    a. Medicine = propylthiouracil or methimazole, both of which block thyroid production of hormone
    b. Drug therapy induces remission in 1mo to 2yr (up to 50% of time), so life-long therapy is not necessary
    c. Radioiodine is first line for Grave's: radioactive iodine is concentrated in the gland & destroys it, resolving the diffuse hyperthyroid state
    d. If the above fail → surgical excision (of adenoma or entire gland)
12. Thyroid storm is the most extreme manifestation of hyperthyroidism
    a. Not a separate disease entity in & of itself
    b. Due to exacerbation of hyperthyroidism of above causes
    c. Precipitated by surgery, infection, & anesthesia
    d. Causes high fever, dehydration, cardiac arrhythmias, high output cardiac failure, coma & 25% mortality rate

e. Tx
    (1) β-blockers and IV fluids are first priority to restore hemodynamic stability
    (2) Give propylthiouracil (PTU) to inhibit iodination of more thyroid hormone
    (3) After PTU on board, give iodine-containing product which will feedback inhibit further thyroid hormone release—make sure the PTU is on board first, or the iodine can cause an initial INCREASE in hormone release before it feed back suppresses release

E. Hypothyroid
1. General
    a. Causes include Hashimoto's, subacute thyroiditis, Riedel's thyroiditis, silent thyroiditis
    b. Si/Sx = **cold intolerance**, weight gain, **low energy**, husky voice, mental slowness, constipation, thick/coarse hair, puffiness of face/eyelids/hands (**myxedema**), prolonged relaxation phase of deep tendon reflexes
    c. Myxedema due to accumulation of hyaluronic acid (hydrophilic) glycosaminoglycan & water in every organ
2. Hashimoto's disease
    a. Autoimmune lymphocytic infiltration of the thyroid gland
    b. 8:1 ratio in women to men, usually between ages of 30 and 50
    c. Other autoimmune diseases often accompany (systemic lupus erythematosus, rheumatoid arthritis, Sjögren's, etc.: **Schmidt's syndrome** = Hashimoto's + endocrine disorders such as diabetes or Addison's disease)
    d. Dx by hypothyroid Sx/Si & labs, also look for antimicrosomal (antithyroid peroxidase antibodies) antibodies
    e. Tx by life-long Synthroid
    f. Fine-needle aspirate → lymphoid follicles with germinal centers & **Hurthle** cells (follicular epithelial cells with basophilic cytoplasmic inclusions)
    g. Minority of glands → fibrous with parenchymal obliteration
3. Subacute thyroiditis
    a. Seen following flu-like illness with sore throat & fevers
    b. Pain often exists in jaw/teeth, can be confused with dental disease, aggravated by swallowing or turning head
    c. Early inflammation leads to spillage of T_4, looks like hyperthyroid, only late leads to hypothyroid
    d. Elevated erythrocyte sedimentation rate is characteristic

e. Disease is most often self-limiting & resolves without consequences after weeks to months
f. Usually does not progress to the stage of clinical hypothyroidism
g. Tx with aspirin, only with cortisol in very severe disease

4. Riedel's thyroiditis
   a. A very rare idiopathic disorder where entire thyroid gland is replaced by fibrous tissue
   b. Can be confused with malignancy
5. Myxedema coma
   a. **The only emergency hypothyroid condition**
   b. Spontaneous or precipitated by cold exposure, infection, analgesia, sedative drug use, respiratory failure, or other severe illness
   c. Si/Sx = overt hypothyroidism, stupor, coma, convulsive seizures, hypotension, hypoventilation
6. Neonatal hypothyroidism = cretinism
   a. Presents with respiratory difficulties, cyanosis, persistent jaundice, poor feeding, hoarse crying, macroglossia, & mental retardation
   b. Tx = lifetime thyroxine

F. Malignancy
1. Terms *hot* & *cold* used to describe nodules, refer to whether or not the nodules take up iodine (i.e., are they functionally active or not)
2. Hot nodules are rarely cancerous, usually seen in elderly, soft to palpation, ultrasound (Utz) shows cystic mass, thyroid scan shows autonomously functioning nodule
3. Cold nodule
   a. Has a greater potential of being cancerous
   b. Usually seen in young adult males & in children
   c. Nodule is firm to palpation, often accompanied by vocal cord paralysis, Utz shows solid mass
4. Papillary CA
   a. **The most common cancer of thyroid**
   b. Good prognosis (Px), 85% 5-yr survival, spread is indolent, via lymph nodes
   c. Pathologically distinguished by **ground glass Orphan Annie nucleus & psammoma bodies** (other psammoma body dz = serous papillary cystadenocarcinoma of ovary, mesothelioma, meningioma)

5. Medullary CA
    a. Has intermediate prognosis
    b. Cancer of parafollicular "C" cells that are derived from the ultimobranchial bodies (cells of branchial pouch 5)
    c. Secretes calcitonin, can Dx & follow dz with this blood assay
6. Follicular CA
    a. Poor Px, commonly blood-borne metastases to bone & lungs
7. Anaplastic CA
    a. Has one of the poorest Px of any cancer (0% survival at 5yr)

VI. Growth Hormone Axis

A. Physiology
1. GH ⇒ liver, ↑ insulin growth factor (IGF) production, IGF feedback inhibits GH secretion from pituitary
2. Somatotropin secreted by hypothalamus stimulates GH
3. IGF binding proteins are GH dependent, increased in acromegaly, decreased in hypopituitary

B. Axis testing
1. Give insulin to cause hypoglycemia, should → ↑ GH (arginine infusion does the same)
2. L-dopa & clonidine ⇒ ↑ GH, much safer test, use it in elderly
3. GHRH ⇒ ↑ GH
    a. If not, Dx = 1° pituitary disease
    b. If GHRH corrects deficiency, Dx = hypothalamic dysfunction
    c. Obesity & type II diabetes will diminish this response
4. Give glucose (OGTT), should see drop in GH, if not Dx = acromegaly that shows either no change in GH or even paradoxical increase
5. Check IGF levels, if ↑↑ → Dx of acromegaly, note that low levels are not diagnostic, because of overlap with normal population

C. Acromegaly
1. Almost always due to pituitary adenoma secreting ↑ GH
2. If secretion begins in childhood, prior to skeletal epiphyseal closure, leads to gigantism
3. If secretion begins after epiphyseal closure, leads to acromegaly
    a. Classic presentation is an adult whose glove, ring, or shoe size acutely changes

   b. Other Si/Sx = coarsening of skin/facial features, prognathism, voice deepening, joint erosions
   c. Often see peripheral neuropathies due to nerve compression, headaches & bitemporal hemianopsia due to pituitary enlargement
4. Dx is by clinical findings as well as serum GH or IGF levels/testing as described above
5. Tx = surgery or radiation to ablate the enlarged pituitary

VII. Calcium Disorders

A. Calcium physiology
   1. 3 calcium fractions are 1) ionized, 2) protein bound, 3) phosphate & citrate complexed
      a. Ionized & complexed calcium is filtered (60%), protein bound is not
      b. Of the protein-bound fraction, albumin binds 90%
      c. Acidosis → ↓ binding, alkalosis → ↑ binding: HCO_3^- Tx for acidosis can cause tetany due to ↓ free serum Ca
   2. Phosphate has the same 3 fractions, but less is protein bound so 90% is filtered
   3. **The renal tubule is THE dominant factor in calcium homeostasis, bone resorption is second**
B. Hormone regulation
   1. ↓ Calcium ⇒ secretion of parathyroid hormone (PTH) from chief cells of parathyroid gland (see Figure 9.9)
   2. PTH ⇒ ↑ renal resorption of Ca, ↓ resorption of phosphate, ↑ 1-α-hydroxylase (1α-OH-lase) in kidney ⇒ ↑ 1,25-OH-vitD ⇒ ↑ Ca & phosphate absorption in intestine: PTH also inhibits 24α-OH-lase
   3. PTHrp acts similarly, can be ectopically produced in lung, breast, renal, islet cell, pheochromocytoma & T-cell cancers
   4. Most hormones/cytokines act directly on osteoclasts, indirectly on osteoblasts via osteoclasts
   5. IL-1 & IL-6 stimulate osteoclast activity & differentiation
   6. Vitamin D deficiency in children causes rickets, in adults osteomalacia
   7. Calcitonin is secreted by the parafollicular cells of the thyroid, major action is to inhibit bone resorption when serum calcium levels are normal

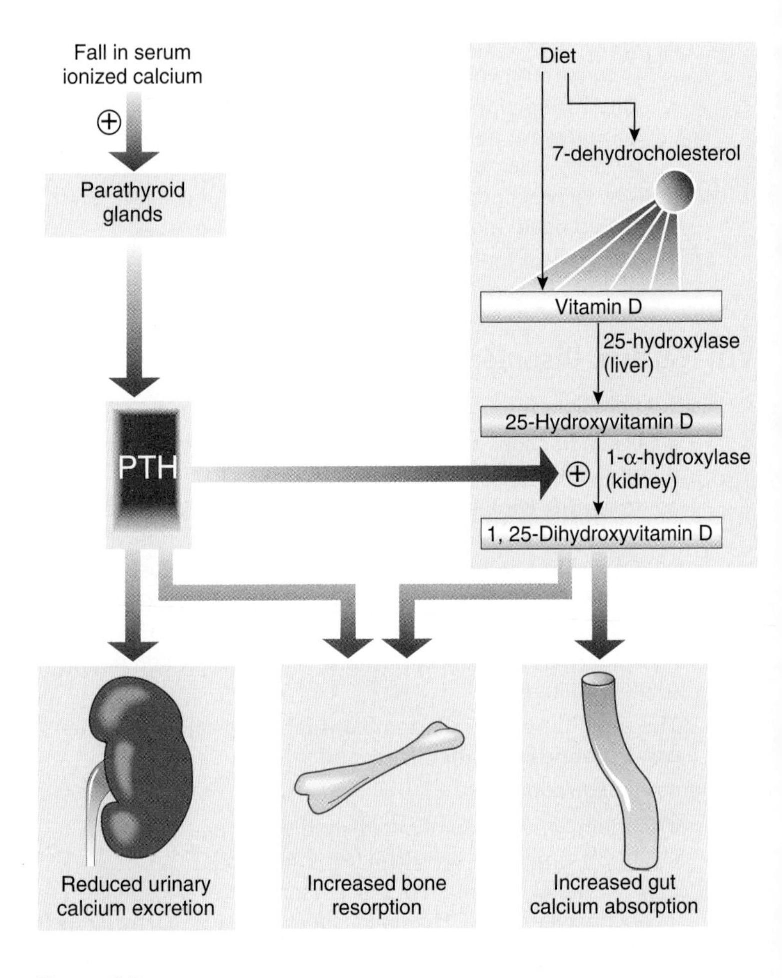

Figure 9.9
Calcium metabolism (From Axford JS. Callaghan CA. Medicine. 2nd ed. Oxford: Blackwell Science, 2004.)

C. Hypercalcemia

1. Sx = altered mentation, constipation, anorexia, nausea/vomit, polyuria/polydipsia, nephrolithiasis, bradycardia, 1° AV block (do NOT give digitalis to such patients!)
2. Major causes of hypercalcemia are hyperparathyroidism & cancer

3. 1° hyperparathyroidism patients have mild/no Sx, PTH levels ↑↑, Ca usually ≤ 12
4. Cancer patients have bad Sx, PTH minimal, Ca usually ≥12
5. If PTH levels are elevated in malignancy, there are 3 possible causes
   a. Concomitant 1° hyperparathyroidism
   b. Tumor makes PTH
   c. Tumor makes PTHrp (cross-reacts with test)
6. Other causes (make up less than 10% of all cases)
   a. Thyrotoxicosis, sarcoidosis, renal failure, drugs (vitamin D, thiazide, lithium, estrogens & antiestrogens, androgens for breast cancer Tx, aminophylline, vitamin A, aluminum toxicity)
   b. Rare: pheochromocytoma, VIP-producing tumor, familial hypocalciuric hypercalcemia, other granulomatous diseases, milk-alkali syndrome, hypophosphatemia, MEN I/II
   c. Milk-alkali = excessive Ca antacid intake, often 2° to self-medication of heartburn or ulcer, Dx by Hx and combination of hypercalcemia + metabolic alkalosis, & often azotemia–cessation of Ca intake reverses
   d. Familial hypocalciuric hypercalcemia = early onset age, frequently hypermagnesemia, autosomal dominant with 100% penetrance, ↑ PTH, hypocalciuria, often aSx
   e. Granulomatous disease causes it by increased 1-α-OHase production by granuloma monocytes, leading to increased 1,25-OH-vit D production
7. Tx
   a. **First hydrate to euvolemia, THEN give loop diuretic then give bisphosphonate**
   b. Bisphosphonate most useful for malignancy-associated hypercalcemia, and is the most effective agent to reduce calcium levels, but it takes 48 to 72 hours to work
   c. Calcitonin can also be given, which has rapid onset (within hours), but is not very effective

D. Hypocalcemia
   1. Causes are 1) hypoparathyroidism, 2) renal failure, 3) vitamin D deficiency, 4) hypomagnesemia
   2. Hypoparathyroid: most common cause is idiopathic autoimmune, can also be congenital parathyroid aplasia (DiGeorge's syndrome), Wilson's disease & hemochromatosis due to gland infiltration, granulomatous dz/infection & thyroidectomy

3. Hypomagnesemia is VERY common cause of hypocalcemia—causes hypocalcemia by 1) inhibiting PTH release & target action, 2) 1-α-OH-lase is Mg dependent
4. Sx = peripheral paresthesias, muscle cramp, seizure, altered mentation, ↑ QT interval
5. **Look for Chvostek's sign** (tap facial nerve anterior to ear causes facial muscle twitch) & **Trousseau's sign** (inflate BP cuff above systolic BP for 3 minutes causes carpal spasm)
6. Tx = calcium supplements with Mg if appropriate

E. Osteoporosis [see Musculoskeletal, Section I.A]

VIII. The Multiple Endocrine Neoplasia Syndromes

A. MEN Type I (Wermer's Syndrome)
1. Hyperplasia or tumors of parathyroid, adrenal cortex, pancreas & pituitary
2. **The 3(4) Ps: P**ituitary (**P**rolactinoma most common), **P**arathyroid, **P**ancreatoma (most often gastrinoma causing Zollinger-Ellison syndrome)

B. MEN Type IIa (Sipple's Syndrome)
1. Pheochromocytoma, medullary CA of the thyroid, hyperparathyroidism due to hyperplasia or tumor
2. This is the only type with both thyroid CA & parathyroid tumor
3. Associated with mutation of the *ret* oncogene

C. MEN Type IIb ("MEN Type III")
1. Pheochromocytoma, medullary CA & multiple mucocutaneous neuromas, particularly of the GI tract
2. Only type that does not include hyperparathyroidism
3. Like MEN IIa, associated with mutation of *ret* oncogene (interesting note: Hirschsprung's disease is a congenital colonic atresia 2° to failure of myenteric plexus neuronal development & is associated with loss of function mutations in the *ret* oncogene, see Gastroenterology and Liver, Section IV.A)

IX. Paraneoplastic Syndromes

A. ACTH
1. Ectopic vs. Cushing's, ectopic ACTH secretion will not suppress cortisol secretion when excess dexamethasone is administered

2. Bronchial carcinoid tumors or thymomas that contain CRH-like material will suppress their ACTH at high doses of dexamethasone

B. Vasopressin (ADH)
   1. Lung cancer (most often oat cell) or any thoracic lesion that affects the right atrial baroreceptors can lead to SIADH
   2. SIADH causes hyponatremia, renal sodium loss, hypervolemia, high urine osmolality

C. Human chorionic gonadotropin (HCG)
   1. Seen in malignant melanoma, adrenocortical CA, breast, renal, lung, gastric & colon cancer

D. Calcitonin
   1. Seen in lung cancer, colon cancer, breast, pancreas, gastric cancer & medullary thyroid cancer

E. Erythropoietin
   1. Seen in hepatocellular CA, causes polycythemia

F. Growth hormone
   1. Seen in bronchial carcinoid tumor & pancreatic tumor
   2. Causes acromegaly

G. Hypoglycemia
   1. Seen in mesenchymal tumors including fibrosarcoma, neurofibroma, spindle cell CA, insulinoma, leiomyosarcoma, hepatic CA, leukemia

H. Hypercalcemia
   1. Most common cause of symptomatic hypercalcemia is malignancy, seen in lung cancers most often
   2. 5 mechanisms
      a. PTH-related peptide (PTHrp)
      b. Cytokines that mobilize calcium (TNF-α/β, prostaglandins)
      c. Solid tumors may rarely secrete PTH
      d. Metastatic bone disease directly stimulates bone resorption
      e. Production of vitamin D seen in T-cell lymphoma, also seen in leiomyoblastoma, Hodgkin's disease & plasma cell tumor

10. MUSCULOSKELETAL

I. Metabolic Bone Diseases

A. Osteoporosis
   1. ↓ synthesis or ↑ resorption of bony matrix protein
   2. Associated with postmenopausal (↓ estrogen), physical inactivity, ↑ cortisol, hyperthyroid, Ca^{2+} deficiency
   3. Results in fractures (particularly hip & vertebrae leading to kyphosis), but not delayed fracture healing, so patients should be encouraged to resume activity as soon as possible
   4. Estrogen halts bone loss, but also can help add bone density
   5. Calcitonin also halts the process but does not reverse it—calcitonin also relieves bone pain, but its effects wear off after chronic use
   6. Bisphosphonates (pamidronate & alendronate) act as pyrophosphate analogues, stabilizing & ↑ bone density
   7. Ca supplements ↓ rate of bone loss, every osteoporosis patient should take Ca if their dietary intake is not = 1–1.5 g/day

B. von Recklinghausen's disease (Osteitis Fibrosa Cystica)
   1. Diffuse osteolytic lesions caused by hyperparathyroidism
   2. Characteristic "**brown tumor**" of bone, osteolytic cysts turn brown due to hemorrhage (see Figures 10.1 and 10.2)
   3. Can mimic osteoporosis on x-rays

C. Osteomalacia
   1. Defective calcification of osteoid matrix due to vitamin D deficiency in **adults**
   2. Again, x-rays show diffuse radiolucency, mimicking osteoporosis
   3. Called "renal osteodystrophy" if secondary to renal disease

D. Rickets
   1. Vitamin D deficiency in **children**, causing ↑ epiphyseal plate thickening
   2. Multiple skeletal defects & short stature
      a. **Craniotabes** (thinning of occipital & parietal bones)
      b. **Rachitic rosary** (costochondral thickening looks like string of beads)
      c. **Harrison's groove** (depression along line of diaphragmatic insertion into rib cage)
      d. **Pigeon breast** = pectus carinatum (sternum protrusion)

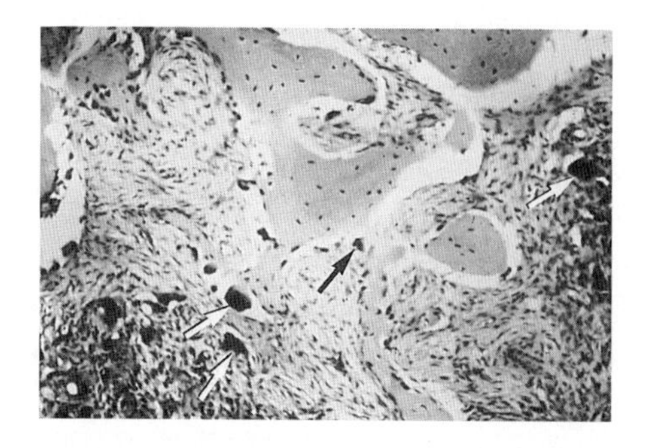

Figure 10.1 Iliac Crest Bone Biopsy of a Patient with Osteitis Fibrosa Cystica
This shows replacement of trabecular bone tissue by fibrous tissue and osteoclasts (arrow). (From Axford JS. Medicine. Oxford: Blackwell Science, 1998.)

E. Scurvy
1. Vitamin C deficiency causes impaired osteoid matrix formation (can't hydroxylate lysine/proline)
2. See subperiosteal hemorrhage (painful), **bleeding gums**, multiple ecchymoses, osteoporosis, & **"woody leg" from hemorrhage into soft tissues**

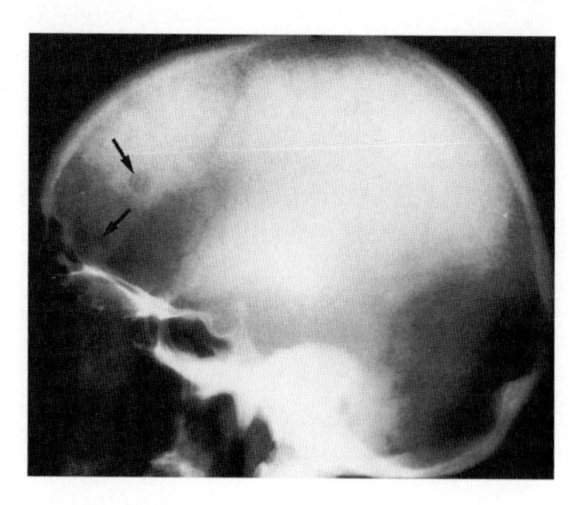

Figure 10.2 Skull Radiograph of a Patient with Primary Hyperparathyroidism
This shows mottling of the skull vault ("salt and pepper" appearance) and larger lytic lesions called "brown tumors" (arrows). (From Axford JS. Medicine. Oxford: Blackwell Science, 1998.)

F. Paget's bone disease (Osteitis Deformans)
   1. Bone disease (dz) due to ↑ activity of both osteoblasts & osteoclasts
   2. Most common in elderly, may be of viral etiology (osteoclastic inclusions)
   3. Most commonly involves spine, pelvis, skull, femur, tibia
   4. Can involve only one bone or many (monostotic vs. polystotic)
   5. 3 morphologic phases: a) osteolytic phase, b) mixed phase, c) late phase
      a. Osteolytic phase → osteoclast activity dominates over osteoblast
      b. Mixed phase → balance, see characteristic **mosaic** pattern of bone
      c. Late phase → ↑ bone density with prominent mosaic pattern (see Figure 10.3)
   6. Complications: fractures/pain (see Figure 10.4), ↑ output cardiac failure (lesions highly vascular), ↓ hearing, osteosarcoma (1% of cases)

G. Differential of metabolic bone disease—see Table 10.1

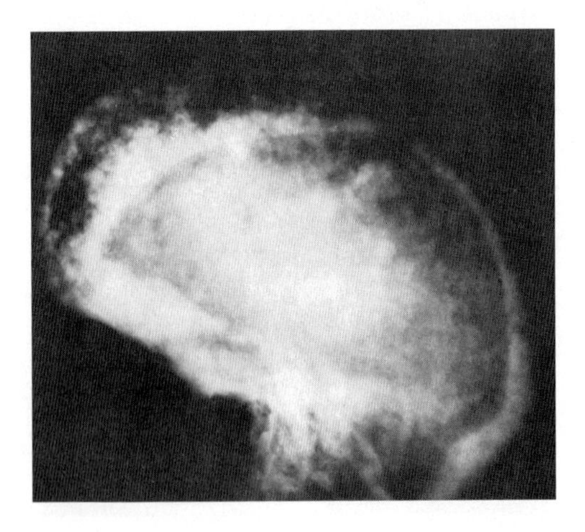

Figure 10.3
Thickening of the cavarum of the skull in Paget's disease. (From Duckworth T. Lecture Notes on Orthopaedics & Fractures. 3rd ed. Oxford: Blackwell Science, 1995.)

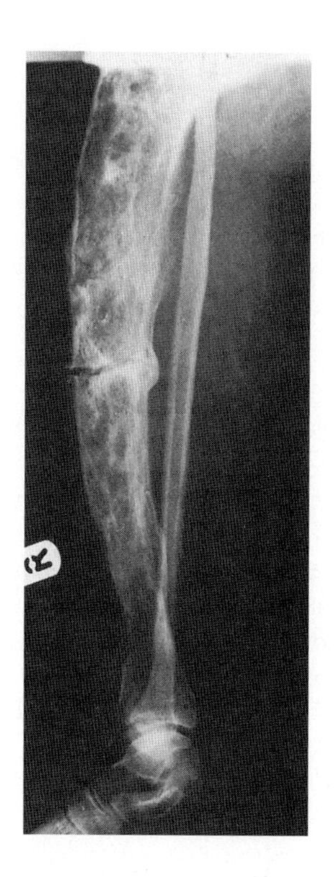

Figure 10.4
Paget's disease showing deformity of the tibia and pseudo-fractures. (From Duckworth T. Lecture Notes on Orthopaedics & Fractures. 3rd ed. Oxford: Blackwell Science, 1995.)

Table 10.1 Differential Diagnosis of Metabolic Bone Disease

Disease	Serum Calcium	Urinary Calcium	Alk. Phosphatase
Osteoporosis/Scurvy	N	N	N
von Recklinghausen's	↑	↑	↑
Osteomalacia/Rickets	↓/N	↓	↑/N
Paget's	N	↓	↑↑↑↑

II. Nonneoplastic Bone Diseases

A. Achondroplasia
   1. Very common cause of dwarfism, autosomal dominant
   2. Early sealing off between epiphysis & metaphysis, causes shortening/thickening of bones
   3. Symptoms (Sx) = leg bowing, hearing loss, sciatica, infantile hydrocephalus
   4. Patients can live normal lifespans

B. Fibrous Dysplasia
   1. Idiopathic replacement of bone with fibrous tissue, 3 types: a) monostotic, b) polystotic, c) McCune-Albright's
      a. Monostotic patients (pts) are often asymptomatic (aSx), but can suffer spontaneous fractures
      b. Polystotic are associated with severe skeletal deformity
      c. McCune-Albright's syndrome
         (1) Caused by G-protein abnormality resulting in hyperparathyroidism, hyperadrenalism, & acromegaly
         (2) **Triad = polystotic fibrous dysplasia, precocious puberty, café-au-lait spots**

C. Aseptic avascular necrosis
   1. Bone infarction usually due to idiopathic disruption of arterial blood supply
   2. Can be secondary (2°) to trauma, embolism, the bends, sickle cell anemia, steroid use
   3. Different name depending upon site of affect
      a. Legg-Calve-Perthe = head of femur
      b. Osgood-Schlatter disease = tibial tubercle
      c. Köhler's bone disease = the navicular bone

D. Osteogenesis imperfecta
   1. Congenital disorder causing diffuse bone weakness
   2. Due to gene mutations resulting in defective collagen synthesis
   3. Multiple fractures secondary to minimal trauma = brittle bone disease
   4. **Classic sign = blue sclera**, due to translucent connective tissue over choroid
   5. Variable expressivity/severity depending upon mutations

E. Osteopetrosis (Marble Bone or Albers-Schönberg disease)
   1. Markedly increased skeletal density due to osteoclastic failure

2. In spite of increased bone density, leads to multiple fractures due to diminished perfusion of thickened bone
3. Also causes anemia due to decreased marrow space, & blindness/deafness/cranial nerve dysfunction due to narrowing & impingement of neural foramina
4. Autosomal recessive variant is fatal in infancy, also there is a less severe dominant variant

F. Pyogenic osteomyelitis
1. In children is usually 2° to hematogenous spread from elsewhere
2. *Staphylococcus aureus* most common, also *Streptococcus agalactiae* (group B Strep), or *Escherichia coli* in newborns
3. **Sickle cell anemics frequently infected by *Salmonella***
4. In adults occurs after compound fracture or surgery
5. In IV drug users it will frequently be caused by *Pseudomonas*
6. Usually involves the bone metaphysis, often distal head of femur, proximal of tibia, proximal of humerus
7. Can cause ischemic necrosis due to compression of vasculature
8. Necrotic bone (**sequestrum**) acts as a foreign body & nidus for persistent infection
9. **Involucrum** is a sleeve of new bone surrounding the necrotic area
10. **Brodie's abscess** = wall of granulation tissue surrounding the involucrum
11. May be complicated by 2° or reactive amyloidosis
12. **X-ray → periosteal elevation, can lag onset of dz by weeks**

G. Histiocytosis X
1. Occurs in bone, in addition to multiple sites throughout the body
2. Proliferation of histiocytic cells resembling Langerhans skin cells
3. **Birbeck granules are pathognomonic** = tennis-racket-shaped cytoplasmic structures, seen on electron microscopy
4. 3 common variants
   a. Letterer-Siwe disease
      (1) Acute, aggressive, disseminated variant, usually fatal in infants & small children
      (2) Signs/symptoms (Si/Sx) = hepatosplenomegaly, lymphadenopathy, pancytopenia, lung involvement, recurrent infections

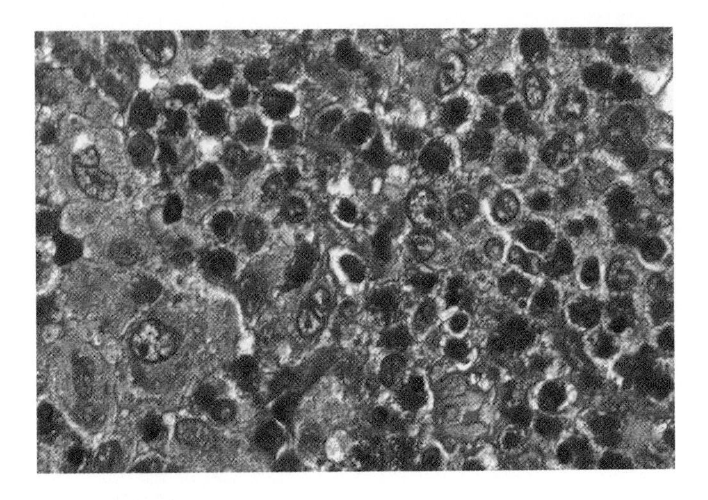

Figure 10.5 Eosinophilic Granuloma
A photomicrograph shows large, plump histiocytes (Langerhans cells) with vesicular, occasionally grooved nuclei and eosinophils. (From Rubin E, Gorstein F, Rubin R, et al. Rubin's Pathology: Clinicopathologic Foundations of Medicine. 4th ed. Baltimore: Lippincott Williams & Wilkins, 2005.)

b. Hand-Schüller-Christian disease
   (1) Chronic progressive variant, presents prior to 5 years old
   (2) Histiocytic infiltration of bone (skull), liver, spleen, etc.
   (3) **Classic triad = skull lesions, diabetes insipidus, exophthalmos**
c. Eosinophilic granuloma (see Figure 10.5)
   (1) This variant has the best prognosis (Px), rarely fatal, sometimes spontaneously regresses
   (2) Extraskeletal involvement generally limited to lung
   (3) See ordinary inflammatory cells, particularly eosinophils, mixed with histiocytes

III. Bone Tumors

A. Benign
   1. Osteochondroma is the most common benign bone tumor, usually in men younger than 25
      a. Growth covered by cartilage cap, may be hamartoma
      b. Usually originates from long bone metaphysis, particularly common are lower end of femur & upper end of tibia
      c. Rarely may transform to chondrosarcoma

2. Giant cell tumors also common, peaks in either sex aged 20–40
   a. Histologic appearance: → spindle shaped cells mixed with numerous multinucleated giant cells
   b. Usually at epiphyseal end of long bones, more than 50% in knee
   c. Classic **soap bubble** appearance on x-ray
   d. Benign but locally aggressive, often recurs after surgical removal

B. Malignant tumors
1. Osteosarcoma (osteogenic sarcoma) is the most common primary malignant bone tumor
   a. Peaks in men aged 10–20, usually in metaphysis of long bones, often distal femur & proximal tibia
   b. Causes pain, swelling, fractures, 2- to 3-fold increase in serum alkaline phosphatase
   c. **Codman's triangle,** lifting of periosteum by expanding tumor, and "sunburst pattern" are characteristic x-ray findings
   d. Paget's bone disease, radiation, bone infarcts, retinoblastoma predispose to osteosarcoma
2. Chondrosarcoma = malignant cartilaginous tumor, peaks in men aged 30–60
3. Ewing's sarcoma = extremely anaplastic small cell tumor resembling malignant lymphoma ("onion skinning" is classic x-ray finding)
   a. Peaks in young boys under 15, metastasizes VERY early, responds well to chemotherapy
   b. May mimic acute osteomyelitis
   c. 11:22 translocation like neuroectodermal tumors (neural crest tumors) & is probably related
4. Multiple myeloma (see Figures 10.6 and 10.7)
   a. Malignant clonal neoplasm of plasma cells producing whole antibodies (Abs) (e.g., IgM, IgG, etc.), light chain Abs, or no Abs (just ↑ B cells)
   b. Usually patients (pts) >40 years old, African Americans have 2:1 incidence compared to whites
   c. **Pt presents with bone pain worse with movement, affecting back & ribs**
   d. Other Si/Sx = **lytic bone lesions visible on x-ray**, pathologic fractures, **hypercalcemia**, renal failure, anemia, frequent infections by encapsulated bacteria, ↓ **anion gap**

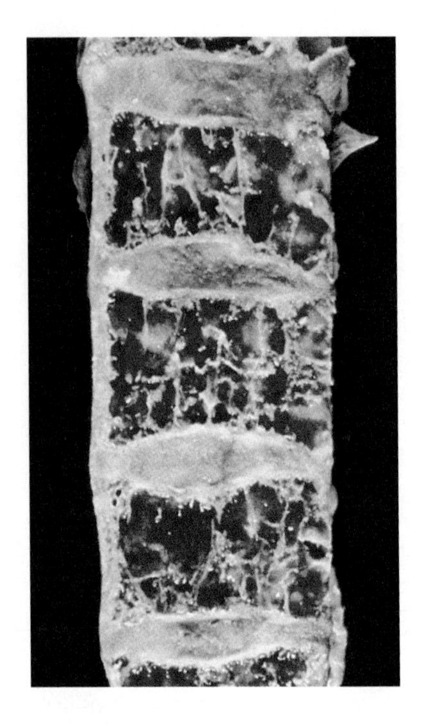

Figure 10.6 Multiple Myeloma
Multiple lytic bone lesions are present in the vertebra. (From Rubin E, Gorstein F, Rubin R, et al. Rubin's Pathology: Clinicopathologic Foundations of Medicine. 4th ed. Baltimore: Lippincott Williams & Wilkins, 2005.)

(Abs positively charged, unseen cations cause ↑ anions making anion gap appear ↓)

e. **Hyperviscosity syndrome**
   (1) Due to sludging secondary (2°) to ↑ serum Ab concentration
   (2) Si/Sx = vascular occlusion, stroke/central nervous system (CNS) dysfunction, retinopathy, congestive heart failure (CHF), coagulopathy, **erythrocyte sedimentation rate (ESR) > 100**

f. **Bence-Jones proteinuria**
   (1) Classic finding of antibody light chains in the urine
   (2) **Urine dipsticks do NOT detect light chains,** can use sulfosalicylic acid test in lieu of dipstick to screen

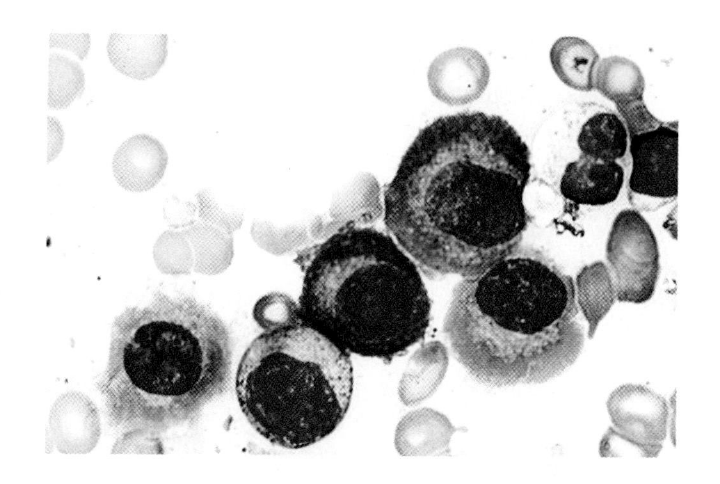

Figure 10.7 Multiple Myeloma
A smear of a bone marrow aspirate shows a cluster of three neoplastic plasma cells. (From Rubin E, Gorstein F, Rubin R, et al. Rubin's Pathology: Clinicopathologic Foundations of Medicine. 4th ed. Baltimore: Lippincott Williams & Wilkins, 2005.)

(3) Diagnosis (Dx) = 24-hr urine collection → protein electrophoresis
(4) Light chain deposition causes renal amyloidosis

g. Dx
  (1) Serum/urine protein electrophoresis (SPEP/UPEP)
    (a) Both → tall electrophoretic peak called "M-spike" due to ↑ Ab compared to normals
    (b) SPEP → M-spike if clones make whole Ab
    (c) UPEP → spike if clones make light chains only
    (d) **Either SPEP or UPEP will almost always be ⊕**
  (2) Dx made with ⊕ SPEP/UPEP & any of ↑ plasma cells in bone marrow, ⊕ osteolytic bone lesions, ⊕ Bence-Jones proteinuria

h. Treatment (Tx)
  (1) Radiation given for isolated lesions
  (2) Chemo added for metastatic disease
  (3) Palliative care important for pain
  (4) Px relatively poor despite Tx

IV. Arthropathy/Connective Tissue Disorders

A. Rheumatoid arthritis (RA)

1. An autoimmune disorder of unknown etiology → **symmetric inflammatory arthritis**
2. Female-male = 3:1, patients are commonly **HLA-DR4⊕**
3. Knees, feet, metacarpophalangeal (**MCP**) & proximal interphalangeal (**PIP**) joints are commonly affected
4. Pathology
    a. Dysregulated inflammation → leukocyte infiltration into joint
    b. Subsequently synovium hypertrophies into the joint, causing erosion of the joint cartilage & bone
5. Si/Sx = symmetric arthritis worse in morning, arthralgia, fevers, weight loss, pleural effusions (serositis), anemia of chronic dz, Baker's cyst in popliteal fossa (mimics deep vein thrombosis)
6. Joints develop flexion contractures & become deformed (ulnar deviation of digits)
7. Subcutaneous nodules are characteristic of RA, but are present in <50% of patients
8. Rheumatoid factor (RF)
    a. RF = IgM anti-IgG
    b. Present in >70% of RA patients, may take months to years of disease before it appears
    c. Is not specific for RA, can be positive in almost any chronic inflammatory state & may be present in 5–10% of healthy geriatric patients
9. ESR is elevated in >90% cases, but is not specific for RA
10. Dx is clinical, no single factor is sufficient
11. Felty's syndrome = splenomegaly + neutropenia, often with thrombocytopenia, develops in 2% of RA patients
12. Tx = NSAIDs for the vast majority of patients
13. Refractory patients take gold salts, penicillamine, chloroquine, all of which are associated with severe side effects, including glomerulonephritis & renal failure
14. TNF antagonists markedly improve symptoms, even in patients refractory to standard therapy

B. Systemic lupus erythematosus

1. Systemic autoimmune disorder, female-male = 9:1
2. Si/Sx include fever, polyarthritis, skin lesions, hemolytic anemia, thrombocytopenia, splenomegaly, pleural effusions,

pericarditis (serositis), Libman-Sacks endocarditis, nephrosis or nephritis, thrombosis & a variety of neurologic disorders

3. Labs
   a. **Antinuclear antibody (ANA) sensitive (>98%) but not specific**
   b. **Anti-double-stranded-DNA (anti-ds-DNA) antibodies are 99% specific but less sensitive**
   c. Anti-Smith (anti-Sm) antibodies are highly specific but not sensitive
   d. Anti-Ro antibodies are ⊕ in 50% of ANA-negative lupus, so they are good fail-safe if clinical suspicion of lupus is high, but ANA is negative
   e. Antiribosomal P & antineuronal antibodies correlate with risk for cerebral involvement of lupus (lupus cerebritis)
   f. Antiphospholipid autoantibodies cause false-positive laboratory test results in SLE
      (1) **SLE patients frequently have false ⊕ RPR/VDRL tests for syphilis due to anticardiolipin antibodies**
      (2) **SLE patients frequently have elevated partial thromboplastin time (PTT) (lupus anticoagulant antibody)**
         (a) PTT is falsely ↑ because the lupus anticoagulant antibody binds to phospholipid, which initiates clotting in the test tube
         (b) **Despite the PTT test & the name *lupus anticoagulant antibody*, SLE patients are THROMBOGENIC, because antiphospholipid antibodies cause coagulation in vivo**
4. **Mnemonic for SLE diagnosis:** DOPAMINE RASH
   a. **D**iscoid lupus = characteristic circular, erythematous macules with scales, postinflammatory central depigmentation
   b. **O**ral aphthous ulcers (can be nasopharyngeal as well)
   c. **P**hotosensitivity
   d. **A**rthritis (typically hands, wrists, knees)
   e. **M**alar rash = classic butterfly macule on cheeks
   f. **I**mmunologic criteria = anti-ds-DNA, anti-Sm Ab, anti-Ro Ab, anti-La Ab (⊕ ANA is a separate criteria)
   g. **N**eurologic changes = psychosis, personality change, seizures
   h. **E**SR rate is almost always elevated (**Note:** this is not 1 of the 11 diagnostic criteria, but it is a frequent laboratory finding)

i. **R**enal disease → nephritic or nephrotic syndrome
j. ANA⊕
k. **S**erositis (pleurisy, pericarditis)
l. **H**ematologic dz = hemolytic anemia, thrombocytopenia, leukopenia

5. Drug-induced SLE
   a. Drugs = procainamide, hydralazine, sulfonamides, INH, cephalosporin
   b. **Lab → antihistone antibodies**, differentiating from idiopathic SLE
   c. Resolves upon cessation of offending drug
6. Tx = NSAIDs, prednisone, cyclophosphamide depending on severity of dz
7. Px = variable & difficult to predict over long term, but 10-yr survival is excellent, **renal dz is a poor Px indicator**

C. Sjögren's syndrome (SS)
1. An autoinflammatory disorder associated with **HLA-DR3**
2. Classic triad of Sjögren's
   a. **Keratoconjunctivitis sicca** = dry eyes (see Head and Neck, Section III.C.2.b)
   b. **Xerostomia** = lack of salivary secretions, often due to parotitis
   c. **Inflammatory arthritis**, usually less severe than pure RA
   d. Concomitant presence of 2 of the triad is diagnostic
3. Some variants affect only the eyes or mouth (primary [1°] SS)
4. Associated systemic Sx = pancreatitis, fibrinous pericarditis, cranial nerve (CN) V sensory neuropathy, renal tubular acidosis, 40-fold ↑ in lymphoma incidence
5. Lab → ANA⊕, anti-Ro/anti-La Ab⊕ ("SSA/SSB Abs"), 70% are RF⊕, 70% have ↑ ESR, anemia/leukopenia
6. Tx = steroids, cyclophosphamide for refractory disease

D. Behçet's syndrome
1. Multisystem inflammatory disorder that chronically recurs
2. Classically presents with painful oral & genital ulcers
3. Also can see arthritis, vasculitis & severe neurologic lesions
4. Tx = prednisone during flare-ups

E. Seronegative spondyloarthropathy
1. Osteoarthritis
   a. **Arthritis** caused by joint wear & tear

b. The most common arthritis, results in wearing away of joint cartilage causing ↑ joint friction & subsequent bone damage
c. Si/Sx = pain & crepitation upon joint motion, ↓ range of joint motion, can have radiculopathy due to cord impingement
d. **X-ray → osteophytes (bone spurs) & asymmetric loss of joint space**
e. Physical examination → **Heberden's nodes** (distal interphalangeal [DIP] swelling 2° to osteophytes) & **Bouchard's nodes** (proximal interphalangeal [PIP] swelling 2° to osteophytes)
f. **Note: RA affects metacarpophalangeal & PIP joints, osteoarthritis affects PIP & DIP joints**
g. Tx = nonsteroidal anti-inflammatory drugs (NSAIDs), muscle relaxants, joint replacement (third line)
h. **Isometric exercise to strengthen muscles around joint has been shown to improve Sx**

2. Ankylosing Spondylitis
   a. A rheumatologic condition most commonly found in **HLA-B27⊕** males (male-female = 3:1)
   b. Rheumatoid Sx are often localized to **spine & sacroiliac joint**, leading to complete fusion of adjacent vertebral bodies
   c. **If sacroiliac joint is not affected, it is not ankylosing spondylitis!**
   d. Systemic manifestations include uveitis & **cauda equina syndrome** [see Appendix A, Section I.B.5], upper lobe pulmonary cysts & 1° heart block with aortic insufficiency
   e. Dx = x-ray signs of spinal fusion (classic "**bamboo spine**"), clinical history & negative rheumatoid factor
   f. Tx = NSAIDs & strengthening of back muscles
3. Reiter's syndrome
   a. Also seen more frequently in males, **about 75% of these patients are HLA-B27⊕**
   b. Presents as nongonococcal urethritis (often chlamydial), conjunctivitis, reactive arthritis & uveitis
   c. Classic dermatologic Sx = **circinate balanitis** (serpiginous, moist plaques on glans of penis) & **keratoderma blennorrhagicum** (crusting papules with central erosion, **look like mollusk shell**)
   d. Tx = erythromycin (for *Chlamydia* coverage) + NSAIDs for arthritis

4. Psoriatic arthritis
   a. Presents with **nail-pitting** & **DIP** joint involvement
   b. Occurs in up to 10% of patients with psoriasis
   c. Psoriatic flares may exacerbate arthritis, & vice versa
   d. Tx = ultraviolet light for psoriasis & gold/penicillamine for arthritis
5. Inflammatory bowel disease can cause seronegative arthritis
6. Disseminated gonococcal infection can cause **monoarticular** arthritis

F. Scleroderma (Progressive Systemic Sclerosis = PSS)
1. Systemic fibrosis affecting virtually every organ, female-male = 4:1
2. Can be diffuse disease (PSS) or more benign CREST syndrome
3. **CREST syndrome**
   a. **C**alcinosis = subcutaneous calcifications, often in fingers (see Figure 10.8)
   b. **R**aynaud's phenomenon, often the initial symptom (see Figure 10.9)
      (1) Raynaud's = vasospasm of end-arterioles, frequently affecting digits
      (2) Digits change colors from **white** → **blue** → **red**
         (a) White = pallor due to vasospasm

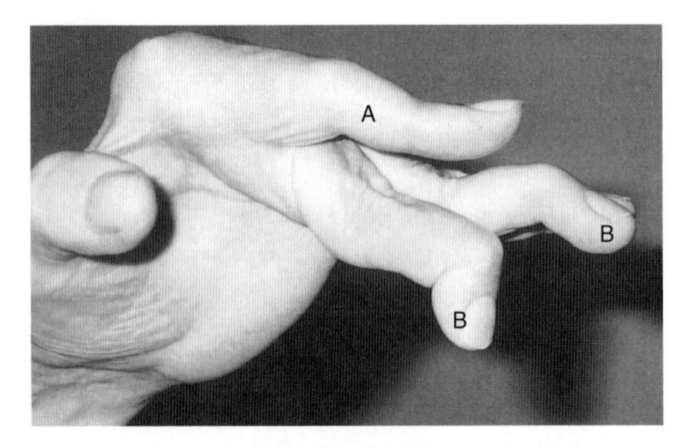

Figure 10.8 Rheumatoid Arthritis
A. Boutonniere and **B.** Swan neck deformities of severe rheumatoid arthritis. (From Berg D. Advanced Clinical Skills and Physical Diagnosis. Oxford: Blackwell Science, 1999.)

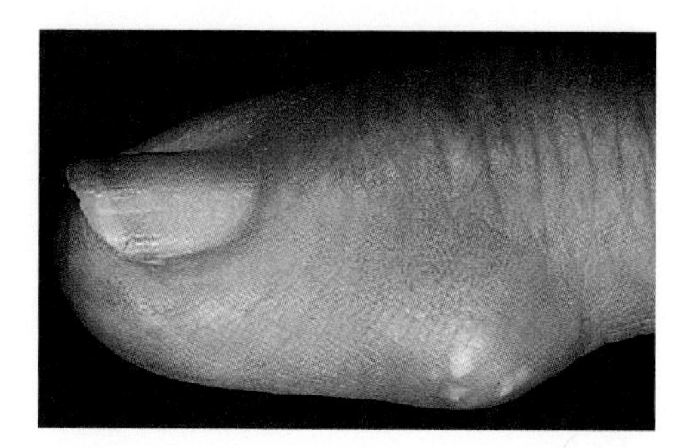

Figure 10.9
Subcutaneous and periarticular calcium deposits may occur and can be extremely painful. (From Axford JS. Callaghan CA. Medicine. 2nd ed. Oxford: Blackwell Science, 2004.)

        (b) Blue = cyanosis due to prolonged vasospasm
        (c) Red = reactive hyperemia when vasospasm ends
    (3) Cold initiates (e.g., waking up in morning) & heat resolves (pts use hair dryers on hands & feet)
   c. **E**sophagitis
    (1) Dysfunctional lower esophageal sphincter causes chronic reflux
    (2) Esophageal strictures develop, Barrett's metaplasia occurs in 1/3 of patients
   d. **S**clerodactyly = fibrosed skin causes immobile digits & rigid facies (in severe cases affects limbs as well) (see Figure 10.10)
   e. **T**elangiectasias occur in mouth, on digits, face & trunk (see Figure 10.11)
4. Systemic Sx = tendonitis, severe flexion contractures, biliary cirrhosis, lung fibrosis causing dyspnea, myocardial fibrosis, renal artery fibrosis causing malignant hypertension
5. Laboratory = ⊕ ANA in 95%, anti-Scl-70 has ↓ sensitivity but ↑ specificity, anticentromere is 80% sensitive for CREST syndrome
6. Tx = immunosuppressives for palliation, none are curative

G. Marfan's disease
1. Defect in the fibrillin gene causes connective tissue abnormality
2. Bones develop into tall, thin body habitus, digits are characteristically long & slender
3. Patients have both pectus excavatum & scoliosis

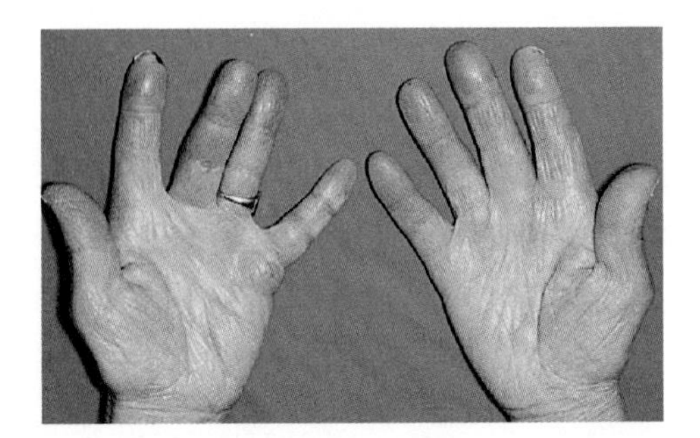

Figure 10.10 Raynaud's Disease
Cyanosis of the fingers due to arterial vasoconstriction, which in this patient has resulted in an area of infarction of the left forefinger. (From Axford JS. Callaghan CA. Medicine. 2nd ed. Oxford: Blackwell Science, 2004.)

4. Cardiac involvement includes progressive aortic valve dilation leading to regurgitation, aortic dissection & mitral valve prolapse
5. **Hallmark is joint laxity, also optic lens dislocations & blue sclera**—lens dislocation upward in Marfan's as opposed to downward in homocystinuria

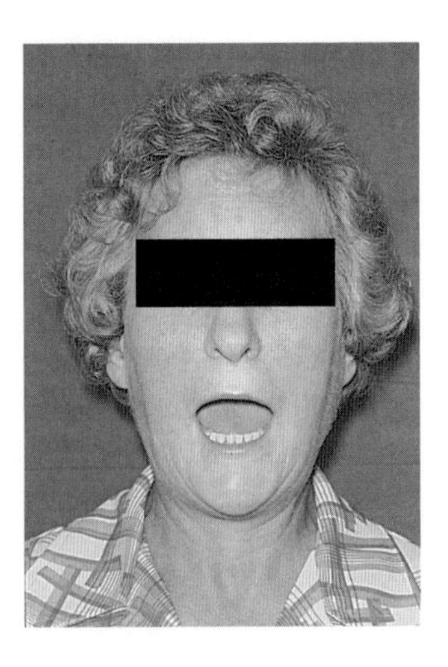

Figure 10.11
Scleroderma may cause thickening of the skin around the mouth and an inability to open the jaw fully. (From Axford JS. Medicine. Oxford: Blackwell Science, 1998.)

H. Ehlers-Danlos syndrome
   1. Autosomal dominant defect in collagen synthesis, variable expressivity
   2. Si/Sx = loose joints & **pathognomonic loss of skin elasticity**
   3. Also look for mitral regurgitation murmur, genu recurvatum of knee (fixed in hyperextension), aortic dilation (↑ risk of rupture)

I. Sarcoidosis
   1. Diffuse, systemic disorder of unknown etiology, which may be infectious or autoimmune in nature
   2. **African Americans are 3x more likely to develop than whites**, peaks in 20s–40s
   3. 50% pts present with incidental finding on CXR in an asymptomatic (aSx) person
   4. Other presentations include fevers, chills, night sweats, weight loss, cough, dyspnea, rash, arthralgia, blurry vision (uveitis)
   5. 90% of patients develop abnormal CXR at some point
   6. **Classic CXR finding is bilateral hilar adenopathy, sarcoidosis should be suspected in ANY patient with this finding on CXR**
   7. Can affect ANY organ system
      a. CNS → CN palsy, classically CN VII (can be bilateral)
      b. **Eye → uveitis (can be bilateral), this classic Sx mandates immediate Ophtho consult & aggressive Tx (see below)**
      c. Cardiac → heart blocks, arrhythmias, constrictive pericarditis
      d. Lung → typically a restrictive defect
      e. GI → ↑ AST/ALT, CT → granulomas in liver, cholestasis
      f. Renal → nephrolithiasis (granulomas secrete 1-α-hydroxylase, causing ↑ production of 1,25-OH-vit D → hypercalcemia)
      g. Endocrine → classic cause of diabetes insipidus due to pituitary involvement, ↑ vitamin D as above
      h. Hematologic → bone marrow involvement & splenic sequestration causes anemia, thrombocytopenia, leukopenia
      i. Derm → various rashes, including erythema nodosum [see Dermatology, Section III.D.12]
   8. Dx is clinical; however, finding of **noncaseating granulomas on Bx (often of lymph nodes) is HIGHLY suggestive if no other explanation is found for the granulomas** (e.g., fungal infections)
   9. Laboratory: 50% pts have ↑ angiotensin converting enzyme level—used to follow Tx (will ↓ with Tx) but not Dx due to ↓ sensitivity

10. Tx = prednisone (first line), but 50% pts spontaneously remit, so only Tx if dz affects a potentially dangerous organ system (e.g., eyes, heart, and kidneys)

J. Mixed connective tissue disease (MCTD)
   1. Syndrome with Si/Sx overlapping SLE, scleroderma & polymyositis, but **characterized by ⊕ anti-U1 ribonucleoprotein (RNP) antibody, which defines the disease**
   2. Commonly onsets in women in teens & 20s
   3. Can involve any organ system with any autoimmune phenomenon, but **anti-U1 RNP seems to actively protect against nephropathy**, which is a rare complication
   4. Tx = steroids, azathioprine

K. Gout
   1. **Monoarticular arthritis** due to urate crystal deposits in joint
   2. Precursor is hyperuricemia
      a. Urate is breakdown product of purine metabolism
      b. Hyperuricemia can be due to overproduction or underexcretion (overproduction → >800 mg/dL urate in urine)
      c. Higher the urate level, the more likely gout is to develop; however, **most people with hyperuricemia never get gout**
      d. **Gout develops after 20–30 years of hyperuricemia, often precipitated by sudden changes in serum urate levels**
      e. Gout in teens → 20s likely genetic (see below)
   3. Causes of overproduction
      a. 1° (genetic enzyme defects)
         (1) X-linked 5′-phosphoribosyl-1-pyrophosphate (PRPP) synthetase **hyperactivity** (regulates first, rate-limiting step in purine synthesis)
         (2) X-linked hypoxanthine phosphoribosyltransferase (HPRT) **deficiency** (Lesch-Nyhan syndrome)
            (a) HPRT regulates purine salvage pathway
            (b) Purines synthesized by salvage pathway feedback inhibit PRPP synthetase
            (c) See Appendix B for Lesch-Nyhan
      b. 2° (acquired) due to idiopathic, alcohol (contains lots of purines), hemolysis/neoplasia/psoriasis (↑ cell turnover)
   4. Under excretion of urate via kidney (<800 mg/dL urine urate) due to idiopathic, kidney dz, drugs (aspirin, diuretics, alcohol)
   5. Si/Sx of gout = painful monoarticular arthritis affecting distal joints (often first metatarsophalangeal joint, where disease is

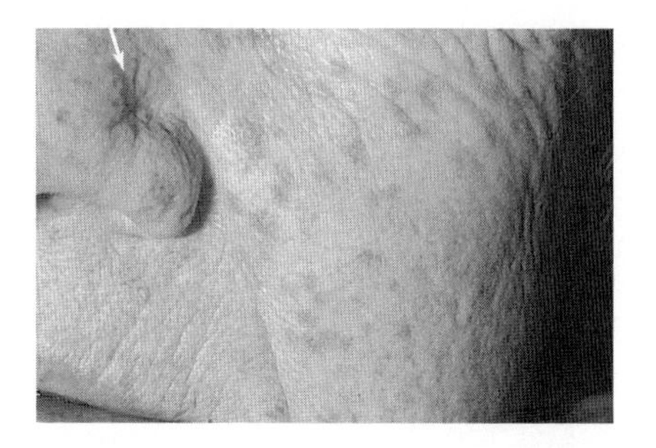

Figure 10.12
Telangiectasia in a patient with systemic sclerosis. (From Axford JS. Medicine. Oxford: Blackwell Science, 1998.)

called "**podagra**"), **overlying skin erythema can mimic cellulitis** (see Figure 10.12)

6. Disease course: some people never suffer more than 1 attack, those that do develop chronic tophaceous gout, with significant joint deformation (**classic rat-bite appearance to joint on x-ray**) & toothpaste-like discharge from joint through the skin
7. Dx
   a. Often based on clinical triad of monoarticular arthritis, hyperuricemia, ⊕ response to colchicine (see below)
   b. To differentiate from pseudogout (see below), needle tap with analysis of crystals in joint must be performed
   c. **Beware—an acute attack can be precipitated by a sudden fall in serum urate levels, so pts do not always have a high urate level during an acute attack**
8. Acute Tx = colchicine (inhibits neutrophil inflammatory response to urate crystals) & NSAIDs (not aspirin!)
9. **Maintenance Tx**
   a. Do not start unless patient has more than 1 attack
   b. Overproducers → allopurinol (inhibits xanthine oxidase)
   c. Underexcreters → probenecid/sulfinpyrazone (block urate reuptake into kidney tubules→ ↑ urate excretion)
   d. **Always start on patients still taking colchicine, because sudden ↓ in serum urate precipitates an acute attack**
10. Pseudogout
    a. Caused by calcium pyrophosphate dihydrate (CPPD) crystal deposition in joints & articular cartilage (chondrocalcinosis) (see Figure 10.13)
    b. Mimics gout very closely, seen in persons age 60 or older,

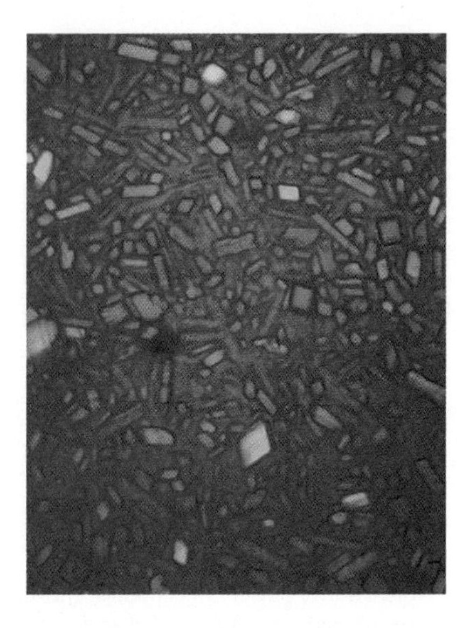

Figure 10.13 CPPD Dihydrate Crystals (Extracted from Synovial Fluid)
These are pleomorphic, rectangular, and weakly positively birefringent. The axis of slow vibration is from bottom left to top right. (From Axford JS. Medicine. Oxford: Blackwell Science, 1998.)

often affects larger, more proximal joints

c. Can be 1° or 2° to metabolic dz (hyperparathyroidism, Wilson's dz, diabetes, hemochromatosis)
d. Dx → microscopic analysis of joint aspirate
e. Tx = colchicine & NSAIDs

11. Microscopy
    a. **Gout → needle-like negatively birefringent crystals** (see Figure 10.14)
    b. **"P"seudogout → "P"ositively birefringent crystals** (see Figure 10.15)

V. Muscle Diseases

A. Muscle physiology
1. Type 1 muscle → slow, sustained movement, ↑ mitochondria & oxidative enzymes
2. Type 2 muscle is for fast, short-duration movement, ↑ ATP-ase & glycogen

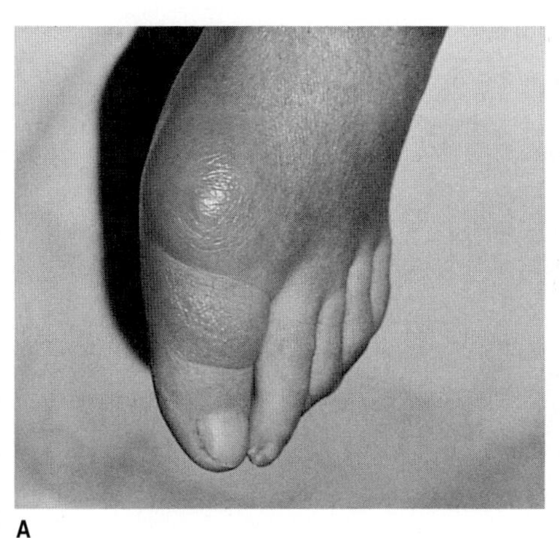
A

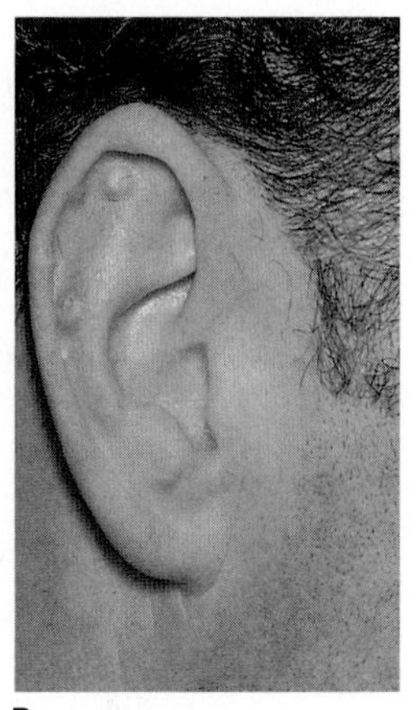
B

Figure 10.14 Gout
A. Acute gouty arthritis affecting the big toe. This is extremely painful! **B.** Urate crystal deposition in the cartilage of the ear. (From Axford JS. Medicine. Oxford: Blackwell Science, 1998.)

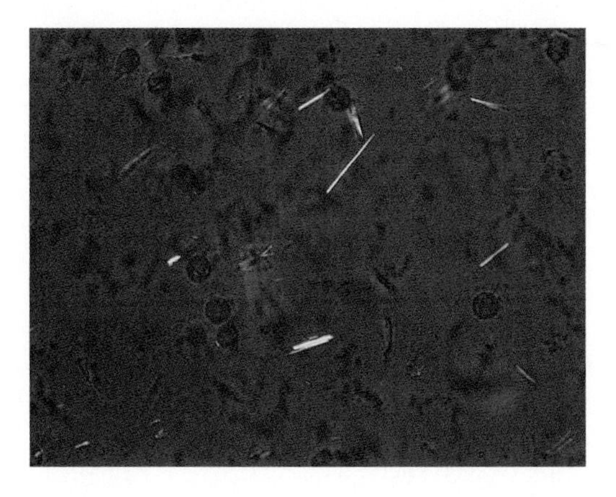

Figure 10.15. Gout
Synovial fluid microscopy under compensated polarized light showing the slender needle-shaped and negatively birefringent urate crystals. The axis of slow vibration is from bottom left to top right. (From Axford JS. Medicine. Oxford: Blackwell Science, 1998.)

3. Muscle fiber function is conditioned by nerve supply
4. Diseases of muscle are divided into 2 groups: neurogenic & myopathic
5. Neurogenic diseases
    a. Affect anterior horn cells, the axons, or at the termination of nerve on the muscle
    b. **See distal weakness, no pain, fasciculations present**
    c. Muscle biopsy can show atrophy of both types of fibers, in groups & clusters, with loss of mosaic pattern
6. Myopathic diseases
    a. Affect the muscle primarily
    b. **See proximal weakness, variable pain, absent fasciculations**, small polyphasic potentials on electromyography (EMG)
    c. Inflammatory myopathy (polymyositis), see scattered necrotic fibers, multiple foci of lymphocytes throughout endomysium

B. Muscular dystrophy
1. Duchenne's is an **X-linked** lack of dystrophin
    a. Sx commence at 1 year of age
    b. See **progressive proximal weakness**, immobilization, muscle wasting & muscle contractions
    c. Death occurs in 10s-20s, most often due to pneumonia
    d. See ↑ creatine phosphokinase (CPK), **calf muscle hypertrophy,** & waddling gait
    e. Gower's maneuver is the characteristic way pts pick themselves off the floor by using arms to help legs
2. Becker's
    a. Similar to Duchenne's, but less severe disease
    b. Abnormality in dystrophin (molecule is truncated & less functional)

C. Metabolic myopathies
1. Glycogenoses: glycogen-cleaving enzymes deficient, resulting in glycogen accumulation in various muscles
    a. Type I = von Gierke's
        (1) Deficiency in glucose-6-phosphatase → accumulation of glycogen in liver
        (2) Si/Sx = hepatomegaly & hypoglycemia
    b. Type II = Pompe's
        (1) Lysosomal acid maltase deficiency (α-glucosidase)
        (2) Glycogen accumulates in liver, heart & muscle

(3) Si/Sx = cardiomegaly, muscle hypotonia, splenomegaly, death before age 3 due to cardiorespiratory failure

c. Type III = Cori's
   (1) Deficiency in debranching enzyme, amyloglucosidase, accumulates glycogen same as above
   (2) Si/Sx = stunted growth, hepatomegaly, hypoglycemia

d. Type V = McArdle's
   (1) Deficiency in muscle glycogen phosphorylase, glycogen accumulates in vesicles in muscle
   (2) Si/Sx = painful muscle cramps & muscle weakness following exercise

D. Polymyositis
1. An autoinflammatory disorder of muscles & sometimes skin (dermatomyositis)
2. Female-male = 2:1, bimodal occurrence, in young children & geriatric populations
3. Sx = symmetric weakness/atrophy of proximal limb muscles, muscle aches, dysphonia (laryngeal muscle weakness), dysphagia (esophageal dysfunction)
4. Dermatomyositis presents with red-to-purple rash over face & neck called a "heliotropic rash"
5. Dx = proximal muscle weakness, ANA⊕, ↑ serum creatine kinase, muscle biopsy → inflammatory changes
6. Main DDx = scleroderma
7. Tx = steroids (using CK to follow effectiveness), but can also use methotrexate or Cytoxan for resistant disease

E. Neoplasia
1. Rhabdomyosarcoma
   a. Most common in children in head, neck & urogenital area
   b. Occurs in conjunction with tuberous sclerosis (see Neurology, Section VI.D)
   c. Tx = surgical excision & radiation, but often fails due to rapid spread of the tumor

F. Myasthenia gravis (MG)
1. Caused by autoantibodies that block the postsynaptic acetylcholine receptor
2. The antibody blockade inhibits propagation of the action potential to the postsynaptic skeletal muscle
3. Most common in women in 20s–30s or men in 50s–60s
4. **MG often associated with thymomas & thyroid diseases, as well as other autoimmune diseases (e.g., lupus)**

5. Sx = **muscle weakness worse with use** (frequently patients complain of weakness at the end of the day)
   a. Classically affects facial muscles, causing diplopia or ptosis, altered smile, dysphagia
   b. Also causes proximal limb weakness
   c. Eventually can cause respiratory failure
6. Course can exacerbate or remit
   a. Often acutely exacerbated by infections
   b. Severe exacerbation called "crisis," can be fatal
7. Dx
   a. Tensilon screening test = trial of edrophonium (short-acting anticholinesterase inhibitor) → immediate ↑ in strength
   b. More definitive test is electromyelography with repetitive nerve stimulation, causing a >15% reduction in evoked action potential responses in stimulated muscle
8. DDx
   a. **Lambert-Eaton syndrome**
      (1) Disorder seen in patients with small cell lung CA
      (2) Caused by autoAbs to **pre**synaptic calcium channels
      (3) Mimics myasthenia symptomatically
      (4) Differs from MG in that Lambert-Eaton causes ↓ reflexes, autonomic dysfunction (xerostomia, impotence) & **Sx improve with muscle use (action potential strength increases upon repeated muscle stimulation)**
   b. Aminoglycoside use can exacerbate Sx in MG patients, or induce mild myasthenia Sx in normal people
   c. Penicillamine can induce mild myasthenia, but it is reversible with cessation of drug use
9. Tx = anticholinesterase inhibitors (e.g., pyridostigmine) first line
   a. Steroids, cyclophosphamide, azathioprine for ↑ severe dz
   b. Plasmapheresis temporarily alleviates Sx by removing the blocking antibody
   c. Resection of thymoma can be curative in patients with both the neoplasm & myasthenia
   d. In addition, even in pts with no thymus neoplasm, resection of a normal thymus causes symptomatic improvement in 85% of patients, & may be curative in up to 35%

11. HEMATOLOGY

I. Introduction

A. Embryology

1. Hematopoiesis begins in yolk sac during first month
2. At third month it begins in liver & spleen
3. Fourth month hematopoiesis begins in the bone marrow
4. At birth, liver & spleen hematopoiesis ↓↓

B. Hematopoiesis

1. 3 stages: 1) proliferation of stem cells, 2) differentiation of blast cells, 3) maturation to final cell type
2. Common stem cell (preblast) expresses CD34 surface protein
3. CD34+ cells differentiate into 1) myeloid & 2) lymphoid blasts
4. Mutations in stem cell → myeloproliferative dz (see Section V)
5. Mutations in blast cell → acute leukemias (see Section VI)
6. Myelopoiesis (see Figure 11.1)
   a. Myeloblast differentiates → progenitors of 1) erythrocyte, 2) megakaryocyte, 3) mast cell, 4) monocyte, & 5) granulocyte
   b. Granulocyte matures → neutrophil, eosinophil, basophil (see Figure 11.2)
   c. 90% of neutrophils die within marrow, last 6 hours in circulation
   d. Monocyte circulates for 6–10 hours, then matures in tissue
   e. Megakaryocytes become multinucleate due to endomitotic reduplication (nucleus multiplies without cell division), matured cells split off platelets, which circulate for 7 days
   f. Proerythrocyte nucleus shrinks & then is extruded, with Wright stain cytoplasm first → blue during RNA transcription, then → pink as hemoglobin is translated
   g. Mature RBCs circulate for 120 days (see Figure 11.2)
7. Lymphoid blast matures → B cells, T cells, natural killer cells

C. Disorders

1. ↑ risk infection if absolute neutrophil count $<1000/mm^3$
2. **All blood cell disorders are of 3 general types**
   a. Altered production: clonal proliferation or bone marrow failure

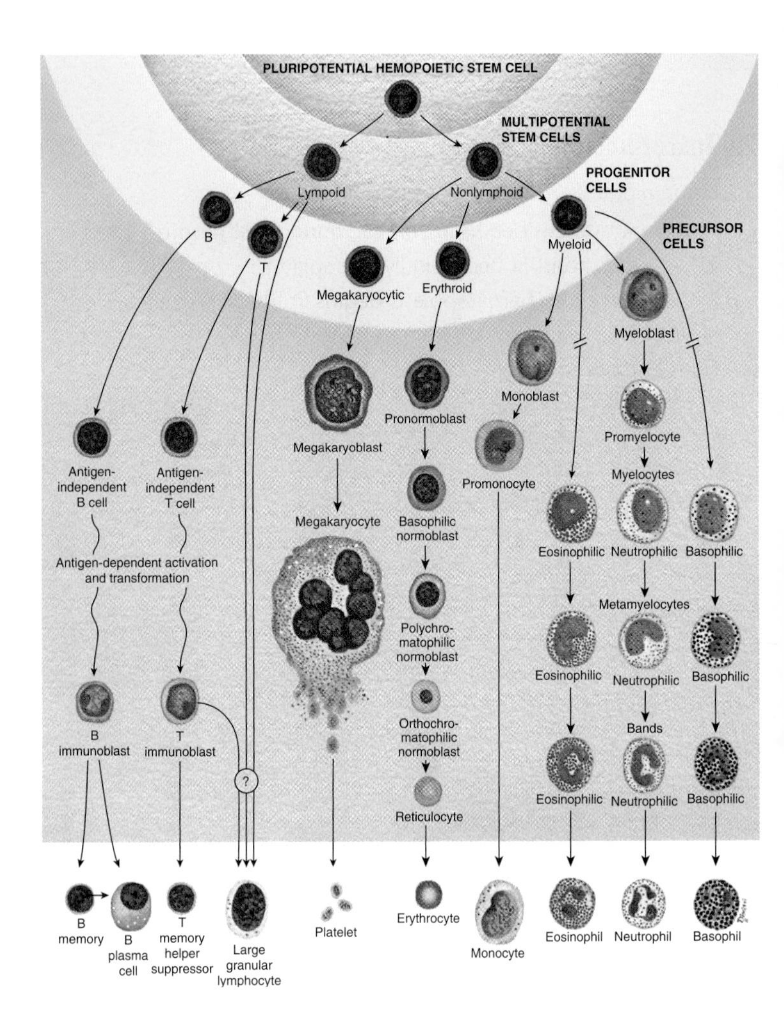

Figure 11.1
Cellular differentiation and maturation of the lymphoid (left) and myeloid (right) components of the hematopoietic system. Only the precursor cells (blasts and maturing cells) and identifiable by light microscopic evaluation of the bone marrow. (From Rubin E, Gorstein F, Rubin R, et al. Rubin's Pathology: Clinicopathologic Foundations of Medicine. 4th ed. Baltimore: Lippincott Williams & Wilkins, 2005.)

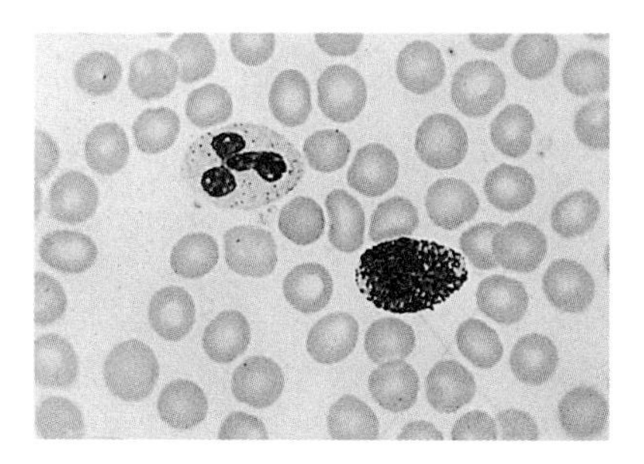

Figure 11.2
Normal blood films. (From Hughes-Jones NC, Wickramasinghe SN. Lecture Notes on Haematology. 6th ed. Oxford: Blackwell Science, 1996.)

    b. Altered destruction: can be ↑ **or** ↓ (↓ apoptosis → cancer)
    c. Qualitative (the cells don't work right)
3. Loss of adhesion allows cells to invade various anatomical sites, this is typical of leukemia/lymphoma
4. Myelodysplasia = preleukemic, increased numbers of abnormal myeloid blasts in marrow but not yet in peripheral blood
5. Blasts in periphery are typical of acute leukemias
6. Lymphocytic disorders are called "lymphocytic leukemia" if cells are in blood, "lymphoma" if they are parenchymal
7. **Acute leukemias onset 5–10 years after prior chemotherapy or radiation therapy given for other malignancies**

D. Biopsies
1. Marrow smear, clot section, bone marrow biopsy
2. Biopsy is the best for marrow architecture
3. Percent cellularity of marrow that should be found on normal biopsy can be estimated by the formula (100% − age)

II. Transfusion Medicine

A. Blood groups—The ABO system
1. ABO is one of 20 or so identified blood groups
2. Blood group O actually possess an antigen (Ag) called "H," which can rarely induce antibody (Ab)
3. AB antigens are **polysaccharide moieties** on RBCs, endothelium, epidermal cells, intestinal cells, leukocytes, & platelets
4. AB Ags elicit IgM antibodies, causing intravascular hemolysis

5. Group O cells & group AB plasma are universal donors (technically must be Rh negative, see below)
6. Incompatible donated plasma is quickly diluted while donated cells are exposed to high concentrations of Ab, so plasma donation is much less sensitive to reactions than cell donations
7. Group AB recipient is universal, since they do not make anti-AB antibody
8. If patient is O type, only O type blood can be safely given
9. If patient is AB, A or B can be used, as well as O packed cells
10. Rh is a **protein antigen** (contrast to AB Ags), determined by D & CcEe loci, but only D is measured to determine Rh positivity
11. Rh antigens elicit IgG antibodies, causing extravascular hemolysis

B. Agglutination
   1. Direct Coombs' test
      a. Test for any autoimmune hemolysis
      b. Patient's (Pt's) RBCs tested with Coombs' reagent = antihuman IgG
      c. If the pt is hemolyzing, the Coombs' reagent binds to the pt's IgG that is attached to the pt's own RBCs, causing agglutination
      d. Cell's zeta potential (negative) repels other cells, so the Coombs' reagent is needed to bridge across the negative potential for agglutination to occur
      e. Direct test looks for IgG, which crosses placenta, rarely agglutinates cells, is optimal at 37 °C, is not naturally occurring
   2. Indirect Coombs' test
      a. The patient's serum is added to foreign cells
      b. Used to diagnose atypical, unexpected antibodies in the patient's serum & for pretransfusion compatibility
      c. Indirect looks for IgM, which cannot cross placenta, agglutinates cells, works at 4–20 °C, & naturally occurs
      d. Indirect also finds IgG directed at unusual epitopes
   3. Reliability of compatibility following cross-match is 99.99%

C. Blood products
   1. Whole blood is rarely given for volume loss
   2. Packed red blood cells (PRBCs) are used for most transfusions

3. Fresh-frozen plasma contains all clotting factors except platelets
4. Cryoprecipitate has factors VIII, vWF, IX, fibrinogen: given for deficiencies of these factors, as well as for uremic bleeding
5. Rh immune globulin (RhoGAM): has IgG anti-Rh, given at 28wk & within 72hr of delivery to block sensitization in an Rh-negative woman who delivers an Rh-positive baby
6. Packed platelets given for thrombocytopenic bleeding

D. Hazards

1. **Intravascular hemolysis is invariably due to ABO incompatibility**
2. Signs/symptoms (Si/Sx) = fever, chills, facial flushing, chest/back pain, heat/pain at infusion site, dyspnea, hypotension, agitation, hemoglobinuria
3. Diagnosis (Dx) = free hemoglobin in urine/serum, Coombs' test, retest ABO match
4. Immediate reactions due to clerical errors, due to ABO incompatibility, can be life-threatening
5. Treatment (Tx) = STOP INFUSION, treat with diuretics plus fluid load to try to prevent acute tubular necrosis & oliguric renal failure
6. Nonhemolytic reactions include fever, urticaria, anaphylaxis, volume overload, citrate toxicity, hyperkalemia, acidosis, endotoxin, air embolism, hypothermia, hemosiderosis & DIC
7. Above often due to anticoagulants (citric acid) or to rapid infusion
8. Infections: HIV, HBV, HCV all screened for and very rarely transmitted

III. Anemias

A. Aplastic anemia

1. Failure of hematopoiesis → ↓ **counts of erythrocytes, neutrophils, & platelets** (lymphocytes spared due to long life)
2. Si/Sx = pancytopenia, petechiae/hemorrhage, pallor, weakness, infection
3. Laboratory = anemia, neutropenia, thrombocytopenia, hypocellular bone marrow

4. Causes
   a. Usually idiopathic
   b. Other = drugs (chloramphenicol), toxins (benzene, etc.), infections (parvovirus B19 is most common, also hepatitis B or C), radiation, paroxysmal nocturnal hemoglobinuria
5. Prognosis (Px) = 90% die within 1 year with transfusions & antibiotics
6. 50–70% of bone marrow transplant (BMT) patients will be cured of disease
7. In non-BMT candidates, can try antithymocyte globulin (ATG) with or without addition of growth factors (e.g., Neupogen, GM-CSF)

B. Megaloblastic anemia
   1. Impaired DNA synthesis with normal RNA & protein synthesis
   2. Causes = B_{12} deficiency, folate deficiency, chemotherapy
   3. **Pathognomonic blood smear → hypersegmented neutrophils** (see Figure 11.3)
   4. In cirrhosis blood smear → "spur cells" (acanthocytes), with large spikes protruding from membrane like cowboy spurs
   5. Folic acid deficiency
      a. Look for megaloblastic anemia with glossitis
      b. Causes can be dietary, ↑ requirements (pregnancy, hemolytic anemia, tumors), drugs (methotrexate, dilantin), or malabsorption due to intestinal resection
      c. Dx: ↓ blood folate, along with characteristic changes in marrow & smear noted above

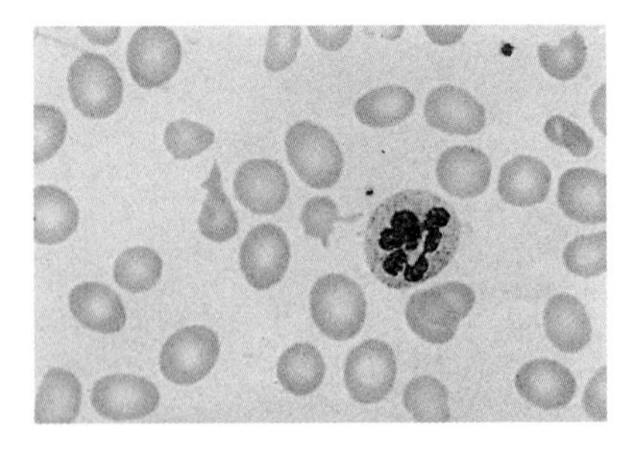

Figure 11.3
Hypersegmented neutrophil in severe pernicious anemia; also note ovalocytes. (From Hughes-Jones NC, Wickramasinghe SN. Lecture Notes on Haematology. 6th ed. Oxford: Blackwell Science, 1996.)

6. B_{12} (cyanocobalamin) deficiency
   a. Si/Sx = megaloblastic anemia with neuropathies (secondary [2°] to defective myelin synthesis)
   b. Often due to lack of intrinsic factor (needed by mucosal cells in terminal ileum for B_{12} absorption)
   c. Causes include autoimmune (pernicious anemia), gastrectomy (chief cells secrete intrinsic factor), ileal resection (↓ uptake), enteritis (blocks uptake) & intestinal tapeworm (*Diphyllobothrium latum*) that metabolizes the B_{12}
   d. Dx = megaloblastic marrow, macrocytic blood picture, ↓ serum B_{12} levels, gastric analysis (achlorhydria is seen in pernicious anemia)
   e. Serum methylmalonic acid & homocysteine levels are more sensitive than pure folate & B_{12} levels
      (1) Both methylmalonic & homocysteine ↑ in B_{12} deficiency
      (2) Only homocysteine elevated in folate deficiency
   f. Schilling test
      (1) Give radioactive B_{12} orally, then nonradioactive B_{12} intramuscularly, collect urine 24 hours
      (2) Normal people will excrete 7–22% of the initial oral B_{12}
      (3) Low urinary levels are seen in defective GI absorption
      (4) If low, repeat test & give oral intrinsic factor with B_{12} to assess change (this will ↑ urinary excretion of oral dose if problem is due to lack of intrinsic factor production)
      (5) If this is also low give oral antibiotic with B_{12} to assess change (this will ↑ urinary excretion if problem is parasitic)
      (6) If antibiotics do not help either, the problem is likely one of absorption in the small bowel

C. Microcytic anemia
   1. Result from ↓ hemoglobin production or impaired function
   2. Iron deficiency anemia (most common anemia in the world)
      a. Iron physiology
         (1) 50 mg of iron/100mL of blood, total body iron 50 mg/kg in males, 30 mg/kg in females
         (2) Males require 1 mg/day, menstruating females require 2 mg/day
         (3) Iron is transported via transferrin to marrow, used by developing RBCs to make hemoglobin & is stored in macrophages

(4) Amount of iron the plasma can bind at any one time is limited by plasma transferrin content = total iron binding capacity (TIBC)

(5) Ferritin is a measure of the total body iron stores

b. Peripheral smear shows hypochromia, microcytosis

c. Laboratory: ↓ iron, ↑ TIBC, ↓ ferritin, marrow stains show ↓↓ iron

d. **Iron deficiency anemia is not a final diagnosis: the cause of the iron deficiency MUST be found**

e. **Iron deficiency anemia in the elderly is due to colon cancer until proven otherwise**

f. Blood loss must be ruled out in all adult cases, in children dietary causes are common

g. Most common cause worldwide is intestinal hookworm infection, suspect in immigrants from Third World

3. Anemia of chronic disease

a. Idiopathic, may be result of aberrant cytokine patterns

b. Laboratory: ↓ iron, ↓ **TIBC**, ↑ **ferritin**, marrow iron increased, can be a normocytic/normochromic

c. Note that despite the ↓ iron, the body does not try to ↑ TIBC—this paradox is not readily explainable

d. **Characteristic laboratory finding is ↓ TIBC**

4. Sideroblastic anemia

a. Problem is in accessing stored iron in mitochondria in the marrow

b. Look for ringed sideroblasts on iron stain of bone marrow

c. Laboratory: ↑ **iron**, N/↑ TIBC, ↑ ferritin

d. **Characteristic laboratory finding is elevated serum iron**

5. Lead poisoning

a. Causes a hypochromic microcytic anemia due to lead inhibition of heme synthesis

b. Associated systemic Sx include encephalopathy (worse in children), seizures, ataxic gait, **wrist/foot drops**, renal tubular acidosis

c. Classic Dx findings

(1) **Bruton's lines** = blue/gray discoloration at gumlines

(2) **Basophilic stippling of red cells (blue dots in red cells)**

(3) X-rays show increased epiphyseal density of long bones

d. Tx = chelation with dimercaprol (BAL) &/or EDTA

6. Hemolytic anemias
   a. Intravascular hemolysis characterized by cell fragments on blood smear (see Figure 11.4), ↓ haptoglobin & ⊕ hemosiderin in urine
   b. Extravascular hemolysis characterized by spherocytes on blood smear (haptoglobin can fall in severe disease [dz])
   c. Extrinsic (extracorpuscular) hemolysis
      (1) Coombs'⊕: antibodies to RBC due to incompatible blood transfusion or autoimmune hemolytic anemia (warm mediated by IgG, cold mediated by IgM)
      (2) Mechanical destruction
         (a) Disseminated intravascular coagulation (DIC)
         (b) Thrombotic thrombocytopenic purpura (TTP)
         (c) Hemolytic–uremic syndrome (HUS)
         (d) Artificial heart valve
      (3) Infectious agents—malaria, *Clostridium*
      (4) Altered plasma components: lipids (see acanthocytes on smear), or hypophosphatemia
      (5) Toxins & drugs (penicillin, α-methyldopa, quinidine)
   d. Intrinsic (intracorpuscular) hemolysis
      (1) Membrane defects include hereditary spherocytosis, hereditary elliptocytes, which are due to congenital defect in cytoskeleton proteins, resulting in very osmotically fragile cells
         (a) Tx = Folate supplementation & splenectomy
      (2) Paroxysmal nocturnal hemoglobinuria is caused by an acquired defect of the *PIG-A* gene, which inhibits

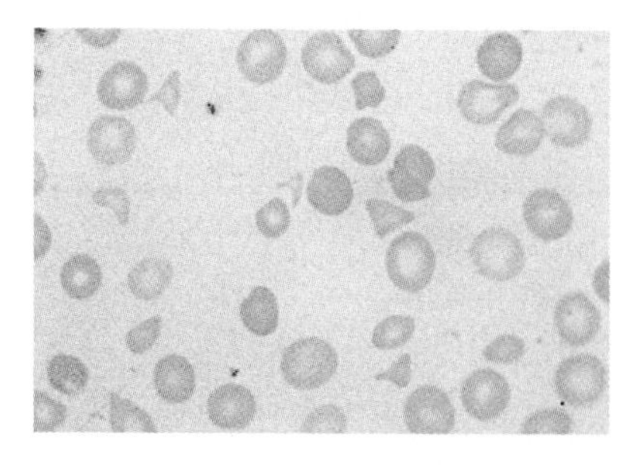

Figure 11.4
Schistocytes in patient with malfunctioning aortic valve. (From Hughes-Jones NC, Wickramasinghe SN. Lecture Notes on Haematology. 6th ed. Oxford: Blackwell Science, 1996.)

GPI-anchoring of a variety of cell-surface proteins, including decay accelerating factor (DAF, or CD55) and membrane inhibitor of reactive lysis (MIRL, or CD59), both of which protect host cells from bystander destruction by activated complement cascade

(3) Enzyme deficiency (e.g., G6PD, protein kinase deficiency)

7. Hemoglobinopathies
   a. Thalassemias (quantitative hemoglobin defects) (see Table 11.1)
      (1) β-thalassemia: ↓ production of β chains
         (a) Usually Mediterranean or black ethnicity
         (b) Homozygous β-/β- = Thalassemia Major (Cooley's anemia)
            (i) Electrophoresis → ↓↓↓ Hgb A, ↑ Hgb A2, ↑ **Hgb F**
            (ii) Si/Sx → hepatosplenomegaly, anemia, frontal bossing due to extramedullary hematopoiesis, hypercellular marrow, iron overload (2° to transfusions), recurrent infxn, early death
            (iii) Smear → marked anisocytosis & poikilocytosis with ↑ reticulocytes, microcytic hypochromic RBCs, with many target cells
         (c) Heterozygous = Thalassemia Minor
            (i) Electrophoresis → ↓ Hgb A, ↑ Hgb A2(γ), **N Hgb F**
            (ii) Patients are often asymptomatic, can see silent anemia, smear shows target cells & microcytic/hypochromic RBC

Table 11.1 α-Thalassemias

# Alleles Affected/ Name of Disease		Characteristic	Blood Smear
4	Hydrops fetalis	Fetal demise, total body edema	Bart's β_4 Hgb precipitations
3	Hgb H disease	Disease caused by precipitation of β-chain tetramers	Intraerythrocytic inclusions
2	α-Thal. Minor	Usually clinically silent	Mild microcytic anemia
1	Carrier state	No anemia, asymptomatic	No abnormalities

(2) α-thalassemia: ↓ production of α chains
   (a) Usually seen in Africans, Mediterraneans, & Asians
   (b) **4** α-chain genes, 2 alleles on both chromosomes

b. Sickle cell anemia (qualitative defect in hemoglobin)
   (1) Sickle S type (the most common type)
      (a) HgS tetramer: single amino acid substitution of valine for glutamine
      (b) Exposes hydrophobic residue, which is then buried by hemoglobin polymerization
      (c) Polymerized tetrads cause the sickling of the cell (see Figure 11.5)
      (d) Sickle cells clog microcapillaries → vaso-occlusive findings, pain crisis, myocardiopathy, infarcts of bone/CNS/lungs/kidneys, priapism, & autosplenectomy due to splenic infarct
      (e) Autosplenectomy → ↑susceptible to encapsulated bacteria
      (f) **Intravascular hemolysis episodes can cause gallstones in children, teens & young adults**
      (g) Heterozygotes may live approximately normal life spans, will have only rare sickle crises
   (2) Sickle C type
      (a) Substitution of lysine for glutamine
      (b) Homozygous CC causes mild chronic anemia, less severe than sickle S

D. Peripheral blood smear findings—see Table 11.2

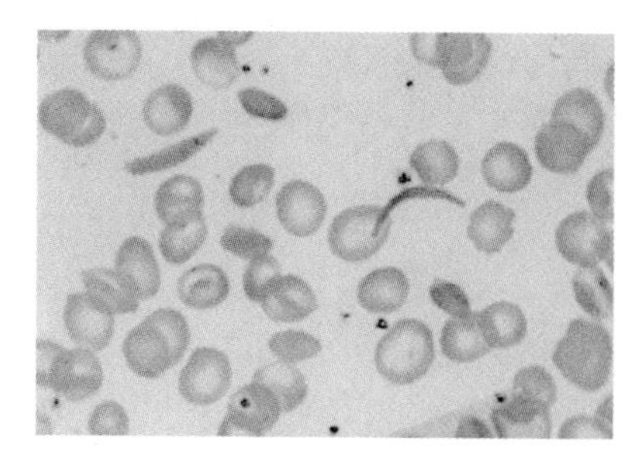

Figure 11.5
Sickle cell anemia. (From Hughes-Jones NC, Wickramasinghe SN. Lecture Notes on Haematology. 6th ed. Oxford: Blackwell Science, 1996.)

Table 11.2 Peripheral Blood Smear in Anemia

Condition	Peripheral Blood Smear
Folate/B_{12} deficiency	Megaloblasts & hypersegmented neutrophils
Liver disease	Megaloblasts & target cells, cirrhosis → "spur cells" (acanthocytes)
Microcytic anemia	Microcytes, hypochromic
Lead poisoning	Microcytes, hypochromic, basophilic stippling of RBCs
Uremia	Burr cells (echinocytes)
Coombs'⊕ hemolysis	Microspherocytes
DIC/TTP/HUS	Schistocytes, helmet cells (PT/PTT ↑ only in DIC)
Thalassemia	Poikilocytosis, microcytic, hypochromic, ↑↑↑ target cells
Sickle cell	Sickle cells, rod-shaped sickle C crystals in sickle C disease
Abetalipoproteinemia	Spur cells (acanthocytes)
Asplenia	Howell-Jolly bodies
G6PD deficiency	Heinz bodies

IV. Coagulation Disorders

A. Thrombocytopenia
1. Presents with petechiae, epistaxis, CNS bleeds, GI bleeds
   a. Bleeding time elevated at counts <50,000
   b. Clinically significant bleeds start at counts <20,000
   c. CNS bleeds occur with counts <10,000
2. Caused by stem cell failure, increased destruction, splenic sequestration
3. Stem cell failure caused by leukemia, aplastic anemia, alcohol (can be mild intake), paroxysmal nocturnal hemoglobinuria
4. Destruction
   a. Idiopathic thrombocytopenic purpura (ITP)
      (1) An autoimmune disorder of autoantibody-mediated platelet destruction

(2) **In children follows upper respiratory infection & is self-limiting, in adults it is chronic**

(3) Si/Sx = petechiae, purpura, epistaxis, **with normal white & red cell morphology on peripheral blood smear**

(4) Tx = steroids (first line), splenectomy (second line) helps 50% of those who fail steroids, immunosuppressives (azathioprine, cyclophosphamide) are third line

b. Thrombotic thrombocytopenic purpura (TTP)

(1) An idiopathic systemic disease of acutely falling platelet counts that can be fatal

(2) **Classic pentad of TTP**

(a) Intravascular hemolytic anemia

(b) Renal failure → proteinuria, hematuria, ↑ creatinine

(c) Thrombocytopenia

(d) Neurologic changes (focal & nonfocal)

(e) Fever

(3) Histopathology

(a) **Characteristic pathology → platelet-fibrin thrombi in capillaries**

(b) **Peripheral smears: fragmented RBCs (schistocytes)**

(4) Tx = plasma exchange or intravenous immunoglobulin until disease (dz) abates, typically several days

(5) Dz is fatal without treatment

c. Drug-induced thrombocytopenia

(1) Heparin, sulfonamides, sulfonylureas, valproate, etc. can induce destruction

(2) Reverses within several days of ceasing drug intake

d. Hemolytic–uremic syndrome (HUS)

(1) Usually in children, often caused by *Escherichia coli* O157:H7

(2) Si/Sx

(a) Glomerular sclerosis causing acute renal failure

(b) Bloody diarrhea & abdominal pain, seizures

(c) **Fulminant thrombocytopenia with hemolytic anemia is highly suggestive**

(3) Tx = dialysis helps children, but adults may be refractory & Px is much poorer

e. Evan's syndrome

(1) IgG autoantibody mediated hemolytic anemia & thrombocytopenia

Table 11.3 Differential Diagnosis of Platelet Destruction

Study	Autoantibody (Drug-Induced, Evan's Syndrome, Lymphoma)	DIC	TTP/HUS
Blood smear	Microspherocytes	Schistocytes (+)	**Schistocytes (+++)**
Coombs' test	⊕	–	–
PT/PTT	Nml	↑↑↑	Nml / ↑

(2) Often have pancytopenia due to multiple autoantibodies
(3) Associated with collagen-vascular dz, TTP, hepatic cirrhosis, leukemia, sarcoidosis, Hashimoto's thyroiditis
(4) Tx = prednisone & intravenous immunoglobulin

f. Lymphoma & leukemia
   (1) Can produce antiplatelet antibodies
   (2) Also induce splenic sequestration

g. Disseminated intravascular coagulation (DIC)
   (1) Platelets trapped in fibrin mesh deposited in blood vessels
   (2) Dx = ↑ fibrin-split products, ↓ fibrinogen, ↑ PT/PTT

h. Differential diagnosis of platelet destruction—see Table 11.3

5. Splenic sequestration
   a. Trapping of platelets in reticuloendothelial cells of spleen
   b. Caused by portal hypertension, lymphoma, leukemia, massive infection, chronic inflammation

B. Platelet dysfunctions
   1. von-Willebrand factor (vWF) deficiency
      a. **This is the most common inherited bleeding disorder (more common than hemophilia!!!)**
      b. Three different types, most commonly autosomal dominant
         (1) Type I due to ↓ secretion of functional vWF
         (2) Type II due to secretion of dysfunctional vWF
         (3) Type III is autosomal recessive, dysfunctional vWF
      c. vWF secreted by endothelial cells, binds platelet surface receptor GpIb (see Bernard-Soulier syndrome below), bridging platelet to subendothelial matrix to initiate stasis

d. vWF deficiency presents with episodic ↑ **bleeding time & ecchymoses, with normal prothrombin time/partial thromboplastin time (PT/PTT)**
e. Stress affects vWF level & can exacerbate disease course
f. Due to mild, episodic nature of the disorder, it may go undiagnosed well into adult life
g. Dx = vWF levels & ristocetin-cofactor test (measures platelet aggregation induced by ristocetin binding of vWF)
h. Tx = DDAVP (↑ vWF secretion, only used in type I vWF, actually harmful in type II), or cryoprecipitate for pts with acute, severe dz

2. Bernard-Soulier syndrome
   a. Autosomal recessive defect of platelet GpIb receptor (binds to vWF)
   b. Presents with chronic, severe mucosal bleeds & **giant platelets on blood smear**
   c. Tx = platelet transfusion
3. Glanzmann's thrombasthenia (GT)
   a. Autosomal recessive defect in GpIIbIIIa platelet receptor that binds fibrinogen, inhibiting platelet aggregation
   b. Presents with chronic, severe mucosal bleeds
   c. Tx = platelet transfusion
   d. New anticoagulant drugs, called gpIIbIIIa antagonists (abciximab, eptifibatide, tirofiban), mimic GT & cause anti-coagulation by inhibiting the gpIIbIIIa receptor
4. Aspirin & uremia are acquired causes of platelet dysfunction

C. Hemophilia

1. Hemophilia A
   a. An X-linked deficiency in factor VIII, the most common hemophilia type
   b. Many mutations, causing variable penetrance of the disease (variable disease severity)
   c. Presents with hemarthroses (bleeding into joint), easy bruisability with minor trauma
   d. **Laboratory → ↑ PTT, normal PT, normal bleeding time,** ↓ factor VIII levels
   e. Can be acquired due to circulating antifactor VIII antibody
      (1) Differentiate genetic from acquired by adding patient's serum to control serum
      (2) If circulating antibody is present, mixed serum also has ↑ PTT

(3) If genetic, the mixed serum will have a normal PTT (control serum's factor VIII is enough despite dilution)

f. Tx = recombinant factor VIII (first line), can use cryoprecipitate

2. Hemophilia B (Christmas disease)
   a. X-linked factor IX deficiency, also with variable dz severity
   b. **Laboratory: ↑ PTT, normal PT, normal bleeding time,** low factor IX levels, normal VIII levels
   c. Disease presentation is identical to hemophilia A, must distinguish by specific factor levels
   d. Tx = factor IX concentrate

D. Clotting factor synthesis (see Figure 11.6)
   1. Disorder can be due to liver disease (liver makes all clotting factors) or vitamin K deficiency

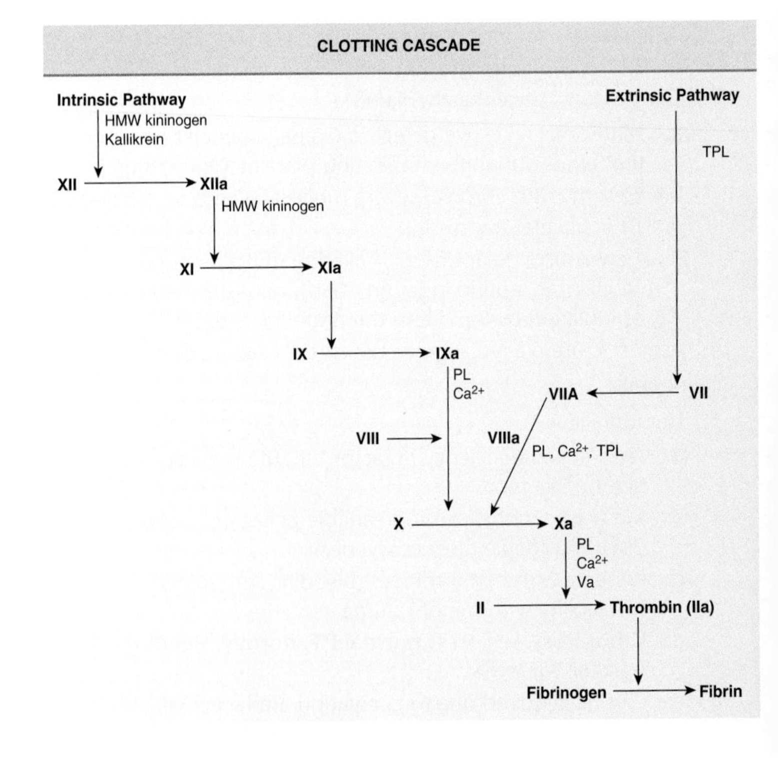

Figure 11.6
HMW = high molecular weight, TPL = tissue thromboplastin, PL = platelet phospholipid.

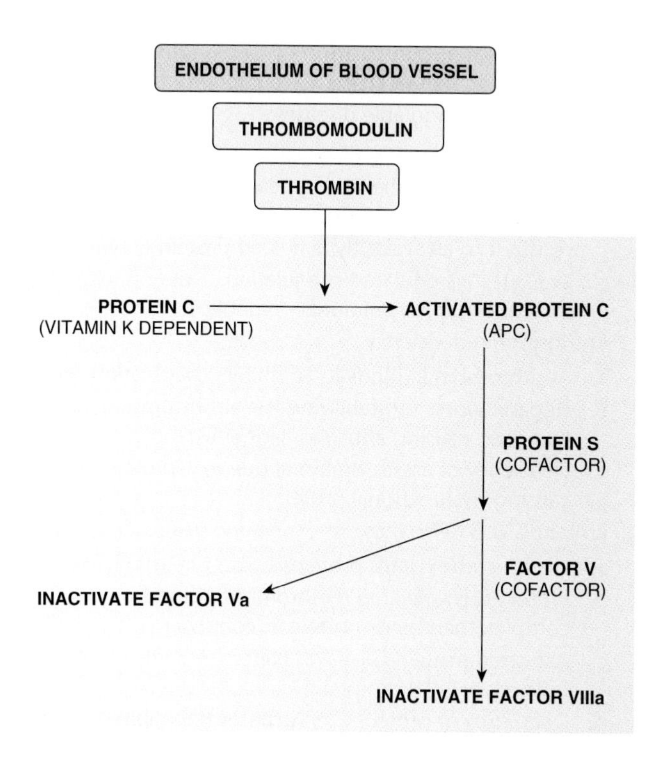

Figure 11.7
Schematic representation of vitamin K dependent mechanism of protein C inhibition of coagulation cascade.

2. Vitamin K necessary cofactor for γ-glutamyl-carboxylase, which carboxylates factors II, VII, IX, X, as well as protein C & S, so that they can interact with calcium (see Figure 11.7)
3. Liver dz & vitamin K deficiency thus affect both intrinsic & extrinsic pathways, so PT & PTT will both be elevated (but PT more so)
4. Coumadin
   a. Acts as a vitamin K analogue to inhibit carboxylation of factors II, VII, IX, X, as well as proteins C & S
   b. INR (pt's PT/control PT) should be >2 for Coumadin anticoagulation
   c. **Clinical Pearl: because Coumadin also interferes with protein C synthesis, & protein C has a very short half-**

life, initial administration of Coumadin can cause a fulminant skin necrosis 2° to capillary thrombosis

E. Congenital hypercoagulable diseases
   1. Factor V Leiden disease
      a. Most common inherited hypercoagulable state
      b. Due to amino acid substitution in factor V, causing it to be resistant to cleavage by activated protein C (APC)
      c. Leads to dysregulated coagulation, ↑ risk of deep venous thrombosis &/or pulmonary embolism
   2. Antithrombin deficiency
      a. Antithrombin III binds to & inhibits coagulation proteins
      b. Heparin works by stabilizing the antithrombin-coagulant complex, causing anticoagulant effect
      c. Deficiency of antithrombin III due to ↓ protein or mutation causing dysfunctional protein
   3. Protein C & S deficiency
      a. Liver γ-carboxylates proteins C & S (vitamin K–dependent)
      b. Protein C is activated by thrombin, thrombomodulin complex then binds protein S (cofactor)
      c. Activated protein C cleaves factors V & VIII, inhibiting further coagulation
      d. Deficiency of protein C or S causes uninhibited coagulation
      e. Coumadin may exacerbate, because it further lowers protein C levels by blocking vitamin K–dependent γ-carboxylation
   4. List of hypercoagulable states—see Table 11.4

V. Myeloproliferative Diseases

A. General characteristics
   1. Caused by clonal proliferation of a myeloid stem cell → excessive production of mature, differentiated myeloid cell lines
   2. There are 4 subtypes: 1) polycythemia vera, 2) thrombocythemia, 3) myelofibrosis, 4) chronic myeloid leukemia
   3. All can transform into acute leukemias

B. Polycythemia vera
   1. Rare disease, peak onset at 50–60 years, male predominance
   2. Si/Sx = headache, vertigo, diplopia, retinal hemorrhages, strokes, angina, claudication (all due to vascular sludging), early satiety, splenomegaly, gout, **pruritus after showering,** plethora

Table 11.4 Hypercoagulable States

Primary (Inherited)		Secondary (Acquired)
Antithrombin III deficiency	Prolonged immobilization	L-asparaginase
Protein C deficiency	Pregnancy	Diabetes mellitus
Protein S deficiency	Surgery/Trauma	Hyperlipidemia
Factor V Leiden deficiency	Oral contraceptives	Anticardiolipin Ab
Dysfibrinogenemia	Homocystinuria	Lupus anticoagulant
Plasminogen (activator) deficiency	Malignancy	DIC
Heparin cofactor II deficiency	Smoking	Vitamin K deficiency
Homocystinemia	Nephrotic syndrome	

3. Tx: phlebotomy to palliate, prognosis (Px) is good
4. **5% of pts progress to leukemia, 20% to myelofibrosis**
5. Differential diagnosis (DDx) for ↑ hematocrit = primary (1°) polycythemia & secondary (2°) erythrocytosis
   a. 1° can be vera or relative (fluid loss), distinguish by normal RBC mass (radioactive test) & signs of hypovolemia (tenting, orthostatic changes, dry mucosa, etc.)
   b. 2° due to high altitude, COPD, CHF, high-affinity hemoglobin, carbon monoxide poison (cigarettes), blood doping
   c. 1° vs. 2° differentials—see Table 11.5

C. Essential thrombocythemia (ET)
   1. Clonal proliferation of megakaryocytes resulting ↑ platelet counts
   2. **Because there are numerous causes of 2° thrombocytosis, ET is a diagnosis of exclusion!**
   3. Causes of 2° thrombocytosis include iron deficiency, any inflammatory disease (chronic infection, collagen-vascular, inflammatory bowel disease, etc.) & malignancy (common in chronic myelogenous leukemia, but can be seen in many cancers)

Table 11.5 Polycythemia Vera versus Reactive Polycythemia

Sign/Test	Polycythemia Vera	Secondary Erythrocytosis
O_2 saturation	Normal	Decreased
Erythropoietin levels	Markedly diminished	Increased
Splenomegaly	+	–
Platelet count	Increased	Normal
Neutrophil count	Increased	Normal
Basophil count	Increased	Normal

4. Si/Sx = platelet count >5 × 10^5 cells/μL, splenomegaly, factitious hyperkalemia (see Nephrology, Hyperkalemia Algorithm), **ecchymoses/bleeding but not typically thrombosis**
5. Tx is only necessary if pt is symptomatic
    a. Platelet exchange (apheresis) used in emergent setting
    b. Hydroxyurea & interferon-α are longer-term options
    c. Anagrelide is now the first-line Tx for ET patients, mechanism is unknown but it somehow decreases platelet synthesis from megakaryocytes
6. Px is good unless dz progresses to myelofibrosis or acute leukemia (less than 5% → leukemia)

D. Idiopathic myelofibrosis
1. Typically affects patients ≥50 years old
2. Clonal proliferation of unknown cell type leading to fibrosis of bone marrow → extramedullary hematopoiesis
3. Si/Sx = massive hepatomegaly, massive splenomegaly, blood smear → teardrop cells, nucleated red cells & immature white cells, gout, anemia often with ↑ white count & platelets (early)
4. Dx is by exclusion, but combination of extramedullary hematopoiesis & hypercellular marrow on Bx are keys
5. DDx = polycythemia vera, leukemia, myelophthisic disorders (invasion of bone marrow by multiple myeloma, lymphoma, metastatic carcinoma, sarcoidosis, tuberculosis, etc.)
6. Tx = symptomatic (splenectomy, antibiotics, allopurinol, etc.)
7. Px = very poor, median 5yr before total marrow failure, can also progress to a refractory acute leukemia

E. Chronic myelogenous leukemia (see below, Section VI.C)

VI. Leukemias

A. Acute lymphoblastic leukemia

1. **Peak age 3–4 years**, most common neoplasm in children
2. Sx: fever, fatigue; Si: anemia, pallor, petechiae, infections
3. Laboratory: Leukocytosis, blasts in peripheral blood (PB), ↓ RBC count, ↓ platelets, **PAS+, CALLA+, TdT+,** marrow bx → ↑ blasts
4. Tx = chemotherapy: induction, consolidation, maintenance—intrathecal chemotherapy during consolidation
5. Px: 80% cure in children (lower in adults), therapy sequelae = growth defects, new cancers, increased rate of sterility

B. Acute myelogenous leukemia—see Table 11.6

1. **Most common leukemia in adults**
2. French American British (FAB) classification = M0 to M7
3. Si/Sx = fever, fatigue, pallor, petechiae, infections, splenomegaly, lymphadenopathy
4. Laboratory: **Myeloperoxidase +, Sudan Black +, Auer Rods,** thrombocytopenia, peripheral blood & marrow biopsy (Bx) → myeloblasts
5. Tx = chemotherapy: induction, consolidation (no maintenance)
6. Px = depends on FAB type, but overall 30% cure, consider allogeneic bone marrow transplant (BMT) for better outcomes

C. Chronic myelogenous leukemia (CML)

1. Presents most commonly in the 50s, can present at any age
2. Sx = fatigue, anorexia, abdominal discomfort, early satiety, diaphoresis, arthritis, bone tenderness
3. Si = leukostasis (WBC $\geq 1 \times 10^5$) → dyspnea, dizzy, slurred speech, diplopia, confusion, retinal hemorrhage, papilledema
4. Laboratory: neutrophilia, thrombocytosis, **Philadelphia chromosome⊕** [see below], peripheral blood → cells of all maturational stages
5. Tx in chronic phase = reduction of WBC count with hydroxyurea or interferon (IFN)-α, or brand new Tx with drug-designed tyrosine kinase inhibitor, signal transduction inhibitor (STI)-571, which specifically blocks the oncogenic tyrosine kinase protein formed by the *bcr:abl* translocation
6. **Blast crisis = acute phase, leads to death in 3–6mo, mean time to onset = 3–4yr, only BMT can prevent**

Table 11.6 Acute Myelogenous Leukemia Subtypes

Subtype	Stain/Karyotype	Special Characteristics
M0: Minimal differentiated		
M1: Myeloblastic	+ Auer rod, + Sudan Black, + myeloperoxidase	
M2: Myeloblastic with differentiation	++ Auer rod, + Sudan Black, +++ myeloperoxidase	Prominent splenomegaly, ⊕ **chloromas** (green tumors made up of the blasts)
M3: Promyelocytic	+++ Auer rod, ↑ granular, +++ myeloperoxidase 15:17 translocation → retinoic acid receptor	**DIC common; Tx = all trans retinoic acid (ATRA) to induce blast differentiation, followed by consolidation chemotherapy**
M4: Myelomonocytic	+ myeloperoxidase	Subtype involves eosinophils
M5: Monocytic		CNS, **gingival involvement**
M6: Erythroblastic		Often preceded by myelodysplasia
M7: Megakaryoblastic		

7. Must differentiate from a "leukemoid" reaction to a severe infection (see Table 11.7)
8. Philadelphia chromosome (Ph chromosome)
   a. Present in >90% of CML patients, **it is pathognomonic**
   b. Shortened chromosome 22—translocation of *abl* from 9 to *bcr* on 22
   c. *bcr:abl* alters growth regulation, fusion protein has constitutive tyrosine kinase activity that acts to promote cell cycling
   d. Translocation ALSO present in lymphocytes (except for long-lived memory cells)

Table 11.7 Differential for CML versus Leukemoid Reaction

Test/Sign	CML	Leukemoid Reaction
Philadelphia chromosome	⊕	–
Maturation of peripheral cells	**Blasts** with marked left shift	Left shift with fewer blasts
WBC count	Very high	High (usually less than 1×10^5)
Leukocyte alkaline phosphatase	**Low**	**High**
Basophilia	⊕	–
Platelet counts	Very high	High
Splenomegaly	Present	Absent
Arthritis/Uricemia	⊕	–
Myeloid:Erythroid marrow ratio	Greater than 10:1	Less than 10:1
Serum B_{12}	Increased	Normal
Malaise	+/–	+++

e. **Even pts without Ph chromosome invariably have *bcr:abl* translocation on a scale too small to be seen by karyotype**

D. Chronic lymphocytic leukemia (CLL)
1. Increasing incidence with age, causes 30% of leukemias in US
2. 95% are memory B-cell types (a form of blood-borne lymphoma) **expressing the CD5 protein as a surface marker**
3. Si: organomegaly, +/– anemia, later stages see thrombocytopenia due to autoimmunity
4. Laboratory: normal morphology lymphocytosis of blood & marrow, monoclonal antibodies (check lambda vs. kappa light chain to determine monoclonality), autoimmune hemolysis (Coombs'⊕, ↑ indirect bilirubin, ↓ haptoglobin, spherocytosis) (see Figure 11.8)
5. Anemia occurs due to autoimmunity, splenomegaly, bone marrow infiltration, chemotherapy

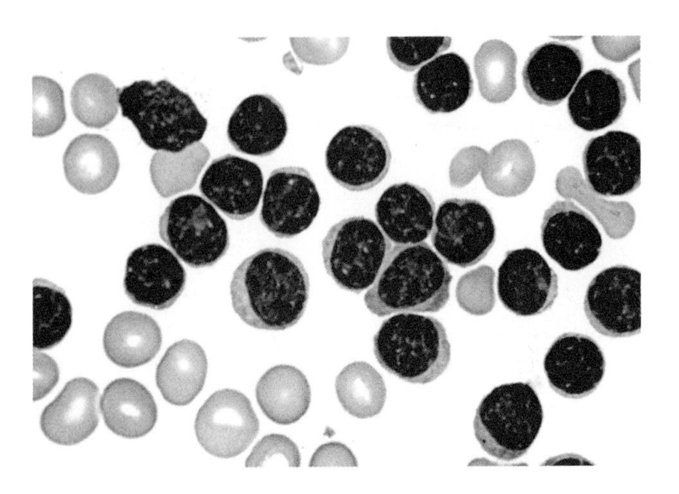

Figure 11.8 Chronic Lymphocytic Leukemia
A smear of peripheral blood exhibits numerous small-to-medium sized lymphocytes. A smudge cell is seen upper left. (From Rubin E, Gorstein F, Rubin R, et al. Rubin's Pathology: Clinicopathologic Foundations of Medicine. 4th ed. Baltimore: Lippincott Williams & Wilkins, 2005.)

6. **Tx: early therapy does NOT prolong life, infection is #1 cause of death, treatment is palliative**
7. Two staging systems, Rai & Binet, involving number of nodes involved & associated organomegaly
8. Chromosome 12 & 14 abnormalities noted
9. *bcl-1* translocated from 11 next to Ig heavy chain promoter on 14
10. Differential: viral infection, but leukocytes won't be small, resting cells
11. Other presentations of similar leukemias
    a. Hairy cell leukemia (B-cell subtype)
        (1) Si/Sx = pancytopenia, erythema nodosum, characteristic hairy cell morphology
        (2) Tx: IFN-α, splenectomy
    b. T-cell leukemias
        (1) T-cell subtype of CLL is rare & tends to be less aggressive, not associated with HTLV
        (2) Human T-cell leukemia virus (HTLV)
            (a) HTLV is endemic to Japan & the Caribbean, transmitted like HIV, via placenta, body fluids & sex

(b) Causes endemic T-cell leukemia, different from T-cell CLL

(c) HTLV also causes tropical spastic paraparesis

(i) Insidious paresis in lower extremities only

(ii) Minimal to mild changes in sensation

(iii) Marked lower extremity hyperreflexia, paralysis, & urinary incontinence

(3) $\gamma\delta$ T-cell leukemias can occur in the gut

(4) Large granular lymphocyte leukemia (T-cell subtype)

(a) Cells have mature CD8 or NK cell morphology

(b) Si/Sx = neutropenia, splenomegaly, arthritis, mild leukocytosis, lymphadenopathy, ↑ blood Ca^{2+}

(5) Generally T-cell leukemias involve skin, often present with erythematous rashes

Most Common Leukemias by Age:
Up to age 15 = ALL; age 15–39 = AML; age 40–59 = AML & CML, age 60 & over = CLL

VII. Lymphoma

A. General characteristics

1. Lymphomas are solid tumors of the lymphoid system (lymph node, tonsils, GI tract, spleen, & liver)
2. Present with large nontender, firm, fixed lymph nodes
3. These are differentiated from reactive lymph nodes, which are tender, soft, moveable & smaller
4. Typically lymphoma is not found in bone marrow like leukemia
5. 2 major types of lymphoma are Hodgkin's & non-Hodgkin's

B. Non-Hodgkin's lymphoma (NHL)

1. Description
   a. Histology → diffuse or follicular (nodular)
   b. Grade → low, intermediate, or high, related to degree of differentiation of cell type
   c. Morphology → large or small cell with multiple variants (e.g., cleaved or noncleaved)
2. Follicular vs. diffuse type
   a. Follicular (nodular) type

(1) Rare in children, better Px than diffuse counterpart

(2) Is a B-cell type
(3) Those with small cells do better than large cells

b. Diffuse type
(1) More aggressive than nodular
(2) Either B-cell or T-cell type
(3) Highly aggressive (high grade) are always diffuse

3. Grade
   a. Low grade → small lymphocytic, follicular small cleaved cell, follicular mixed small cleaved
   b. Intermediate grade → follicular large cell, diffuse small cleaved cell, diffuse mixed/small/large cell types
   c. High grade
      (1) The most aggressive NHLs; all are histologically diffuse types
      (2) Types
         (a) Immunoblastic type seen in immunocompromised
         (b) Lymphoblastic involves mediastinum & bone marrow, is TdT positive & has T-cell markers
         (c) **Small Noncleaved cell = Burkitt's lymphoma**
            (i) B-cell type, closely linked to Epstein-Barr virus
            (ii) African Burkitt's (endemic) involves jaw bones
            (iii) US form involves abdomen more commonly
            (iv) **Classic histologic description is the "starry sky pattern,"** caused by dark background of densely packed lymphocytes (sky) with light colored spots in them caused by scattered macrophages (the stars)
            (v) Translocation of *c-myc* from chromosome 8 to chromosome 14 Ig heavy chain locus
4. Cutaneous T-cell lymphoma (CTCL, mycosis fungoides)
   a. Slowly progressive CD4+ T-cell lymphoma of the skin, usually occurring in elderly
   b. **Classic histologic description → cells contain cerebriform nuclei** (nucleus looks like cerebral gyri) (see Figure 11.9)
   c. Often presents with systemic erythroderma, a total body erythematous & pruritic rash, which can precede clinically apparent malignancy by years
   d. Leukemic phase of this disease is called "Sézary syndrome"
5. Angiocentric T-cell lymphoma
   a. 2 subtypes = nasal T-cell lymphoma (lethal midline granuloma) & pulmonary angiocentric lymphoma (Wegener's granulomatosis)

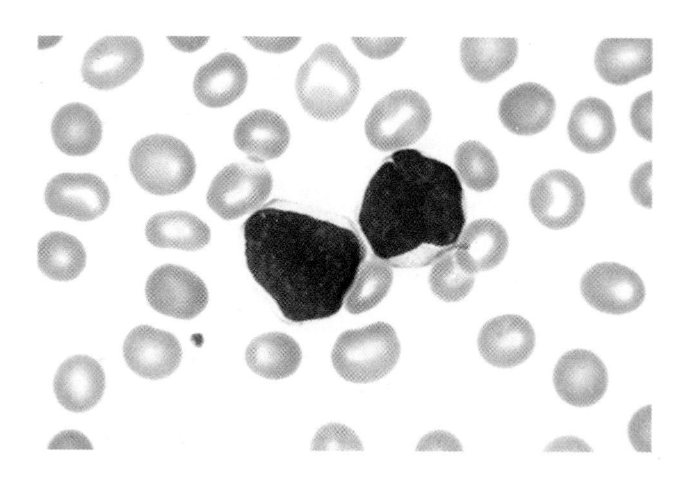

Figure 11.9 Sézary Cells
Two circulating, neoplastic, T-helper cells with irregular nuclei and a thin rim of cytoplasm are seen. (From Rubin E, Gorstein F, Rubin R, et al. Rubin's Pathology: Clinicopathologic Foundations of Medicine. 4th ed. Baltimore: Lippincott Williams & Wilkins, 2005.)

b. Nasal T-cell lymphoma is EBV associated
c. Both are highly lethal, nonresponsive to chemotherapy
d. Classic presentation = large mass that when biopsied is nondiagnostic due to large areas of necrosis within mass
e. Can cause airway compromise by local compression/edema
f. Tx = palliative radiation therapy

C. Hodgkin's lymphoma
1. Occurs in a bimodal age distribution, young men (women for nodular sclerosis type, see below) & geriatric population
2. EBV infection is present in up to 50% of cases
3. Si/Sx resemble inflammatory disorder, **classic Pel-Epstein fevers** (fevers wax & wane over weeks), chills, night sweats, weight loss, leukocytosis, **in some pts sx worsen with alcohol intake**
4. Reed-Sternberg (RS) cells
   a. Possibly the malignant cell of Hodgkin's
   b. **Classically appear as binucleated giant cells ("owl eyes") with eosinophilic inclusions** (see Figure 11.10)
   c. **One variation is Lacunar cell, a mononucleated giant cell**
   d. Dz severity is proportional to number of R-S cells seen in tumor

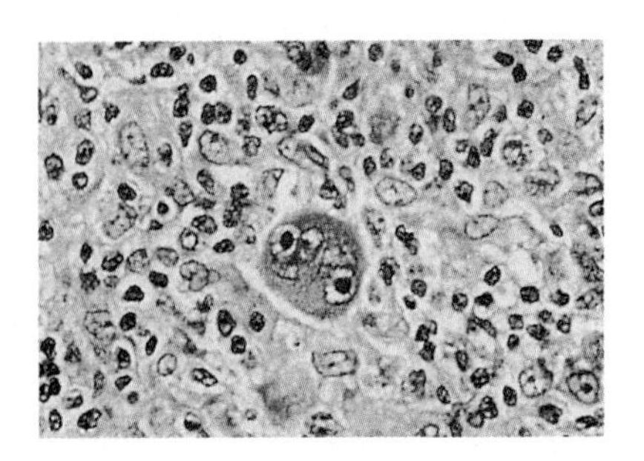

Figure 11.10
Reed-Sternberg cell in patient with Hodgkin's disease.

5. Rye classification contains 4 variants
    a. Lymphocytic predominance is least frequently occurring, a B-cell type
    b. Mixed cellularity
        (1) Most frequently occurring type
        (2) Histology → lymphocytes, eosinophils, RS cells, plasma cells
    c. Nodular sclerosis
        (1) More frequent in women
        (2) Histology
            (a) **Nodular division of lymph nodes by fibrous bands**
            (b) **Lacunar cell RS variant**
    d. Lymphocyte depletion
        (1) Poorest prognosis
        (2) Histology → frequent necrosis, many RS cells
6. Clinical staging more closely linked to Px than histologic type
    a. Stage I = 1 lymph node involved
    b. Stage II = 2 or more lymph nodes on same side of diaphragm
    c. Stage III = involvement on both sides of diaphragm
    d. Stage IV = disseminated, ≥1 organ or extranodal tissue involved
    e. Type A = systemic symptoms absent
    f. Type B = systemic symptoms present (e.g., fever, night sweats, unexpected weight loss >10%)

12. DERMATOLOGY

I. Terminology

1. Macule = flat discoloration, $<$ 1cm in diameter
2. Papule = elevated skin lesion, $<$ 1cm in diameter
3. Plaque = similar to papule but $>$ 1cm in diameter.
4. Vesicle = small fluid containing lesion $<$ 0.5 cm in diameter.
5. Wheal = like a vesicle but occurs transiently as in urticaria (hives)
6. Bulla = large fluid containing lesion, $>$ 0.5 cm in diameter.
7. Lichenification = accentuated skin markings in thickened epidermis, induced by constant scratching
8. Acanthosis = increased thickness of stratum spinosum
9. Keloid = an irregular raised lesion resulting from scar tissue hypertrophy
10. Tinea = fungal infection that can affect scalp (Tinea capitis), body (corpora), inguinal area (cruris), athlete's foot (pedis), nails (onychomycosis)
11. Tinea versicolor is due to *Malassezia furfur* or *Pityrosporum ovale*, found on upper trunk, appear as hypo- or hyperpigmented lesions
12. Petechiae = flat, pinhead, nonblanching, red-purple lesion caused by hemorrhage into the skin: seen in any cause of thrombocytopenia
13. Purpura = flat, nonblanching, red-purple lesion, larger than petechiae, caused by hemorrhage into skin: seen in Henoch-Schönlein purpura (HSP) & thrombotic thrombocytopenia purpura (TTP)
14. Exanthem = rash arising as a cutaneous manifestation of infectious disease (dz)
15. Enanthem = intraoral rash that arises as a manifestation of infectious disease (e.g., Koplik's spots in measles)

II. Histology

A. Layers of skin

1. Epidermis is of ectodermal origin
   a. Stratum corneum
   b. Stratum lucidum, only present in extremely thick skin

   c. Stratum granulosum
   d. Stratum spinosum (prickle cell layer)
   e. Stratum germinativum (basalis)
   f. Melanocytes & Merkel cells are of neural crest origin
2. Dermis is of mesenchymal origin
   a. Papillary dermis
   b. Reticular layer

B. Histologic descriptions
1. Hyperkeratosis = increased thickness of stratum corneum (seen in chronic dermatitis)
2. Parakeratosis = hyperkeratosis with retention of nuclei in stratum corneum & thinning of stratum granulosum (usually seen in psoriasis)
3. Acantholysis = loss of cohesion between epidermal cells (seen in pemphigus vulgaris)
4. Spongiosis = intercellular edema causing stretching & loss of desmosomal attachment, allowing formation of blisters within epidermis (seen in acute & subacute dermatitis)

III. Common Disorders

A. Psoriasis
1. Seen more frequently in certain HLA types, due to some unknown genetic component
2. Pink plaques with silvery scaling **occurring on extensor surfaces such as elbows & knees** (also scalp, lumbosacral, glans penis, intergluteal cleft) & **fingernail pitting**
3. **Köbner's phenomenon** = psoriatic lesions appear at sites of cutaneous trauma (skin scratching, rubbing, or wound)
4. Histology: even elongation of rete ridges, **parakeratosis,** absent granulosa layer, **microabscesses of Munro** (neutrophil aggregates within stratum corneum)
5. **Classic diagnostic sign: Auspitz sign = removal of overlying scale → pinpoint bleeding due to thin epidermis above dermal papillae** (see Figure 12.1)
6. Treatment (Tx) = topical steroids (first line), UV light
7. If psoriasis is refractory to first line, use PUVA (second line)
   a. PUVA = **P**soralens + **UVA** light
   b. Psoralens intercalates into DNA, is activated by UV light to inhibit DNA synthesis
   c. Methotrexate & cyclosporin A for third line

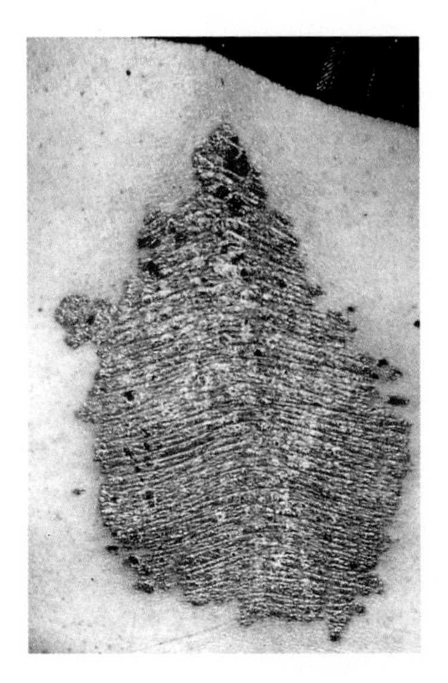

Figure 12.1 Psoriasis
Large plaque on the back with scales and minute bleeding sites (Auspitz sign). (From Berg D. Advanced Clinical Skills and Physical Diagnosis. Oxford: Blackwell Science, 1999.)

B. Eczema (Eczematous Dermatitis)
  1. A group of superficial, pruritic, inflammatory skin disorders
  2. Common etiologies
    a. Chemicals cause contact dermatitis, a delayed-type hypersensitivity (see Figure 12.2)
    b. Atopy = inherited predisposition to asthma, allergies & atopic dermatitis
      (1) Patients have exaggerated allergic-type hypersensitivity
      (2) Atopic dermatitis
        (a) **Atopic dermatitis is an "itch that rashes,"** the eczema is secondary (2°) to scratching the chronic pruritus
        (b) Commonly found on the face in infancy
        (c) Later in childhood can present on the flexor surfaces such as antecubital & popliteal fossa

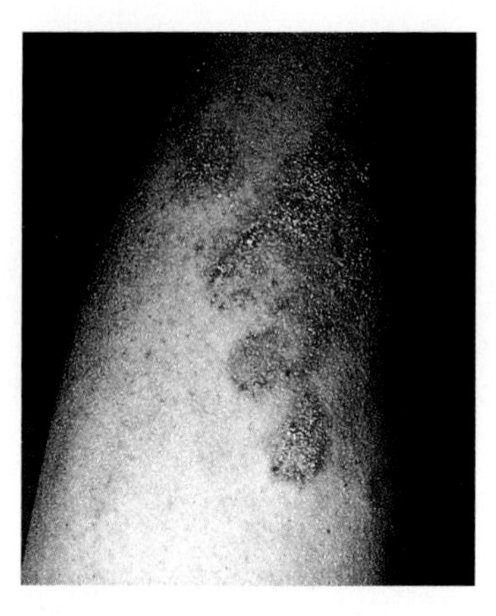

Figure 12.2 Contact Dermatitis
Lower-extremity skin. Extremely pruritic plaques and patches with vesicles and crusting due to recent exposure to the noxious oils of poison ivy. (From Berg D. Advanced Clinical Skills and Physical Diagnosis. Oxford: Blackwell Science, 1999.)

3. Eczema has 3 stages
   a. Acute stage presents with spongiosis & vesicles
   b. Subacute stage presents with erythema, papules, & edema
   c. Chronic stage presents with progressive acanthosis, hyperkeratosis & lichenification
4. Tx = avoid skin irritants, keep skin moist with lotions, steroids & antihistamines can be used for symptomatic relief
5. Steroids have 4 basic strengths
   a. Low potency = 1% hydrocortisone
   b. Moderate potency = 0.1% triamcinolone
   c. High potency = Fluocinonide (Lidex)
   d. Very high potency = Diflorasone
6. Weakest potency can be used on face, genitals, & skin folds to prevent skin atrophy & striae; also used in infants & children to prevent systemic side effects
7. Avoid using fluorinated steroids on face, but consider them for areas of thick skin (palms & soles)

C. Urticaria (Hives)
   1. Very common disorder caused by mast cell degranulation & histamine release, inducing transient, localized edema, pruritus, & erythema

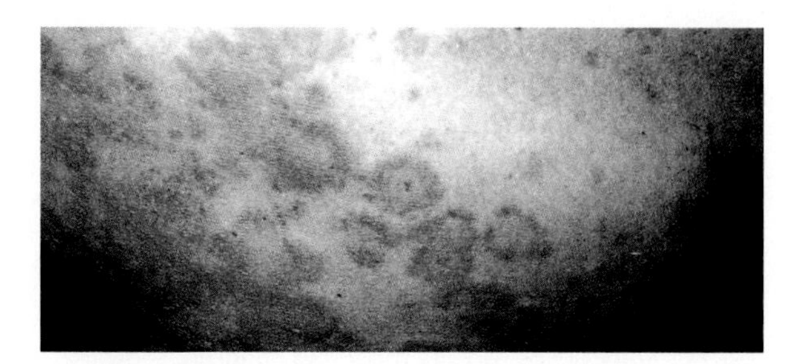

Figure 12.3 Urticaria on Skin of the Left Back
Pruritic papules and plaques are visible, some with an annular (ring-like) pattern. (From Berg D. Advanced Clinical Skills and Physical Diagnosis. Oxford: Blackwell Science, 1999.)

2. Most lesions are IgE-mediated (type I hypersensitivity), but certain chemicals in sensitive patients (pts), as well as inhibitors of prostaglandin synthesis (e.g., aspirin), can also cause IgE-independent reactions
3. Presents with wheals surrounded by erythema, dermographism (can write a word on the skin & it remains imprinted as erythematous wheals) (see Figure 12.3)
4. Urticaria rarely associated with angioedema of face, lips, tongue & respiratory tract
5. Tx = antihistamines & epinephrine

D. Pigmentation
1. Albinism
   a. Melanocytes are present but fail to produce pigment
   b. The oculocutaneous form predisposes to skin cancer
2. Vitiligo
   a. Loss of melanocytes in discrete areas of skin, appearing as depigmented patches
   b. Occurs in all races but is most apparent in darkly pigmented individuals
   c. May be autoimmune in nature
3. Freckle
   a. Also called "ephelis"
   b. Have normal melanocyte number but increased melanin within basal keratinocytes

4. Lentigo (liver spots) are pigmented macules caused by melanocyte hyperplasia that, unlike freckles, do not darken with sun exposure
5. Nevocellular nevus
   a. Common mole, benign tumor derived from melanocytes
   b. Variations of nevi
      (1) Blue nevus: a black-blue nodule present at birth, often mistaken for melanoma
      (2) Spitz nevus: occurs mostly in children, red-pink nodule, confused with hemangioma or melanoma, often having spindle-shaped cells
      (3) Dysplastic nevus: atypical, reddish-pigmented lesion, with dermal fibrosis, dermal lymphocytic infiltration, proliferation of melanocytes, & a marked tendency to transform into malignant melanoma
      (4) Dysplastic nevus syndrome is the autosomal dominant inherited form
6. Melasma (chloasma)
   a. A mask-like hyperpigmentation on face seen in pregnancy
   b. Sunlight accentuates the pigmentation, which eventually fades after delivery
   c. Tx = hydroxyquinone cream (works for any ↑ pigmentation)
7. Hemangioma
   a. Capillary hemangiomas present at birth
      (1) Port-wine stains (purple red on face or neck)
      (2) Strawberry hemangiomas (bright red raised lesions)
      (3) Cherry hemangiomas (small red papule)
      (4) These are all benign & usually disappear on their own
   b. More severe cutaneous hemangiomas occur in neurocutaneous syndromes (see below, Section IV.D)
8. Xanthoma
   a. Yellowish papules, often accumulations of foamy histiocytes
   b. Can be idiopathic or associated with familial hyperlipidemia
   c. If seen on eyelids they are called "xanthelasma"
9. Bronze diabetes = primary (1°) hemochromatosis
   a. Familial defect causing intestinal hyperabsorption of iron
   b. Iron becomes deposited in a variety of organs, but most heavily in liver & pancreas

c. **Classic triad: ↑ skin pigmentation, cirrhosis, diabetes mellitus**
d. Other symptoms (Sx) = cardiomyopathy, pituitary failure, & hepatocellular CA arthropathies
e. **Clinical pearl: hemochromatosis is the likely diagnosis (Dx) in any patient with osteoarthritis involving the metacarpophalangeal (MCP) joints**
f. Characteristic laboratory finding is transferrin saturation (iron/TIBC) ≥50%
g. Tx = phlebotomy, which improves survival if started early

10. Addison's disease causes hyperpigmentation [see Endocrinology, Section III.C.3]
11. Pityriasis
    a. Pityriasis alba
        (1) Areas of hypopigmentation on face or upper extremities differentiated from tinea versicolor by KOH prep
        (2) Tinea versicolor has characteristic "spaghetti & meatball" appearance on KOH prep
    b. Pityriasis rosea = erythematous maculopapular rash appearing on back in a Christmas tree distribution
12. Erythema nodosum
    a. Inflammation of subcutaneous fat (panniculitis) with involvement of adjacent vessels
    b. Caused by immunologic reaction provoked by infection, drugs, or systemic diseases
    c. Characteristic lesions are **tender red nodules occurring on the lower legs** & sometimes forearms
    d. Some patients have painful joints & fever
    e. Usually resolves in 6–8 weeks, Tx directed at underlying cause
    f. Common causes
        (1) Infections = *Mycoplasma, Chlamydia, Coccidioides, Mycobacterium leprae* & others
        (2) Drugs = sulfonamides & contraceptive pills
        (3) Chronic inflammation = inflammatory bowel disease, sarcoidosis, rheumatic fever
        (4) Pregnancy
13. Dermatomyositis
    a. An autoimmune disorder sometimes seen with polymyositis (see Musculoskeletal, Section V.D.4)
    b. Presents with erythematous scaly rash on hands, heliotropic (reddish-purple) patches on eyelids

14. Seborrheic keratosis
    a. Black or brown benign plaques, 3–20 mm diameter
    b. Appear to be stuck onto skin surface
    c. Commonly seen in elderly, & runs in families
    d. Can be mistaken for melanoma
    e. Tx = liquid nitrogen freezing, usually too many to treat
15. Acanthosis nigricans
    a. Black velvety plaques on flexor surfaces & intertriginous areas
    b. Seen in obesity & endocrine disorders (e.g., diabetes)
    c. Can mark underlying malignancy (e.g., GI/GU, lymphoma)
    d. Induced by nicotinic acid, cortisol, estrogens, growth hormone
16. Seborrheic dermatitis
    a. Common disorder of infants & elderly
    b. Signs (Si)/Sx = erythema, scaling, white flaking (dandruff) near sebaceous glands (face, scalp, groin, axilla, external ear)
    c. Dx = clinical & KOH prep to rule out fungal infection
    d. Tx = selenium sulfide shampoo on face & trunk

IV. Cancer

A. Malignant melanoma
   1. Increasing in age-adjusted incidence
   2. Most common in lightly pigmented individuals, sun exposure is an important pathogenic factor
   3. Can arise from melanoma cells or dysplastic nevus cells
   4. Growth can occur in all directions, but usually begins by growing radially or laterally within the epidermis & superficial dermis (papillary zone), from where it does not metastasize (see Figure 12.4)
   5. **Melanomas kill people by high rate of metastasis**
   6. Clinically, lesion removal during lateral growth phase imparts a better prognosis due to far lower rate of metastasis
   7. Vertical growth phase consists of extension into the deep dermis
      a. **Lesions during this phase have a markedly increased capacity to metastasize**
      b. Most important prognostic factor = depth of lesion within dermis

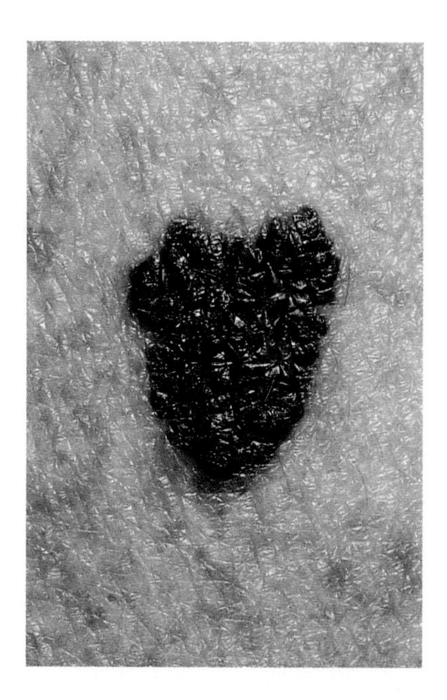

Figure 12.4 Superficial Spreading Melanoma
(From Axford JS. Medicine. Oxford: Blackwell Science, 1998.)

8. 4 types: superficial spreading, acral (nails), lentiginous (Hutchinson freckle), & nodular
9. Nodular melanoma begins with vertical phase, has the worst prognosis (Px)
10. Physical examination focuses on the **ABCDEs**
    a. **A**symmetry: benign lesions are usually symmetrical, melanomas are usually asymmetrical
    b. **B**order: benign lesions have smooth borders, melanomas have irregular borders
    c. **C**olor: benign lesions have only one color, melanomas have more than one color
    d. **D**iameter: benign lesions are usually < 6 mm in diameter, melanoma usually > 6 mm in diameter
    e. **E**levation: melanoma is usually elevated & palpable, especially when malignant
11. Tx = excision & perhaps regional lymph node dissection, consider adjunctive chemotherapy for systemic treatment or prophylaxis (generally not very effective)

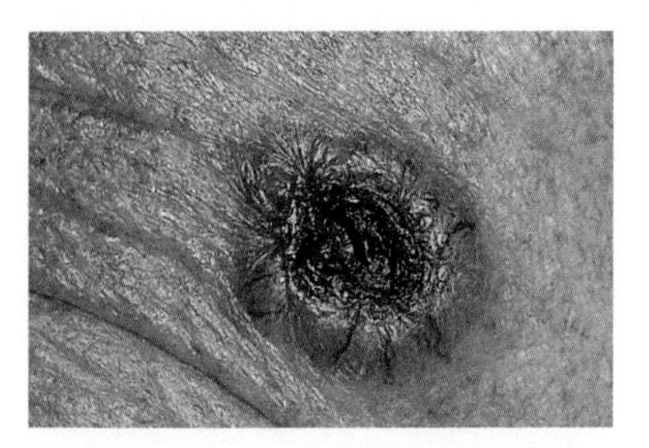

Figure 12.5 Classic Crateriform Basal Cell Carcinoma
Shown here is an ulcerating nodule. (From Axford JS. Medicine. Oxford: Blackwell Science, 1998.)

B. Basal cell carcinoma
   1. **Most common malignant skin tumor**
   2. Typically seen in sun-exposed areas
   3. **Rodent ulcer usually seen on face, with pearly borders & fine telangiectasias** (see Figure 12.5)
   4. Not usually found on lips
   5. Histologically look for palisade arrangement of nuclei & tumor islands
   6. Tx = excision, **these lesions virtually never metastasize**

C. Squamous cell carcinoma
   1. More common in elderly men, mostly occurring on sun-exposed areas
   2. **Actinic keratosis (AK) frequently precedes this form of skin cancer**
      a. AK = rough keratin plaques, usually seen on sun-exposed areas
      b. Lips, scalp, cheeks, & ear are commonly affected (see Figure 12.6)
   3. Squamous CA more likely to metastasize than basal cell CA, but not as likely as melanoma
   4. **Histologically look for keratin pearls**
   5. Tx = AK removal (using cryotherapy) before it converts to squamous cell CA, & excision of squamous cell CA before metastasis

D. Neurocutaneous syndromes (Phakomatoses)
   1. Tuberous sclerosis
      a. Autosomal dominant skin & CNS syndrome (see Neurology, Section VI.D)

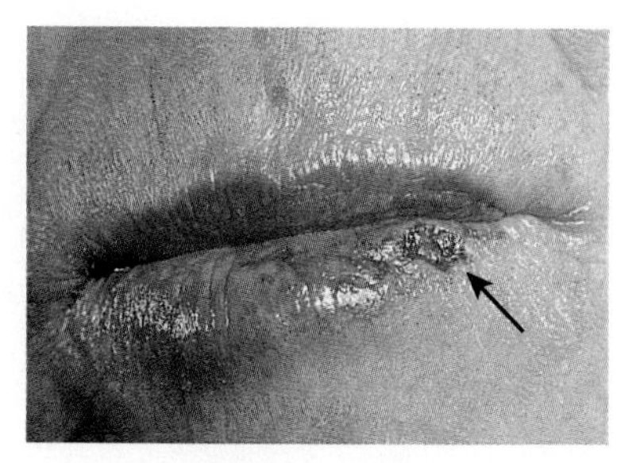

Figure 12.6 Squamous Cell Carcinoma of the Lip (Early Ulcer)
(From Axford JS. Medicine. Oxford: Blackwell Science, 1998.)

b. Skin findings include hypomelanotic macules (hypopigmented, described as ash leaf patches), leathery cutaneous thickening (Shagreen spots), & adenoma sebaceum of the face

2. Neurofibromatosis (NF) [see Neurology, Section IV.C.2]
   a. Autosomal dominant
   b. Presents with café-au-lait spots, neurofibromas, meningiomas, acoustic schwannomas, kyphoscoliosis
   c. NF 2 presents with bilateral acoustic neuromas (CN VIII)
3. Sturge-Weber
   a. No genetic pattern
   b. Presents with port-wine hemangioma of face, in the distribution of the trigeminal nerve, which also involves the meninges
   c. Mental retardation & seizures accompany this disorder
4. von Hippel-Lindau syndrome
   a. Autosomal dominant syndrome of diffuse hemangiomas
   b. ↑ risk of developing renal cell CA, also associated with increased secretion of erythropoietin causing polycythemia

E. Kaposi's sarcoma
1. Endothelial cell cancer caused by human herpes virus 8
2. Appears as red/purple plaques or nodules on skin & mucosa (see Figure 12.7)
3. Frequently also affects GI viscera & lungs
4. **Almost exclusively seen in homosexual AIDS patients (not in AIDS patients who contracted HIV by IV drug abuse)**
5. No effective Tx, although may regress with strong HIV Tx

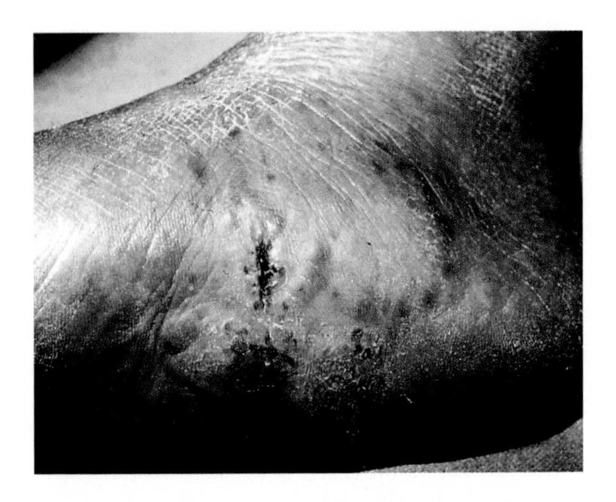

Figure 12.7 Kaposi's Sarcoma, Plantar Aspect of the Foot
Multiple purple papules and nodules are seen, which may become confluent. The patient has an area of bacterial infection associated with the lesions. The patient had AIDS with a CD4 count of 34 at the time of the photograph. (From Berg D. Advanced Clinical Skills and Physical Diagnosis. Oxford: Blackwell Science, 1999.)

V. Blistering Disorders

A. Pemphigus vulgaris (PG)
   1. PG is a rare autoimmune disorder, **affecting 20–40 year olds**
   2. **IgG autoantibodies are directed against an epidermal cement substance** (desmoglein III, a cadherin)
   3. IgG titers correlate with course of disease
   4. Destruction of cement substance leads to intraepidermal acantholysis **with sparing of basal layer**
   5. Demonstrated by classic **immunofluorescence surrounding epidermal cells showing "tombstone fluorescent pattern"** (see Figure 12.8)
   6. PE shows **flaccid epidermal bullae** that easily slough off leaving large denuded areas of skin (Nikolsky's sign), subject to 2° infection
   7. **Can be fatal if not treated**
   8. Tx = steroids

B. Bullous pemphigoid (BP)
   1. Resembles PG but much less severe clinically
   2. Common autoimmune disease affecting **mostly the elderly**

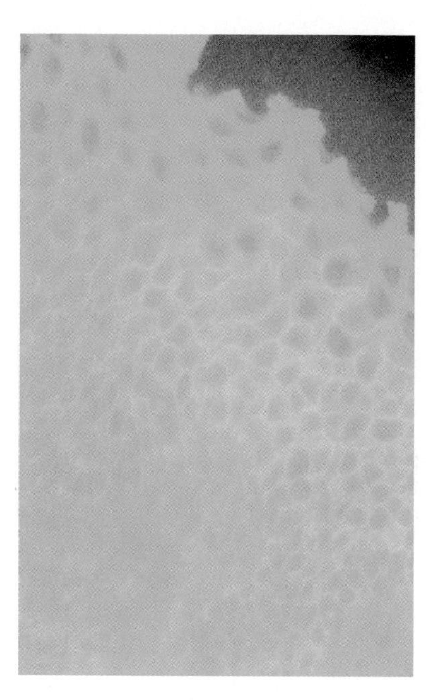

Figure 12.8 Bright Green Immunofluorescence of IgG in the Intercellular Space in a Patient with Pemphigus Vulgaris
(From Axford JS. Medicine. Oxford: Blackwell Science, 1998.)

3. **IgG antibodies directed against an antigen in the epidermal basement membrane**
4. Demonstrated by **immunofluorescence as a linear band along the basement membrane** (lamina lucida layer) (see Figure 12.9)
5. Increased eosinophils can usually be seen in dermis
6. Physical examination shows **hard, tense bullae** that do not rupture easily & usually heal without scarring if uninfected

C. Erythema multiforme

1. Characterized by **target-like lesions** (see Figure 12.10)
2. Caused by a hypersensitivity response to certain drugs or infections, or to systemic disorders such as malignancy or collagen vascular disease
3. Commonly lesions accompany a herpes eruption (prevent eruption of herpes with acyclovir & prevent erythema multiforme)
4. Lesions come in many forms, hence the name "multiforme"

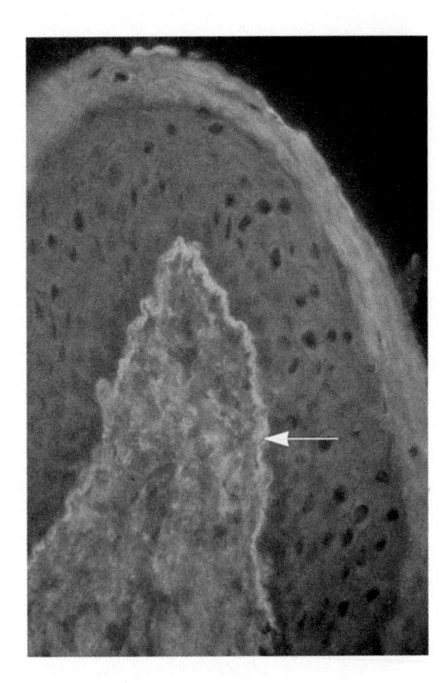

Figure 12.9 Bright Green Immunofluorescence of IgG at the BMZ (arrow) in a Patient with Pemphigoid
(From Axford JS. Medicine. Oxford: Blackwell Science, 1998.)

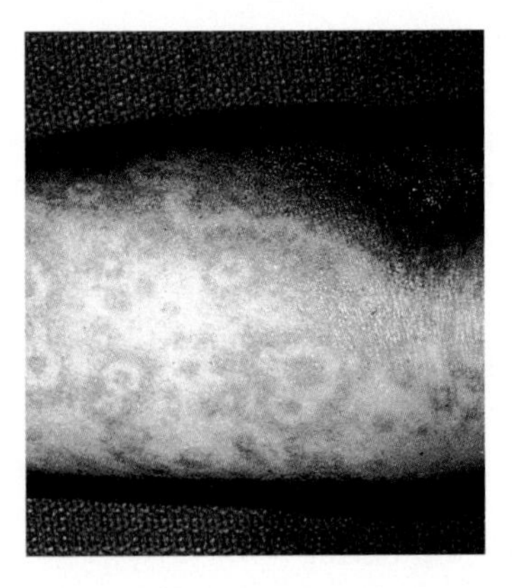

Figure 12.10 Erythema Multiforme, Volar Aspect of the Forearm
Target-shaped erythematous lesions are shown on a patient who was administered TMP/sulfa for a week prior to development of the rash. (From Berg D. Advanced Clinical Skills and Physical Diagnosis. Oxford: Blackwell Science, 1999.)

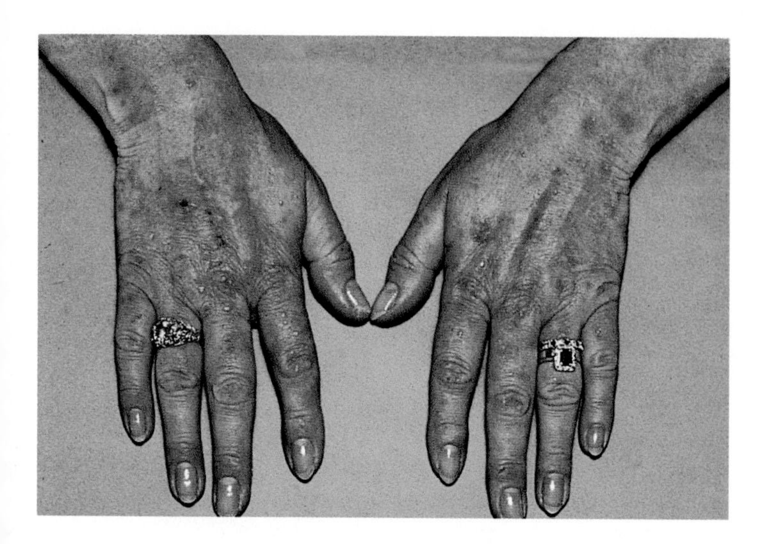

Figure 12.11 Porphyria Cutanea Tarda
Blisters, erosions, and scars are visible on the dorsal aspect of hands. (From Axford JS. Medicine. Oxford: Blackwell Science, 1998.)

5. **A severe febrile form (sometimes fatal) is Stevens-Johnson syndrome, where hemorrhagic crusting also affects lips & oral mucosa**

D. Cutaneous porphyria tarda
1. Autosomal dominant defect in heme synthesis (50% ↓ in uroporphyrinogen decarboxylase activity in RBC & liver)
2. Si/Sx = blisters on sun-exposed areas of face & hands (see Figure 12.11), ↑ facial hair around temples & cheeks, under Woods lamp **urine fluoresces with distinctive orange-pink color due to ↑ levels of uroporphyrins**
3. **No abdominal pain** (differentiates from other porphyrias)
4. Course = remitting/relapsing, exacerbations due to hepatitis virus, hepatoma, alcohol abuse, estrogen, sunlight
5. Tx = sunscreen, phlebotomy, chloroquine, no EtOH

VI. Viral Exanthems

A. Measles (Rubeola)
1. Caused by a **paramyxovirus**
2. Presents with erythematous maculopapular rash, erupts about 5 days after onset of prodromal symptoms

3. **To diagnose measles, use the 3 Cs: cough, coryza, conjunctivitis**
4. **In addition, a high fever must be present**
5. **Koplik spots (white spots on an erythematous base appearing on the buccal mucosa) are pathognomonic,** however will disappear by the time the rash onsets so are often not found upon presentation of patient
6. Measles rash begins on the head & spreads downward, lasting 4–5 days resolving from the head downward

B. Rubella (German Measles)
1. Caused by a **togavirus**
2. **Presents with suboccipital lymphadenopathy** (one of the very few diseases to do this) & maculopapular rash
3. Rash begins on face, then becomes generalized, lasts 5 days
4. Fever may accompany rash on first day only
5. May find reddish spots of various sizes on soft palate

C. Hand, foot & mouth disease
1. Caused by **Coxsackie A** virus
2. Vesicular rash on hands & feet with ulcerations in the mouth
3. Rash clears in about 1 week

D. Roseola infantum (Exanthem Subitum)
1. Caused by **herpes virus 6**
2. Often begins with **abrupt high fever persisting for 1–5 days even though child has no physical signs to account for fever & does not experience malaise**
3. Once high fever drops rash appears
4. Macular or maculopapular rash appears on the trunk, spreads peripherally over entire body
5. Rash often resolves in 24hr

E. Erythema infectiosum (Fifth Disease)
1. Caused by **parvovirus B-19**
2. **Classic finding is "slapped cheeks,"** erythema of the cheeks
3. Subsequently an erythematous maculopapular rash involves the arms & spreads to trunk & legs forming a reticular pattern
4. This disease may be dangerous in sickle cell pts (& other anemias) due to parvovirus B-19's tendency to cause aplastic crises in such patients

F. Varicella (Chicken Pox)
1. Caused by the **varicella-zoster virus,** a type of herpes virus
2. Highly contagious, pruritic "tear drop" vesicles that break & crust over, beginning on face or trunk (centripetal) & spreading toward extremities
3. New lesions appear for 3–5 days & typically take 3 days to crust over, so rash persists for about 1 week
4. **Lesions are contagious until they crust over**
5. Vesicles can be found on scalp & mucous membranes
6. Zoster (shingles) represents a reactivation of an old varicella infection
7. Painful skin eruptions are seen along the distribution of dermatomes that correspond to the affected dorsal root ganglia

G. Verrucae (Warts)
1. Verruca vulgaris = hand wart
2. Verruca plana (flat wart) is smaller than vulgaris, seen on hands & face
3. Verruca plantaris or palmaris appears on soles & palms
4. Human papilloma virus (HPV) types 1–4 cause skin & plantar warts
5. HPV 6 & HPV 11 cause anorectal & genital warts (condyloma acuminatum)
6. HPV 16, 18, 31, 33, 35 cause cervical cancer
7. Condylomata lata are flat warts caused by *Treponema pallidum* (syphilis)

VII. Bacterial Cutaneous Disorders

A. Acne
1. Acne is an inflammatory disease of pilosebaceous unit
2. Caused by *Propionibacterium acnes*
3. Open comedones are termed "blackheads" & closed comedones are termed "whiteheads"
4. Tx = systemic antibiotics, topical antibiotics, Retin-A, benzoyl peroxide, if acne is scarring consider Accutane

B. Impetigo
1. Superficial epidermal infection characterized by honey-crusted lesions (see Figure 12.12)
2. Can be bullous or nonbullous, with nonbullous being the most common

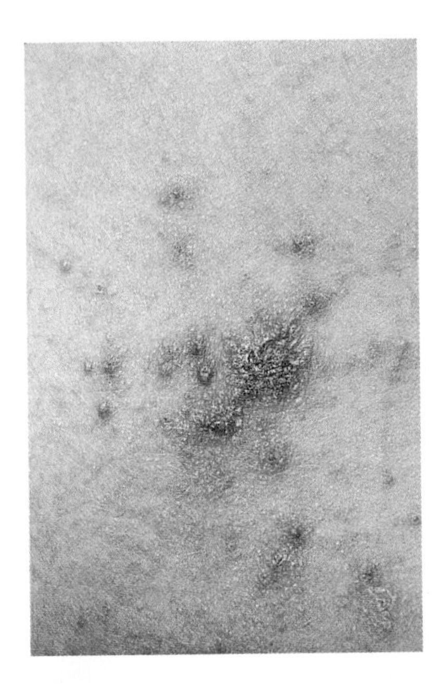

Figure 12.12 Impetigo
Vesicopustules with golden crust are shown. (From Axford JS. Medicine. Oxford: Blackwell Science, 1998.)

3. Vesicles occur most often in children around the nose & mouth
4. Common organisms include *Staphylococcus aureus* & *Streptococcus pyogenes*
5. Blisters produced by a toxin (often epidermolysin)
6. Tx = systemic antibiotics for 7–10 days

C. Scarlet fever
1. *Streptococcus pyogenes* (group A Strep = GAS) is the cause
2. Rash (**"sunburn with goose bumps"**) is erythematous, finely punctate, blanches with pressure, appears initially on trunk becomes generalized within a few hours to several days
3. Sandpaper rough skin, **strawberry tongue,** beefy red pharynx, circumoral pallor
4. **Pastia's lines = rash, worst in the creases of the axillae & groin**
5. Eventual desquamation of hands & feet as rash resolves

6. Systemic symptoms include fever, chills, delirium, sore throat, & cervical adenopathy, all of which appear at same time as rash
7. Complications include rheumatic fever & glomerulonephritis (these can also result from postop GAS wound infection)
8. Tx = Penicillin

D. Hidradenitis suppurativa
1. Plugged apocrine glands (similar to cystic acne) presenting as inflamed masses in groin/axilla, become secondarily infected
2. Tx = surgical débridement & antibiotics

E. Bacillary angiomatosis
1. Red or purple vascular lesions, from papule to hemangioma-sized, located anywhere on skin & disseminated to any organ
2. Almost always seen in HIV patients
3. Caused by *Bartonella henselae* & *Bartonella quintana*
4. Transmission via young cats, flea is thought to be vector
5. Lesions caused by dysregulated angiogenesis
6. Sx = fever, weight loss, abdominal pain, & dysfunction of any organ involved in dissemination
7. Dx = histopathology with visualization of organisms in lesion
8. Tx = erythromycin, highly effective

F. Rose spots
1. Seen in typhoid fever (*Salmonella typhi*)
2. Sx = high fever (often > 103° F), weakness, myalgias, anorexia, headache, abdominal tenderness, splenomegaly, constipation
3. **Rose spots** = small pink papules in groups of 1–2 dozen on trunk, found in 30% of typhoid fever patients
4. Some patients have **classic pulse-fever dissociation** = high fever with relative bradycardia (also seen in brucellosis)
5. **Tx for chronic asymptomatic typhoid fever (carrier state like "Typhoid Mary") is cholecystectomy because *S. typhi* resides in the gallbladder**

VIII. Systemic Diseases

A. Henoch-Schönlein purpura
1. Caused by an IgA-mediated angiitis, related to IgA nephropathy (Berger's disease)

2. Diagnostic rash = **palpable purpura** on legs & buttocks (in children)
3. Associated with abdominal pain, intussusception & glomerulonephritis
4. Tx usually not necessary, benign disorder that only rarely progresses to renal failure

B. Kawasaki's syndrome
1. Vasculitis that affects medium-sized vessels
2. Coronary artery aneurysms are deadly components of this dz
3. Most commonly presents in children 6 months → 4 years, usually in Asians
4. Patients present with high, unresponsive fever for at least 5 days
5. Additional Si/Sx: **CRASH** mnemonic
    a. **C**onjunctivitis
    b. **R**ash, primarily truncal, which can resemble any type of rash previously discussed
    c. **A**neurysms of coronary arteries
    d. **S**trawberry tongue, crusting of lips, fissuring of mouth & oropharyngeal erythema
    e. **H**ands & feet show induration, erythema of palms & soles, desquamation of fingers & toes
    f. Associated Sx = arthritis, diarrhea, hydrops of gallbladder, single node adenopathy (> 1.5 cm in neck)
    g. Laboratory: ↑ ESR, C-reactive protein, **thrombocytosis** (600,000–1,800,000)
6. Tx = ↑ dose aspirin, **steroids contraindicated in these pts**
7. Intravenous immunoglobulin may prevent cardiac disease

IX. Burns

A. First degree
1. Caused by damage limited to the epidermis
2. Appear as painful, reddened skin, will heal on their own without consequence

B. Second degree
1. Caused by damage extending partially into the dermis
2. Present with painful blistering, will heal on their own without consequence

C. Third degree

1. Caused by damage extending throughout the entire dermis
2. Present with blackened, leathery-appearing skin, require skin grafts to heal
3. **Third-degree burns damage cutaneous nerves, so these burns are characteristically painless**
4. Tx = fluid replacement, débride & cleanse area to prevent infection, give tetanus toxoid—do NOT give antibiotics prophylactically, only for specific infection
5. Most common infection is *Pseudomonas*

APPENDIX A. BASIC NEUROLOGY REVIEW

I. Spinal Cord (see Figure A.1)

A. Gray matter = dorsal horn + ventral horn
   1. Dorsal horn = somatosensory processing
   2. Ventral horn = α-motor neurons for striated muscle & γ-motor neurons for muscle spindles

B. White matter (dorsal columns, anterolateral system, corticospinal path)
   1. Dorsal columns carry **proprioception, vibration sense, fine touch**
      a. Skin afferent nerves, cell bodies in dorsal root, ascend in columns
      b. Synapse in nuclei in lower medulla, DECUSSATE
      c. Ascend as medial lemnisci, synapses at VPL nucleus in thalamus
      d. From thalamus travels to primary sensory cortex in parietal lobe, postcentral gyri
      e. Lesion above medulla causes contralateral deficit
      f. Lesion below medulla causes ipsilateral deficit
   2. Anterolateral system carries **pain, temperature, crude touch**
      a. Skin afferent nerves, cell bodies in dorsal root, synapse in dorsal horn of cord
      b. CROSS at same level, ascend in lateral white matter
      c. Synapse in thalamic VPL, axons then sent to primary sensory cortex, postcentral gyri
      d. Lesion above level of entrance to cord causes contralateral deficit
   3. Corticospinal path carries **motor commands**
      a. Axons originate at precentral gyri in parietal cortex
      b. Axons run through internal capsule to cerebral peduncles
      c. Become ipsilateral pyramidal tracts, DECUSSATE in medulla
      d. End up in lateral white matter, lateral corticospinal tract, synapse in anterior horn
      e. Anterior horn neurons send α- & γ-motor neurons to muscles
      f. Lesion above medulla causes contralateral deficit
      g. Lesion below medulla causes ipsilateral deficit

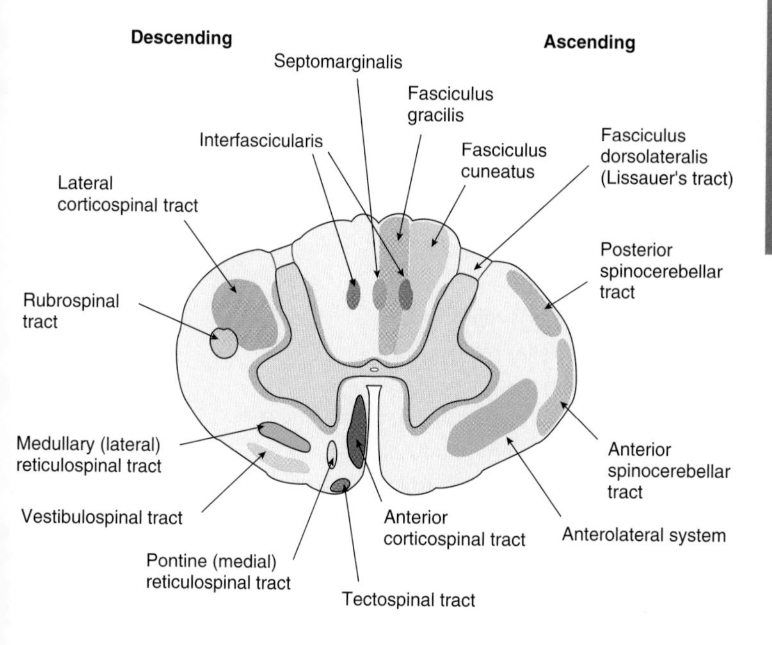

Figure A.1 Ascending and descending spinal tracts
This diagram indicates the size and position of the spinal tracts in the paired funiculi. Ascending tracts are shown on the right side, while descending tracts are shown on the left side. (Reproduced with permission from Pritchard TC and Alloway KD. Medical Neuroscience. Madison, Connecticut: Fence Creek Publishing, 1999:114. © Fence Creek Publishing, LLC.)

4. **Brown Sequard syndrome**
   a. Hemisection of spinal cord below the medulla
   b. Causes ipsilateral motor paralysis (pyramidal path), ipsilateral fine touch loss (dorsal column) & contralateral loss of pain/temperature sense (anterolateral column)
5. **Cauda Equina syndrome**
   a. Syndrome caused by impingement of spinal cord
   b. Symptoms (Sx) include impotence, incontinence, leg weakness, leg paresthesias

C. Reflexes
1. Myotatic reflex = deep tendon reflex (DTR)
   a. In parallel with muscle fibers

b. Ia afferents stimulated by muscle spindle stretch ⇒ synapse of α-motor neurons in anterior horn to contract homonymous muscle—also disynaptic inhibition of antagonists

c. γ-motor neurons contract spindle fibers to stretch spindle ⇒ synapse α-motor neurons of same muscle to maintain tone during contraction when the spindle can no longer sense stretch

d. Nerve roots of DTRs

(1) Biceps reflex = C5

(2) Triceps reflex = C7

(3) Patellar reflex = L4

(4) Achilles reflex = S1

2. Golgi tendon reflex (inverse myotatic reflex)

a. In series with extrafusal fibers

b. Contraction leads to inhibition of homonymous & synergistic muscles & excitation of antagonists

c. Also responds to extreme stretch to protect muscle from overexertion

3. Flexor withdrawal reflex

a. Nociceptive pain fibers are afferent signals

b. Leads to multiple level excitation of flexors & inhibition of extensors on the same side of the body as the pain emanated from

c. Leads to multiple inhibition of flexors & excitation of extensors on contralateral side—this helps the body maintain balance while withdrawing from the nociceptive stimulus

D. Practical anatomy

1. Anterior horn of gray matter swells at C4-T1 (brachial plexus) & L2-S3 (lumbosacral trunk)

2. Spine extends to L1–L2 in adults, subarachnoid space extends to S2

3. Lumbar puncture should be performed between L4 and L5

4. L4–L5 can be approximated at the level of the superior iliac crests

E. Upper vs. Lower motor neuron syndromes

1. Lower motor syndromes ⇒ hyporeflexia, hypotonia, muscle atrophy, fibrillation/fasciculation

2. Upper motor syndromes ⇒ hyperreflexia, hypertonia, +/− atrophy, ! Babinski sign (toes upgoing)

II. Brain Stem

A. Hindbrain

1. Location
    a. Caudally to the decussation of the pyramids at the junction of spinal cord to medulla
    b. Rostrally to the central canal opens into the fourth ventricle
2. Superior cerebellar peduncle forms fourth ventricle roof

B. Midbrain

1. Functional anatomy
    a. Cerebral aqueduct (of Sylvius) connects third & fourth ventricles
    b. Roof of midbrain = the colliculi (see Figures A.2 and A.3)
        (1) The inferior colliculi = auditory goes to medial geniculate of thalamus (**medial = music**)
        (2) Superior colliculi & lateral geniculate nuclei of thalamus process visual information, but do not directly receive information from the optic chiasm (**lateral = light**)
    c. Cerebral peduncles, carrying motor command fibers from internal capsule, sit ventrally
    d. Oculomotor nerve emerges from the interpeduncular fossa
    e. Dorsal to cerebral peduncles sits the substantia nigra
        (1) Pars compacta sits dorsally, these are the dopaminergic neurons destroyed in Parkinson's disease
        (2) Pars reticulata sits ventrally, GABAergic neurons
        (3) Pars compacta receives inhibitory signals from caudate & putamen (striatum), sends stimulatory signals back

C. Cranial nerves–III to XII located in the brain stem

1. Motor nuclei lie close to midline, sensory nuclei tend to lie more laterally
2. CN III lesion = downward/outward eye deviation & ptosis (levator palpebrae superioris)
    a. Associated Edinger-Westphal nucleus damage causes loss of parasympathetic innervation of pupillary constrictor & ciliary muscles, leads to pupillary dilation, loss of accommodation
    b. **Fixed, dilated pupil is classic presentation**
3. CN IV lesion = **contralateral eye deviates up & in (CN IV is the only nerve that crosses the midline)**

4. CN V nucleus is gigantic, understand the corneal reflex & masticator reflex
   a. CN $V_{sensory\ afferents}$ ⇒ main sensory nuclei V ⇒ CN VII ⇒ orbicular oculi muscles
   b. Ia masticator muscle spindle afferents via V_3 ⇒ CN V motor nuclei ⇒ masseter muscle
   c. Lesions of $V_{sensory}$ lead to ipsilateral loss of pain & temperature sensation of face
5. CN VI lesion = medial deviation of eye, may also see CN VII involvement due to proximity of VII nerve to body of VI
6. CN VII lesions of **2 varieties**: nuclear lesions or corticobulbar lesions
   a. CN VII lesions ⇒ are all known as Bell's palsies, paralysis of facial muscles, loss of anterior 2/3 taste, loss of lacrimation & salivation, & can also involve CN VI
   b. Corticobulbar fibers innervate **all cranial motor nuclei bilaterally, except CN VII**
      (1) CN VII fibers to upper facial muscles do receive bilateral corticobulbar innervation
      (2) CN VII fibers to lower facial muscles **only receive contralateral cortical innervation**
      (3) Consequence: **a unilateral lesion of cortex can lead to contralateral lower facial muscle paralysis, while no deficit will be noticed in the upper facial muscles**
7. CN VIII lesions: path is so complex may see no deficit due to redundant innervation
8. CN IX lesions = unilateral loss of swallowing, taste & gag reflex
9. CN X lesions = unilateral loss of palatal elevation, taste & laryngeal dysfunction
10. CN XI lesions = unilateral loss of trapezius, sternocleidomastoid function
11. CN XII lesion = deviation of tongue to **same side as lesion**

D. Skull passageways
   1. Superior orbital fissure ⇒ CN 3, 4, 5_1, 6
   2. Foramen rotundum ⇒ CN 5_2
   3. Foramen ovale ⇒ CN 5_3
   4. Internal auditory meatus ⇒ CN 7, 8
   5. Jugular foramen ⇒ CN 9, 10, 11
   6. Cavernous sinus ⇒ CN 3, 4, 5_1, 6 (all that control extraocular motion)

E. Other brain stem lesions

1. Lesions above caudal medulla ⇒ loss of contralateral pain/temperature (anterolateral tract), loss of discriminatory touch/proprioception (dorsal column/medial lemniscal tract) & loss of contralateral fine digit motor control (pyramidal tract)
2. Lesions of reticular activating systems cause comas
3. Horner's syndrome = lesion of cervical sympathetic chain ⇒ ipsilateral ptosis, miosis, anhydrosis

III. Cerebellum

A. Anatomy

1. Vestibulocerebellum controls balance & proprioception
2. Spinocerebellum controls limb extensions
3. Pontocerebellum controls fine digit movement

B. Lesions

1. Lateral cerebellar lesions cause ipsilateral deficits
2. **Cause abnormal execution of movement (intention tremors)**
3. Vestibulocerebellar lesions cause ↓ equilibrium (detect by Romberg test)
4. Spinocerebellar lesions cause hypotonia & increased extensor reflexes
5. Pontocerebellar lesions cause hypotonia & ataxia

IV. Diencephalon

A. Hypothalamus

1. Location: above optic chiasm, infundibulum, mamillary bodies, so divided into 3 regions: suprachiasmatic, infundibular, mamillary
2. Function–**TAN HATS**
   a. **T**hirst/water balance, **A**deno/**N**eurohypophysis, **H**unger/satiety, **A**utonomic regulation, **T**emperature regulation, **S**ex drive
   b. Lesion of posterior hypothalamus causes poikilothermy (cold-blooded)—i.e., posterior turns on heat when person is cold, anterior cools person down when hot
   c. Lesion of ventromedial hypothalamus causes ventral & medial growth (become fat)—i.e., lesion of satiety zone → to hyperphagia & obesity

d. Lesion of mamillary bodies ⇒ Korsakoff syndrome = confabulations, anterograde amnesia—this is a common lesion in alcoholics, get hemorrhage of the mamillary bodies due to thiamine deficiency

B. Thalamus (see Figures A.2, A.3, A.4, A.5, A.6, and A.7)
  1. Location: lie on either side of third ventricle, attached by massa intermedia
  2. Function
     a. Lateral geniculate = visual (**l = light**), medial = auditory (**m = music**)
     b. Ventroposterolateral (VPL)/VPM = body/facial proprioception, pain, vibration sense
     c. Ventral anterior nuclei = motor
  3. Thalamic relay nuclei are GABAergic

C. Pituitary gland (Hypophyseal gland)
  1. Location: at bottom of infundibular stalk, resting in sella turcica
  2. Neurohypophysis (brain ectoderm) is posterior, adenohypophysis (Rathke's pouch) is anterior

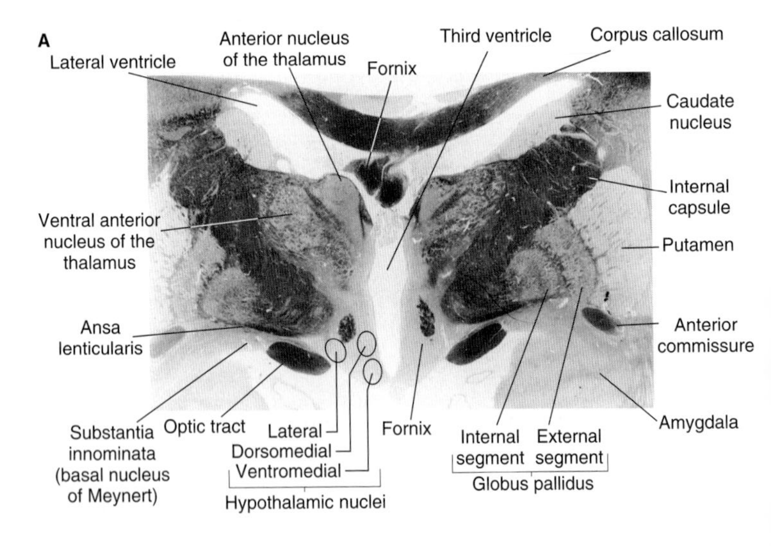

Figure A.2
Coronal section through the rostral thalamus at the level of the anterior thalamic nuclei. (Reproduced with permission from Pritchard TC and Alloway KD. Medical Neuroscience. Madison, Connecticut: Fence Creek Publishing, 1999:175. © Fence Creek Publishing, LLC.)

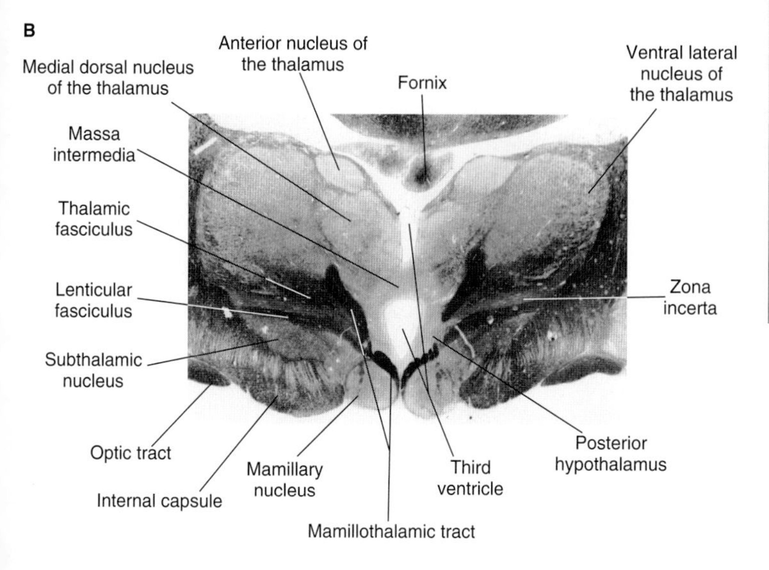

Figure A.3
Coronal section through the thalamus at the level of the medial dorsal nucleus. (Reproduced with permission from Pritchard TC and Alloway KD. Medical Neuroscience. Madison, Connecticut: Fence Creek Publishing, 1999:176. © Fence Creek Publishing, LLC.)

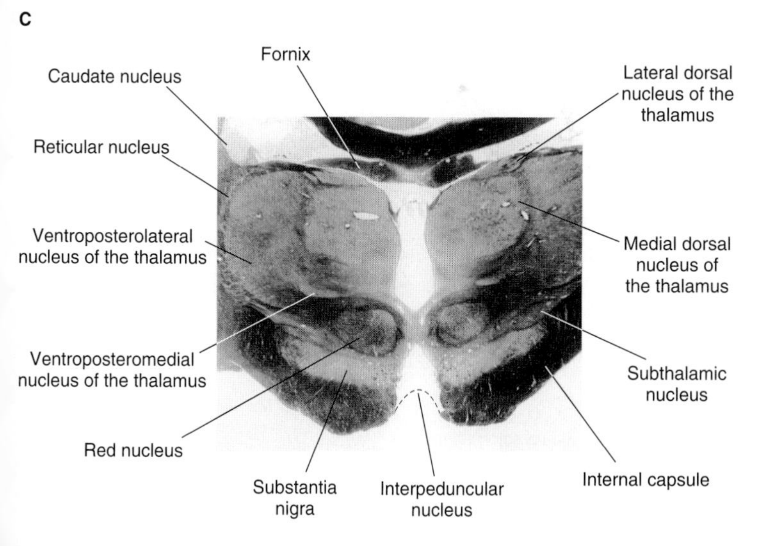

Figure A.4
Coronal section through the thalamus near the rostral limit of the ventroposteromedial nucleus. (Reproduced with permission from Pritchard TC and Alloway KD. Medical Neuroscience. Madison, Connecticut: Fence Creek Publishing, 1999:176. © Fence Creek Publishing, LLC.)

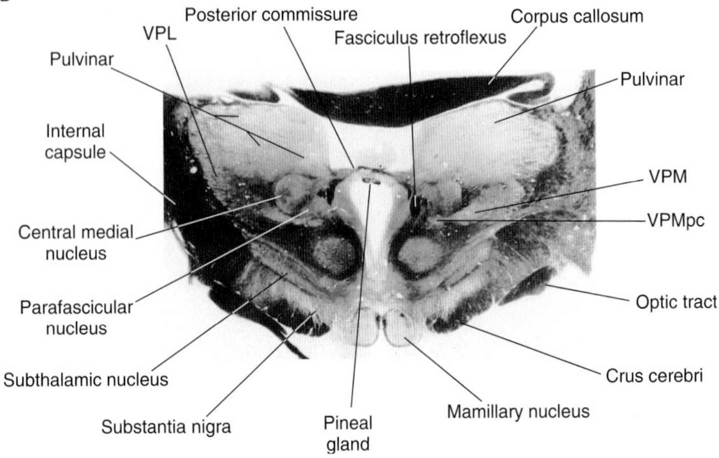

Figure A.5 Coronal section through the caudal thalamus
VPM = ventroposteromedial nucleus; VPMpc = parvocellular division of the VPM nucleus. (Reproduced with permission from Pritchard TC and Alloway KD. Medical Neuroscience. Madison, Connecticut: Fence Creek Publishing, 1999:177. © Fence Creek Publishing, LLC.)

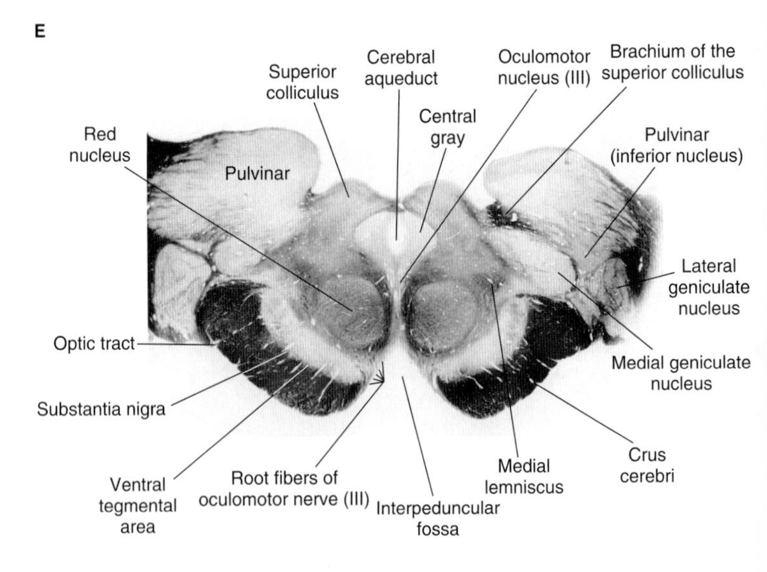

Figure A.6
Coronal section through the diencephalic-mesencephalic junction. (Reproduced with permission from Pritchard TC and Alloway KD. Medical Neuroscience. Madison, Connecticut: Fence Creek Publishing, 1999:177. © Fence Creek Publishing, LLC.)

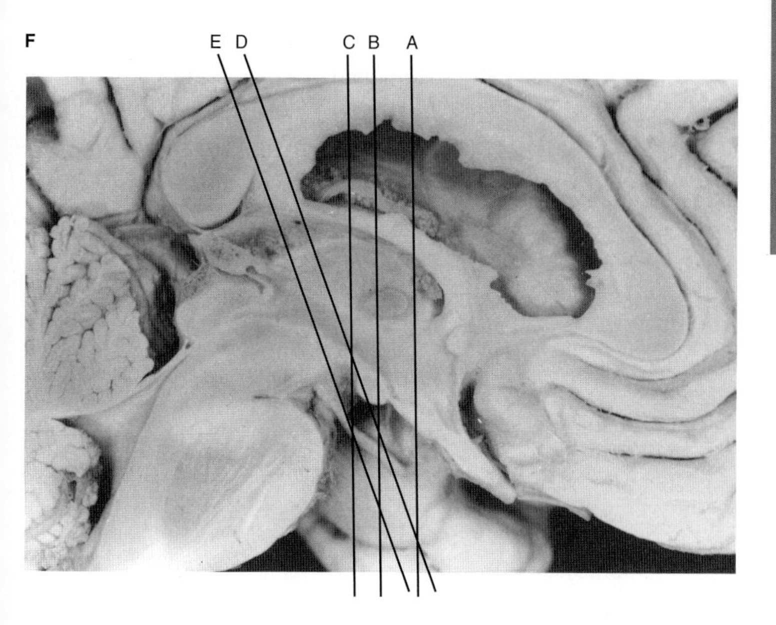

Figure A.7
Midsagittal section of the brain showing planes of section of Figures A-2 through A-6. (Reproduced with permission from Pritchard TC and Alloway KD. Medical Neuroscience. Madison, Connecticut: Fence Creek Publishing, 1999:178. © Fence Creek Publishing, LLC.)

3. Adenohypophysis receives blood supply from capillary loops of a portal system in the median eminence
4. Releasing hormones in the portal system regulate adenohypophyseal secretion, neurohypophysis regulated directly by the neurons

V. Telencephalon

A. Basal ganglia ("Corpus Striatum")

1. Caudate
    a. Location: medial to lateral ventricle (tail wraps around lateral to dorsal tip of ventricles) (see
    b. Separated from thalamus & globus pallidus by internal capsule
2. Putamen (putamen + caudate = striatum)
    a. Location: attached to the rostral head of caudate
    b. Immediately lateral to globus pallidus

3. Globus pallidus (globus pallidus + putamen = lenticular nucleus)
    a. Location: medial to putamen
    b. Separated from thalamus by internal capsule
4. Blood supply
    a. Bulk of supply from lenticulostriate branches of middle cerebral artery
    b. Much of globus pallidus supplied by anterior choroidal branch of internal carotid
5. Interpretation of circuitry
    a. Direct basal ganglia signals → excitation of motor cortex
    b. Indirect basal ganglia signals inhibit motor cortex
    c. Substantia nigra dopamine stimulates signal most of the time
6. Parkinson's disease
    a. Destruction of substantia nigra dopamine producers shuts system down
    b. Signs ⇒ akinesia (limited initiation of movement), bradykinesia, **resting tremor**, rigidity
7. Huntington's disease
    a. Destruction of striatum leads to excessive output signal, less GABAergic inhibition of thalamic-cortical signals
    b. Signs ⇒ choreoathetosis, hyperkinesia, initial hypotonia

B. Internal capsule
1. Location
    a. Anterior limb separates head of caudate & globus pallidus
    b. Posterior limb separates thalamus & globus pallidus
2. Function
    a. Posterior limb contains corticospinal fibers running from cortex to lower motor functions
    b. Lesion causes contralateral hemiplegia, hyperreflexia, spasticity, rigidity (upper motor neuron signs)

C. Cortex
1. Blood supply
    a. Anterior cerebral artery supplies medial gyri
    b. Middle cerebral artery supplies lateral portions of gyri
    c. Posterior cerebral artery supplies occipital lobe
2. Frontal lobe lesions ⇒ ↑ suck/grab response, perseveration, forgetfulness, gaze palsy toward side of lesion (in epilepsy gaze is away from lesion, stroke is toward it), Broca's aphasia
    a. Broca's = expressive aphasia, can't form the words you know, **Broca's is Broken** speech

3. Temporal lobe lesions ⇒ upper quadrant homonymous hemianopia (Meyer's loop), Wernicke's jargon aphasia, autonomic dysfunction, Korsakoff memory disturbances, Klüver-Bucy
   a. Wernicke's aphasia = receptive aphasia, motor speech is fine but planning is bad, causes double-talk nonsense
   b. Korsakoff memory = diminished recent recall
   c. Klüver-Bucy = hyperorality, hypersexuality, disinhibited behavior
4. Parietal lobe lesions ⇒ ↑ avoidance, astereognosis, alexia, ↓ tactile discrimination, ↓ position sense, visual inattention, Gerstmann's syndrome
   a. Astereognosis = unable to recognize objects by palpation
   b. Visual inattention seen on Poppelreder figure examination
   c. Gerstmann's = acalculia, agraphia (can't write), agnosia (can't recognize common objects or faces)
5. Occipital lobe lesions ⇒ visual agnosia, cortical blindness

D. Hippocampus = cingulate gyri, hippocampus, fornix, amygdala
1. Located in the medial temporal lobe, comprised of the dentate gyrus, CA regions (hippocampus), subiculum & entorhinal cortex
   a. Entorhinal cortex inputs information into dentate gyrus
   b. Dentate gyrus sends information to CA regions, then to subiculum
   c. Subiculum sends information to entorhinal cortex & via fimbria to other locations as well
2. Diseases
   a. Temporal lobe epilepsy affects CA1, CA3 & dentate gyrus cells
   b. Alzheimer's affects entorhinal cortex & CA1 field, also other regions
3. Limbic system = cingulate gyri, hippocampus, fornix, amygdala
   a. Functions ⇒ **5 Fs**: feeding, fighting, feeling, flight, sex

VI. Olfaction

A. Anatomy/Lesions
1. Primary (1°) receptor ⇒ olfactory bulb ⇒ primary olfactory cortex ⇒ amygdala, entorhinal cortex, hippocampus
2. Bilateral anosmia can be due to trauma, viral disease
3. Unilateral anosmia is an early sign for a local tumor

VII. Epilepsy

A. Classification
1. Simple seizure = no loss of consciousness
2. Complex = impaired consciousness
3. Partial = seizure begins in a local area, general = total hemisphere dz
4. Absence = generalized seizure with little motor involvement & brief lapse of consciousness
5. Grand mal = generalized tonic clonic seizure
6. EEG spike & slow wave complex signifies ↑ hypersynchronicity

VIII. Neurotransmitters

A. Neurotransmitters
1. Acetylcholine (Ach)
    a. Choline acetyltransferase catalyzes the formation of ACh from acetyl-CoA & choline in the presynaptic terminal
    b. ACh stored in synaptic vesicles with ATP for later release
    c. ACh degraded to acetyl-CoA & choline by acetylcholinesterase
2. Norepinephrine (NE)
    a. Primary transmitter for postganglionic sympathetic neurons
    b. Synthesized in the nerve terminal & released into the synapse to bind with α or β receptors on the postsynaptic membrane
    c. Removed from synapse by reuptake or is metabolized in the presynaptic terminal by MAO & COMT
    d. VMA is a clinically important metabolite (used to measure catecholamine turnover, e.g., in pheochromocytoma)
3. Dopamine (DA)
    a. Predominant in the midbrain neurons, released from the hypothalamus & inhibits prolactin secretion
    b. Metabolized by MAO & COMT
    c. D1 receptors activate adenylate cyclase via a G_s protein
    d. D2 receptors inhibit adenylate cyclase via a G_i protein
    e. At low doses, DA causes dilation of renal vessels
    f. At higher doses, DA induces systemic vasoconstriction via α_1 receptors

4. Serotonin
    a. Present in high concentrations in the brain stem, formed from tryptophan
    b. Is converted to melatonin in the pineal gland
5. Histamine: formed from histidine, present in neurons of hypothalamus
6. Glutamine
    a. Most prevalent excitatory neurotransmitter in the brain
    b. Reacts with the kainate receptor (sodium & potassium ion channel)
7. GABA
    a. Inhibitory neurotransmitter synthesized from glutamate by glutamate decarboxylase
    b. 2 types of GABA receptors are GABA A (increases Cl^- conductance & is the site of action benzodiazepines & barbiturates), GABA B (increases K^+ conductance)
8. Glycine
    a. Inhibitory neurotransmitter found in the spinal cord & brain stem
    b. Increases Cl^- conductance

IX. Cellular Neurobiology

A. Embryologic derivatives
1. Ectoderm → epidermis (including hair, nails), nervous system, adrenal medulla, pituitary
2. Mesoderm → muscle, connective tissue, bone, cardiovascular structures, lymphatics, urogenital structures, serosal lining of body cavities (e.g., peritoneum), spleen, adrenal cortex & dura mater
3. Endoderm → gut tube epithelium & derivatives (e.g., lungs, liver, pancreas, thymus, thyroid, parathyroid)
4. Notochord induces ectoderm to form neuroectoderm (neural plate)
5. Postnatal derivative of notochord is the nucleus pulposus of the intervertebral discs
6. Neural crest cells differentiate to form the autonomic nervous system, dorsal root ganglia, melanocytes, chromaffin cells of adrenal medulla, enterochromaffin cells, pia mater, celiac ganglion, Schwann cells, odontoblasts & parafollicular cells of thyroid

7. Glial cell types: astrocytes, oligodendrocytes, ependyma, microglia

B. Blood-brain barrier (BBB)

1. Formed by 3 structures: arachnoid, choroid plexus epithelium, & intracerebral capillary epithelium
2. Glucose & amino acids cross by carrier-mediated transport mechanism
3. Nonpolar/lipid-soluble substances cross more readily than polar/water-soluble ones
4. BBB has several functions
   a. Maintains a constant environment for neurons in CNS
   b. Protects brain from endogenous or exogenous toxins
   c. Prevents escape of neurotransmitters from CNS
5. Inflammation, irradiation, & tumors may destroy the BBB, permitting entry into the brain of substances that usually are excluded

APPENDIX B. ZEBRAS AND SYNDROMES

Disease	Description/Symptoms
Adrenoleukodystrophy	X-linked recessive defect in long chain fatty acid metabolism due to a peroxisomal enzyme deficiency. Causes rapidly progressing central demyelination, adrenal insufficiency, hyperpigmentation of skin, spasticity, seizures & death by age 12.
Alkaptonuria	Defect of phenylalanine metabolism causing accumulation of homogentisic acid. Presents with black urine, ochronosis (blue-black pigmentation of ear, nose, cheeks) & arthropathy due to cartilage binding homogentisic acid.
Banti's syndrome	"Idiopathic portal HTN." Splenomegaly & portal HTN following subclinical portal vein occlusion. Insidious onset, occurring years after initial occlusive event.
Bartter's syndrome	Kidney disease that causes Na, K, & Cl wasting. Despite increased levels of renin, the blood pressure remains low.
Binswanger's disease	Subacute subcortical dementia caused by small artery infarcts in periventricular white matter. Usually seen in long-standing hypertension, but is rare.
Caisson's disease	Decompression sickness (the "bends") caused by rapid ascent from deep-sea diving. Sx occur from 30min to 1hr = joint pain, cough, skin burning/mottling.
Caroli's disease	Segmental cystic dilation of intrahepatic bile ducts complicated by stones & cholangitis, can be cancer precursor.

(Continued)

Disease	Description/Symptoms
Charcot-Marie-Tooth disease	Autosomal dominant peroneal muscular atrophy causing foot drop & stocking glove decrease in vibration/pain/temperature sense & DTRs in lower extremities. Histologically → repeated demyelination & remyelination of segmental areas of the nerve. Patients may present as children (type 1) or adults (type 2).
Cheyne-Stokes respirations	A central apnea seen in CHF, ↑ ICP, or cerebral infection/inflammation/trauma: cycles of central apnea followed by regular crescendo-decrescendo breathing (amplitude first waxes & then wanes back to apnea): **Biot's** is an uncommon variant seen in meningitis in which the cycles consist of central apnea followed by steady amplitude breathing that then shuts back off to apnea.
de Quervain's tenosynovitis	Tenosynovitis causing pain on flexion of thumb (motion of abductor pollicis longus).
Diamond-Blackfan syndrome	"Pure red cell aplasia," a congenital or acquired deficiency in the RBC stem cell. Congenital disorder is sometimes associated with abnormal facies, cardiac & renal abnormalities. Tx = steroids.
Ellis-van Creveld	Syndrome of polydactyly + single atrium.
Erb's paralysis	"Waiter's tip"–upper brachial plexopathy (C5, 6).
Fabry's disease	X-linked defect in galactosidase, Sx = lower trunk skin lesions, corneal opacity, renal/cardiac/cerebral disease that are invariably lethal in infancy or childhood.
Fanconi's anemia	Autosomal recessive disorder of DNA repair. Presents with pancytopenia, risk of malignancy, short stature, bird-like facies, café au lait spots, congenital urogenital defects, retardation, absent thumb.
Farber's disease	Autosomal recessive defect in ceramidase, causing ceramide accumulation in nerves, onset within months of birth, death occurs by age 2.

(Continued)

Disease	Description/Symptoms
Fibrolamellar carcinoma	Variant of hepatocellular carcinoma. Occurs in young people (20–40yr), is not associated with viral hepatitis or cirrhosis. Has a good Px. Histologically shows nests & cords of malignant hepatocytes separated by dense collagen bundles.
Fitz-Hugh-Curtis syndrome	*Chlamydia* or gonorrhea perihepatitis as a complication of pelvic inflammatory disease. Presents with right upper quadrant pain & sepsis.
Galactosemia	Deficient galactose-1-phosphate uridyl transferase blocks galactose conversion to glucose for further metabolism, leading to accumulation of galactose in many tissues. Sx = failure to thrive, infantile cataracts, mental retardation, cirrhosis. Rarely due to galactokinase deficiency, blocking the same path at a different step.
Gaucher's disease	The most frequent cause of lysosomal enzyme deficiency in Ashkenazi Jews. Autosomal recessive deficiency in β-glucocerebrosidase. Accumulation of sphingolipids in liver, spleen & bone marrow. Can be fatal if very expensive enzyme substitute (alglucerase) not administered.
Hepatorenal syndrome	Renal failure without intrinsic renal dz, occurring during fulminant hepatitis or cirrhosis, presents with acute oliguria & azotemia, typically progressive & fatal.
Holt-Oram syndrome	Autosomal dominant atrial septal defect in association with finger-like thumb or absent thumb, & cardiac conduction abnormalities & other skeletal defects.
Homocystinuria	Deficiency in cystine metabolism. Sx mimic Marfan's = lens dislocation (downward in homocystinuria as opposed to upward in Marfan's), thin bones, mental retardation, hypercoagulability & premature atherosclerosis → strokes & MIs.
Hunter's disease	X-linked lysosomal iduronidase deficiency, less severe than Hurler's syndrome. Sx = mild mental retardation, cardiac problems, micrognathia, etc.

(Continued)

Disease	Description/Symptoms
Hurler's disease	Defect in iduronidase, causing multiorgan mucopolysaccharide accumulation, dwarfism, hepatosplenomegaly, corneal clouding, progressive mental retardation & death by age 10.
Isovalinic acidemia	"Sweaty-foot odor" disease. Caused by a defect in leucine metabolism, leads to buildup of isovaline in the bloodstream, producing characteristic odor.
Kasabach-Merritt	An expanding hemangioma trapping platelets, leading to systemic thrombocytopenia.
Keshan's disease	Childhood cardiomyopathy 2° to selenium deficiency, common in China.
Klippel-Trénaunay-Weber syndrome	Autosomal dominant chromosomal translocation → prematurity, hydrops fetalis, hypertrophic hemangioma of leg & Kasabach-Merritt thrombocytopenia.
Klumpke's paralysis	Clawed hand—lower brachial-plexopathy (C8, T1) affecting ulnar nerve distributions, often presents with Horner's syndrome as well.
Leigh's disease	Mitochondrially inherited dz → absent or ↓↓ thiamine pyrophosphate. Infants or children present with seizures, ataxia, optic atrophy, ophthalmoplegia, tremor.
Lesch-Nyhan syndrome	Congenital defect in HPRT → gout, urate nephrolithiasis, retardation, choreiform spasticity & self-mutilation (patients bite off their own fingers & lips). Mild deficiency → **Kelley-Seegmiller** syndrome = gout without nervous system Si/Sx.
Lhermitte sign	Tingling down the back during neck flexion, occurs in any craniocervical disorder.
Liddle's disease	Disease mimics hyperaldosteronism. Defect is in the renal epithelial transporters. Si/Sx = HTN, hypokalemic metabolic alkalosis.
Li-Fraumeni's syndrome	Autosomal dominant inherited defect of p53 leading to primary cancers of a variety of organ systems presenting at an early age.

(Continued)

Disease	Description/Symptoms
Maple syrup urine disease	Disorder of branched chain amino acid metabolism (valine, leucine, isoleucine). Sx include vomiting, acidosis, & pathognomonic maple-like odor of urine.
Marchiafava-Bignami syndrome	Overconsumption of red wine → demyelination of corpus callosum, anterior commissure & middle cerebellar peduncles. Possibly anoxic/ischemic phenomenon.
Melanosis coli	Overzealous use of laxatives causing darkening of colon, but no significant dz.
Mendelson's syndrome	Chemical pneumonitis following aspiration of acidic gastric juice, patient presents with acute dyspnea, tachypnea & tachycardia, with pink & frothy sputum.
Minamata disease	Toxic encephalopathy from mercury poisoning, classically described from fish eaten near Japanese mercury dumping site.
Molluscum contagiosum	Poxvirus skin infection causing umbilicated papules, transmitted by direct contact, often venereal. The central umbilication is filled with semisolid white material that contains inclusion bodies & is highly characteristic for the disease.
Mönckeberg's arteriosclerosis	Calcific sclerosis of the media of medium-sized arteries, usually radial & ulnar. Occurs in people over 50, but it does NOT obstruct arterial flow since intima is not involved. It is unrelated to other atherosclerosis & does not cause dz.
Munchausen's syndrome	A factitious disorder in which the pt derives gratification from feigning a serious or dramatic illness. Munchausen's by proxy is when the pt derives gratification from making someone else ill (often a mother injures her child for attention).
Niemann-Pick's disease	Autosomal recessive defect in sphingomyelinase with variable age onset (↑ severe dz in younger pt) → demyelination/neurologic Sx, hepatosplenomegaly, xanthoma, pancytopenia.

(Continued)

Disease	Description/Symptoms
Noonan's syndrome	Autosomal dominant with Sx similar to Turner's syndrome → hyperelastic skin, neck webbing, ptosis, low-set ears, short stature, pulmonary stenosis, AS defect, coarctation of aorta, small testes. Presents in males, X & Y are both present.
Peliosis hepatis	Rare primary dilation of hepatic sinusoids. Associated with exposure to anabolic steroids, oral contraceptives & danazol. Irregular cystic spaces filled with blood develop in the liver. Cessation of drug intake causes reversal of the lesions.
Poncet's disease	Polyarthritis that occurs DURING active TB infection but no organisms can be isolated from the affected joints, is thought to be autoimmune-mediated disease.
Pott's disease	Tubercular infection of vertebrae (vertebral osteomyelitis) leading to kyphoscoliosis secondary to pathologic fractures.
Refsum's disease	Autosomal recessive defect in phytanic acid metabolism → peripheral neuropathy, cerebellar ataxia, retinitis pigmentosa, bone disease & ichthyosis (scaly skin).
Rett's syndrome	Congenital retardation secondary to ↑ serum ammonia levels, more common in females, Sx = autism, dementia, ataxia, tremors.
Schafer's disease	Defect in hexosaminidase B, in contrast to the A component of the enzyme that is defective in Tay-Sachs. Px is better for Schafer's.
Schindler's disease	Defect in N-acetylgalactosaminidase.
Sweet's syndrome	Recurrent painful reddish purple plaques & papules associated with fever, arthralgia & neutrophilia. Occurs more commonly in women, possibly due to hypersensitivity reaction associated with *Yersinia* infection. Can also be seen in following URI or along with leukemia. Tx = prednisone, antibiotics if associated with *Yersinia* infection.

(Continued)

Disease	Description/Symptoms
Syndrome X	Angina relieved by rest (typical) with a normal angiogram. Caused by vasospasm of small arterioles unlike Prinzmetal's angina, which is vasospasm of large arteries.
Tay-Sachs disease	Autosomal recessive defect in hexosaminidase A, causing very early onset, progressive retardation, paralysis, dementia, blindness, cherry-red spot on macula & death by 3–4yr. Common in Ashkenazi Jews.
Usher syndrome	Most common condition involving both hearing & vision impairment. Autosomal recessive disorder characterized by deafness & retinitis pigmentosa (a form of night blindness).
Verner-Morrison syndrome	VIPoma = Vasoactive intestinal polypeptide overproduction. Leads to pancreatic cholera, increased watery diarrhea, dehydration, hypokalemia, hypo/achlorhydria.
Xeroderma pigmentosa	Defect in repair of DNA damage caused by UV light (pyrimidine dimers). Patients highly likely to develop skin cancers. Only Tx is avoidance of sunlight.

APPENDIX C. TOXICOLOGY

Toxin	Antidote
Acetaminophen	N-acetylcysteine, charcoal
Acids/Alkalis	Dilution with water, gastric lavage, cortisol for alkali burns of esophagus
Anticholinergics	Physostigmine
Arsenic, mercury, gold, lead	Gastric lavage, dimercaprol (BAL), penicillamine
Aspirin	Dialysis
Benzodiazepines	Flumazenil
Beta-blockers	Glucagon, calcium gluconate
Cadmium	Edetate
Carbon monoxide	100% oxygen
Copper	Penicillamine
Cyanide	Amyl nitrite, sodium thiosulfate
Digoxin	Digoxin Fab-antibodies
Ethylene glycol	Ethanol
Heparin	Protamine
Iron	Deferoxamine
Isoniazid	Pyridoxine
Lead	EDTA, dimercaprol
Methemoglobinemia	Methylene blue
Mushrooms (*Amanita muscaria*)	Physostigmine
Opioids	Narcan
Organophosphates	Atropine, pralidoxime
Paraquat	Gastric lavage, charcoal
Phenobarbital	Sodium bicarbonate

(Continued)

Toxin	Antidote
Quinidine (Torsades des Pointes)	Magnesium IV & isoproterenol
Streptokinase, t-PA	Aminocaproic acid
Theophylline	Beta blockers
Tricyclic antidepressants	Sodium bicarbonate
Warfarin	Vitamin K

APPENDIX D. PEARLS

Amyloid

- 1° amyloid comprised of λ light chains of antibodies (AL)
- 2° amyloid
  - Chronic inflammation → comprised of serum amyloid A (SAA)
  - Renal disease → comprised of β_2-microglobulin

Child Abuse

- Shaken-baby syndrome, look for retinal hemorrhages, coup & countercoup contusions

Death

- Time of death determined by both rigor mortis & livor mortis
  - Rigor mortis = muscle stiffness
  - Livor mortis = gravitation of blood to dependent parts of body

Environmental

- Radiation toxicity
  First hematopoiesis affected (lymphocytes die before other cells)
  Then GI epithelium
  Then CNS
- Teratogens, **mnemonic: Wart**
  Warfarin, **a**lcohol, **A**CE inhibitors, **r**etinoids, **t**halidomide

Laboratory

- Alkaline phosphatase made in both liver & bone, determine source by heat fractionation: **Liver Lives, Bone Burns** = liver fraction is heat stabile, bone fraction is heat labile
- Vasculitis
  C ANCA stains cytoplasm (Proteinase 3), seen in Wegener's
  P ANCA stains perinuclear (myeloperoxidase), seen in polyarteritis nodosa

Neuropathies

- Claw hand is found in ulnar nerve along with median nerve palsy
- Wrist drop is found in radial nerve palsy
- Foot drop is found in peroneal nerve palsy

Nutrition

- Marasmus = total calorie malnutrition
- Kwashiorkor = protein malnutrition

Pharmacology/Toxicology

- The Neuroleptic Rule of 4: dystonia occurs at 4 hr → 4 days, akathisia & extrapyramidal symptoms at 4 days → 4 wk, tardive dyskinesias at 4 mo
- Anticholinergic toxicity → blind as a bat, mad as a hatter, dry as a bone, bloated as a bladder, hot as a hare, red as a beet
- Malignant hyperthermia
  Hereditary hypersensitive ryanodine receptor in sarcoplasmic reticulum of skeletal muscle. Halothane & succinylcholine induce excessive calcium release, causing muscle rigidity, tachycardia & fevers as high as 42° C. Labs show ↑ CPK & K^+. Gold standard test = caffeine-halothane test. Tx = dantrolene
- MAO inhibitors + tyramine (found in cheese & wine) induce hypertensive crisis
- Chloramphenicol causes the lethal gray baby syndrome
- Vancomycin causes Red Man Syndrome (skin turns red)
- Albuterol is used in treatment of hyperkalemia due to β_2 agonist inducing cellular uptake of potassium
- Succinylcholine for intubation paralysis is contraindicated in burns, trauma & neuromuscular diseases d/t induction of massive hyperkalemia & arrhythmias

Prenatal

- α-fetoprotein (αFP) prenatal testing
  Decrease in Down's syndrome
  Increase in multiple gestation, neural tube deficit & duodenal atresia
- Neonatal screening is performed for hypothyroidism, PKU & galactosemia
- Chorionic villi sampling can be performed in the ninth to eleventh week, amniocentesis in the sixteenth to eighteenth week

Shock

- Hypovolemic causes low cardiac output, high pulmonary vascular resistance, low PCWP, decreased blood pressure, decreased urine output, tachycardia
- Cardiogenic causes low cardiac output, high PVR, high PCWP, high CVP, low blood pressure, & tachycardia
- Septic causes high cardiac output, low PVR, increased temperature
- Septic shock induced by LPS stimulation of IL-1, TNF, & other mediators

Surgery

- Causes of postop fever
  Wind atelectasis 24–48 hr postop
  Wound infection
  Water UTI
  Walking DVT
  Wonder drugs—Drug fever

Trauma

- Loss of consciousness differential Dx (**AEIOU TIPS**)
  Alcohol
  Epilepsy, environment (temp)
  Insulin (+/−)
  Overdose
  Uremia (electrolytes)
  Trauma
  Infection
  Psychogenic
  Stroke
- Coma cocktail = dextrose, thiamine, naloxone, & O_2

Radiology Pearls

- Lucent vs. Sclerotic lesions

  On plain film, a lucency is a focal area of bone or tissue that has a decreased density, usually resulting from a pathological process. A lucent bone lesion may appear like a dark, punched-out hole in the surrounding, normal bone. In contrast, sclerotic bone lesions appear denser than the surrounding bone. Thus, a sclerotic mass presents as whiter and more intense than its surroundings.
- Hypodense vs. Hyperdense

  Similar to that on plain films, tissue density on CT can be characterized by how light or dark it appears relative to surrounding, normal parenchyma. Hypodense lesions appear darker than normal tissue and hyperdense lesions are brighter. Air- or fluid-filled lesions such as cysts and abscesses are common hypodense lesions.
- Ring-Enhancement

  This refers to a bright intensity that can be observed surrounding many lesions on both CT and MRI. This usually indicates local edema around a mass lesion and in the brain it can indicate breakdown of the blood-brain barrier.

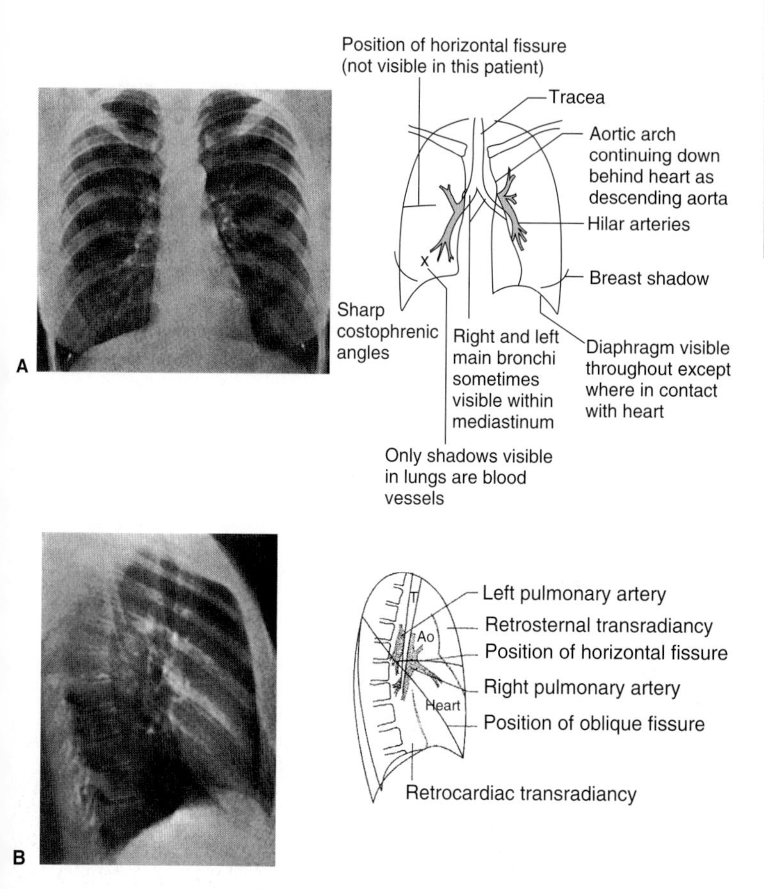

Figure D.1 Normal chest.
A. PA view. The arrows point to the breast shadows of this female patient.
B. Lateral view. Note that the upper retrosternal area is of the same density as the retrocardiac areas, and the same as over the upper thoracic vertebrae. The vertebrae are more transradiant (i.e., blacker) as the eye travels down the spine, until the diaphragm is reached. Ao = aorta; T = Trachea. (From Armstrong P, Wastie M. Diagnostic Imaging. 4th ed. London: Blackwell Science, 1998.)

- Radiopaque

  The more radiopaque an object is, the brighter it appears on plain film. Dental fillings, bullets, and metal prostheses are very radiopaque so they appear white on plain film.

- Radiolucent

  The more radiolucent an object is, the darker it appears on plain film.

APPENDIX E. VITAMINS

Vitamin	Deficiency	Excess
B_1 (thiamine)	Dry beriberi → neuropathy Wet beriberi → high output cardiac failure Either → Wernicke-Korsakoff's syndrome	
B_2 (riboflavin)	Cheilosis (mouth fissures)	
B_3 (niacin)	Pellagra → dementia, diarrhea, dermatitis. Also seen in Hartnup's disease (dz of tryptophan metabolism)	
B_5 (pantothenate)	Enteritis, dermatitis	
B_6 (pyridoxine)	Neuropathy (frequently caused by isoniazid therapy for TB)	
B_{12} (cyano-cobalamin)	Pernicious anemia (lack of intrinsic factor) → neuropathy, megaloblastic anemia, glossitis	
Biotin	Dermatitis, enteritis (caused by ↑ consumption of raw eggs, due to the avidin in the raw eggs blocking biotin absorption)	
Chromium	Glucose intolerance (cofactor for insulin)	
Copper	Leukopenia, bone demineralization	
Folic acid	Neural tube defects, megaloblastic anemia	
Iodine	Hypothyroidism, cretinism, goiter	

(Continued)

Vitamin	Deficiency	Excess
Iron	Plummer-Vinson syndrome = esophageal webs, spoon nails	Hemochromatosis → multiorgan failure (bronze diabetes)
Selenium	Myopathy (Keshan's disease [see Appendix B])	
Vitamin A	Metaplasia of respiratory epithelia (seen in cystic fibrosis due to failure of fat-soluble vitamin absorption), xerophthalmia, night blindness (lack of retinal in rod cells), acne, Bitot's spots, spots, frequent respiratory infections (respiratory epithelial defects)	Pseudotumor cerebri (can be caused by consuming polar bear livers), headache, nausea, vomiting, skin peeling
Vitamin C	Scurvy: poor healing, hypertrophic bleeding gums, easy bruising, deficient osteoid mimicking rickets	
Vitamin D	Rickets in kids, osteomalacia in adults	Kidney stones, dementia, constipation, abdominal pain, depression
Vitamin E	Fragile RBCs, sensory & motor peripheral neuropathy	
Vitamin K	Clotting deficiency	
Zinc	Poor wound healing, decreased taste & smell, alopecia, diarrhea, dermatitis, depression (similar to pellagra)	

QUESTIONS

1. A 30-year-old female presents to your clinic with fever, chills, malaise, and fatigue of 14 days' duration. She has marked petechial hemorrhages in the skin and mucous membranes and splinter hemorrhages beneath the nails. Hematocrit is decreased and the patient has a loud murmur.

   Which of the following is the most likely cause of these symptoms?

   A. *Haemophilus influenzae*
   B. *Streptococcus viridans*
   C. *Candida albicans*
   D. Pneumococci
   E. *Pseudomonas aeruginosa*

2. A 32-year-old female presents with forgetfulness and mental status changes. Physical examination is normal. Laboratory findings include hypoglycemia and increased insulin and C peptide levels.

   Which of the following statements is correct?

   A. C peptide is not increased in an insulinoma.
   B. Insulinoma is the most common islet cell tumor.
   C. Factitious hypoglycemia is occurring from the surreptitious injection of insulin.
   D. CNS abnormalities will not reverse upon glucose administration.
   E. This patient has diabetes.

3. A 61-year-old female has silver scaling plaques that cover her elbows, knees, and lumbosacral area. Her nails are pitted and she states that she must be careful not to scratch herself or a new psoriatic lesion will appear. This patient's greatest concern is that when she peels off an area of scale it results in pinpoint bleeding.

   Which of the following is the colloquial name for this last phenomenon?

   A. Köbner's phenomenon
   B. Microabscesses of Monro
   C. Koplik spots
   D. Auspitz sign
   E. Pastia's lines

4. A 25-year-old male presents to your clinic complaining of "cold feet." On physical examination you discover his blood pressure is 145/97. He has weak pulses below the diaphragm. A chest radiograph reveals notching below the ribs.

   What is the cause of these symptoms?

   A. Pulmonary stenosis
   B. Atrial septal defect
   C. Coarctation of the aorta

D. Eisenmenger's syndrome
E. Ventricular septal defect (VSD)

5. A 61-year-old man has been hospitalized for an acute MI. Six days later he complains of pleuritic chest pain and a cough. On physical examination, he is in mild distress, T 99.8, HR 94, RR 22, BP 145/85. His right lower lung fields have decreased breath sounds, are dull to percussion and decreased tactile fremitus. Heart rate is regular with no audible murmurs. There is no chest wall tenderness and there are no EKG changes. You do a pleural tap and the results are significant for the following.
protein: 2.4g/dL
LDH: 130 IU/L
pH: 7.4
WBC: 500
glucose: 75
specific gravity: 1.015
serum protein: 5 g/dL
serum LDH: 300 IU/L
The *most likely* cause of this patient's pleural effusion and symptoms is
A. nosocomial pneumonia with gram-negative bacilli.
B. congestive heart failure.
C. hypoalbuminemia secondary to liver failure.
D. occult malignancy.
E. esophageal rupture.
F. pulmonary embolus.

6. A 47-year-old female presents to the emergency room with 2 hours of severe substernal chest pain radiating to her left arm. Serial EKGs demonstrate ST segment elevation.
What initial therapy will have the most significant impact on mortality?
A. β-blockers
B. ACE inhibitors
C. Nitrates
D. Thrombolytics
E. HMG CoA reductase inhibitors

7. A 30-year-old male in the ICU under continuous monitoring has a new onset of atrial fibrillation for the last 48 hours. He states he has palpitations, breathlessness, angina, and syncope. Doppler ultrasound shows mitral stenosis with concomitant elevated left atrial pressure and volume. An EKG demonstrates low amplitude undulations punctuated by QRS complexes and T waves.

The initial therapy for this patient should be which of the following?

A. β-blockers
B. Cardioversion
C. ACE inhibitors
D. Furosemide
E. Heparin and coumadin

8. A 5-year-old girl is brought in by her mother because of a new neck mass. She had a bout of otitis media 6 months ago but is otherwise healthy and well nourished, 60% range for height and 55% range for weight with appropriate growth curves. Her mother states that it does not seem to bother the child and she has noticed no changes in her behavior or activity. On examination the mass is midline, nontender, noncompressible, and elevates when the girl swallows and sticks out her tongue.

   The most likely cause of this new mass is

   A. a branchial cleft cyst.
   B. a cystic hygroma.
   C. a dermoid cyst.
   D. a thyroglossal duct cyst.
   E. the thyroid gland.

9. A 35-year-old woman complains of clumsiness and incoordination. She has persistent fatigue for the past 2 weeks. She also notes blurry vision in her right eye and is unable to hold a coffee mug. Her medical history is significant for a tonsillectomy at age 5. She has recently moved to the South because of job relocation. Her eye examination is grossly normal. She has ataxia, hyperactive deep-tendon reflex of the triceps and biceps on the right, and decreased muscular strength on the right. As part of the work-up, a lumbar puncture is performed.

   Which of the following cerebrospinal fluid findings best fits for this patient's condition?

   A. Mononuclear pleocytosis
   B. Decreased protein level
   C. Elevated opening pressure
   D. Decreased total cell count
   E. Proliferation of oligoclonal bands

10. A 25-year-old male comes to your clinic for a sports physical. On physical examination, you note an S_4 heart sound and a sustained apical impulse. The patient is asymptomatic.

    A sustained apical impulse is an indication of which of the following?

    A. Hypertrophic cardiomyopathy
    B. Aortic stenosis

C. Atrial septal defect
D. Tricuspid stenosis
E. Aortic regurgitation

11. A 50-year-old female with a 10-year history of diabetes mellitus presents with microalbuminemia. Kidney biopsy shows focal areas of glomerulosclerosis. Hyaline arteriosclerosis is also present.

    What initial treatment should be used?

    A. ACE inhibitors
    B. β-blockers
    C. Diuretics
    D. Digoxin
    E. Aldosterone

12. A 41-year-old woman notes that she has been tiring easily for 3 months. For the past 2 weeks, she has experienced discomfort in the upper right abdominal area and itchiness all over the body that worsens at night. The patient also has some joint pains that is attributed to arthritic pain, and an OTC pain reliever has helped. She denies any weight loss, fever, chills, or alcohol usage. Her past medical history consists of an appendectomy at age 17. Vital signs are within normal range. She has mild jaundice but no scleral icterus. Abdominal exam shows tenderness at upper left quadrant with no hepatomegaly. CT scan of the abdomen shows no obstruction. Liver function tests (ALT, AST, alkaline phosphatase, GGT) are elevated.

    Which laboratory test will be most helpful in diagnosing her condition?

    A. Antimitochondrial antibodies
    B. Antinuclear antibodies
    C. ESR
    D. MRI of the liver
    E. Liver biopsy

13. A 68-year-old female patient is in your office for a routine physical. Menses began at the age 13, and her menses were regular until menopause at age 47. Her breast history is significant for fibrocystic disease that regressed a few years before menopause. She delivered her daughter by spontaneous vaginal delivery at age 25 and breastfed her baby daughter for 8 months. The patient drinks 4–5 cups of coffee a day, does not smoke, and has an occasional glass of wine with dinner. She has a sister who was diagnosed with breast cancer at age 71 and died at age 75 from a myocardial infarction.

    Which factor in your patient's history puts her at greatest risk for breast cancer?

    A. Her caffeine intake
    B. Her alcohol intake

C. Early menarche
D. Late menopause
E. History of fibrocystic disease
F. Her age
G. A history of breast cancer in a first-degree relative
H. Giving birth at age 25
I. Breast-feeding for 8 months

14. The ER nurse reports that a 21-year-old male alcoholic is confused and acting strangely in his room. He is clumsy and cannot walk without stumbling. While interviewing the patient, he is inattentive and listless. He is oriented to person. His vital signs show mildly elevated temperature, tachycardia, and tachypnea. He looks cachetic and disheveled. He has ataxic gait and fails the Romberg test. Eye examination shows scleral icterus, nystagmus, and weakness on abduction of both eyes.

    Where would you expect to find a lesion on an MRI of this patient?

    A. Pineal gland
    B. Occipital lobe
    C. Medulla
    D. Frontal lobe
    E. Mamillary bodies

15. A 70-year-old man who had a small bowel resection earlier today now has an hourly urine output of 10cc/h. His BUN/Cr ratio is 10:1. Urinalysis shows Una $>$40 mEq/L, FENa $>$1, and Uosm 350. Muddy brown casts are present in the urine.

    What is your diagnosis?

    A. Prerenal azotemia
    B. Acute glomerulonephritis
    C. Acute tubular necrosis
    D. Postrenal azotemia
    E. Focal segmental glomerulosclerosis

16. A 55-year-old patient in the critical care unit is in chronic renal failure. What are the hormonal responses to hypophosphatemia that increase the plasma phosphate concentration toward normal without producing significant effect on plasma calcium concentration?

    A. Increased PTH release
    B. Increased urinary phosphate excretion
    C. Decreased intestinal phosphate absorption
    D. Increased renal vitamin D production

17. A 34-year-old woman complains of fatigue, fever, and muscle pain for the past month. The symptoms are persistent throughout the day, and using an OTC pain reliever has not helped. She also notes

pain in the joints—especially in the knuckles of both hands—and faint red rashes on both cheeks. She works as a nurse and denies any stress at work or at home. She is currently taking hydralazine for hypertension. Her vital signs are normal. Physical examination shows malar rashes and swelling of MCP joints in both hands.

Other than routine laboratory tests, which additional test would be helpful in diagnosing this patient?

A. Antihistone antibodies
B. Anti-mitochondrial antibodies
C. Westergren erythrocyte sedimentation rate (ESR)
D. C reactive protein
E. Activated partial thromboplastin time (PTT)

18. A 17-year-old male with a 10-year history of asthma comes to your office with the complaint of having to use his inhaled beta-agonist medication 4 times a week and at least 2 nights per month. You decide to have your patient begin inhaled corticosteroids and check his lung function in 2 months.

The mechanism of action of inhaled steroids is to

A. inhibit phosphodiesterase and increase amounts of cAMP.
B. stimulate β2-adrenergic receptors.
C. inhibit β1-adrenergic receptors.
D. decrease inflammation.
E. inhibit 5-lipoxygenase (interfering with leukotriene formation).
F. inhibit mast cell degranulation.

19. A patient on an experimental drug develops a toxic reaction and has selective injury to the loop of Henle. Clinically, the patient experiences sodium wasting, hypokalemia, and polyuria.

The acid base balance would show which of the following?

A. Metabolic acidosis
B. Metabolic alkalosis
C. Respiratory alkalosis
D. Respiratory acidosis
E. Normal acid base balance

20. Your patient undergoes left breast biopsy for microcalcifications found by mammography. The pathology report comes back as ductal carcinoma in situ (DCIS). Histologically, the pathologist notes that it arises from the terminal ducts although they are markedly enlarged and is of the comedocarcinoma type. It has not invaded the basement membrane, thus the description "in situ" denotes the specimen has clean margins.

Which of the following do you tell your patient?

A. Even though the margins are clean, because it is DCIS, she is at risk for recurrent ipsilateral breast cancer in the future.

B. Even though the margins are clean, because it is DCIS, she is at risk for recurrent breast cancer in either breast in the future.
C. There is no more risk because the margins were clean and this is not a premalignant lesion.
D. She is lucky that she caught the breast cancer in this stage, while it is still in situ it has probably already metastasized.

21. A 58-year-old farmer comes to you because of multiple lesions on his face and the back of his neck. He is otherwise healthy but looks much older than his stated age because of the decreased elasticity in his facial skin. The lesions he is concerned about are round with pearly borders and fine telangiectasias at the base. A few have ulcerated, which is why he has come to see you.

Which of the following is *true* regarding this most common malignant skin tumor?

A. These are commonly found on the extremities.
B. Actinic keratosis are a frequent precursor to this lesion.
C. These virtually never metastasize.
D. These are not typically due to sun exposure.
E. Histologically, these have characteristic keratin pearls.
F. Seborrheic keratosis are a frequent precursor to this lesion.

22. A 3-year-old boy is brought to your clinic by his parents. Physical exam shows a large flank mass. A biopsy of the mass shows immature stroma, primitive tubules and glomeruli, connective tissue and bone.

Which type of tumor does this child have?

A. Adenoma
B. Renal cell carcinoma
C. Wilms' tumor
D. Transitional cell carcinoma
E. Squamous cell carcinoma

23. A 26-year-old female with congenital spherocytosis and enlarged spleen comes to seek your advice. Her test results are: Hb 12.5, Hct 34, RBC 3.80, reticulocytes 15%, MCV 89, MCH 33, MCHC 37.

Which of the following will be present?

A. Hemoglobinuria
B. Increased pigment stones in the gallbladder
C. Decreased RBC Hb concentration
D. Splenic infarctions and decreased spleen size
E. Decreased RBC osmotic fragility

24. A 52-year-old male with a history of chronic alcoholism presents with signs of liver disease. He has ascites, palmar erythema, and spider telangiectasias. The reason for his visit to you is because he wants to talk to you about his gynecomastia. In addition to his

concerns about the "un-manly" development of his torso, he wants to know what his risk is for breast cancer because his wife was recently diagnosed with invasive ductal cancer and is currently receiving radiation therapy.

Which of the following do you tell him?

A. Because his breasts are as large as his wife's he is at equal risk and should consider mammography every 1 to 2 years.

B. Because the gynecomastia is a result of increased circulating estrogens produced from conversion of androstenedione he is at increased risk; he should therefore begin monthly breast examinations.

C. Although alarming, there is no evidence that gynecomastia is associated with an increased risk of breast cancer. He doesn't have to worry because he is a man, his risk is zero.

D. Although alarming, there is no evidence that gynecomastia is associated with an increased risk of breast cancer. Although breast cancer is uncommon in men, it is not zero. Regardless, ceasing his alcohol intake might result in decreasing breast size.

25. A 23-year-old woman notes that, for the past month, her upper eyelids have become red but are not painful or itching. In addition, she is progressively weaker for the past 3 months. She has difficulty getting up from a chair and has pain in her arms and thighs. This patient never experienced these symptoms before. Her family history is significant for hypertension and diabetes. Vital signs are normal. Her eye exam is normal except for a heliotropic rash on both upper eyelids with some edema. Muscular strength is noticeably weaker on upper and lower limbs, but reflexes are normal. Laboratory tests show normal ESR, normal electrolytes and TSH, and elevated serum creatine kinase. A muscle biopsy is taken.

Which pathological finding would you expect to see on the biopsy?

A. Inflammation of endomysium connective tissue

B. Rimmed vacuoles within myocytes

C. Amyloid deposits within myocytes

D. Normal pathology

E. Inflammation of perimysial connective tissue

26. A 50-year-old radiation therapy technician comes to your clinic with sore throat and 2 days of cough. He has no prior history of hematological disorders. His temperature is elevated to 39°C. The patient's spleen is enlarged 6cm below the costal margin; his liver span is normal. The remaining physical exam is unremarkable. Labs include Hb 12, Hct 40, wbc 83,500 with left shift and 5%

basophils, platelets 250,000. Bone marrow biopsy shows hypercellularity, primarily of the myeloid and megakaryocytic lineages, with a greatly altered myeloid to erythroid ratio.

Which of the following diagnoses explains all of the above?

A. Chronic myelogenous leukemia
B. Acute myelogenous leukemia
C. Hodgkin's lymphoma
D. Non-Hodgkin's lymphoma
E. Acute lymphoblastic leukemia

27. A 60-year-old male with ruddy complexion comes to your clinic complaining of weakness and blood in his stool. On physical examination, he has splenomegaly. Laboratory findings show increased RBC mass, thrombocytosis with a platelet count $>$400,000 cells/μL. Bone marrow examination shows hypercellularity and decreased hematopoietic elements except lymphocytes. Hematocrit is 60%.

What is your diagnosis?

A. Polycythemia vera
B. Chronic myelogenous leukemia
C. Acute lymphoblastic leukemia
D. Iron-deficiency anemia
E. Essential thrombocythemia

28. A 35-year-old woman with a history of peptic ulcer disease presents with worsened abdominal pain, palpitations, dizziness, nausea, and vomiting. She has had multiple episodes of dark stools for the past few hours. She has been treated in the past with proton pump inhibitors that only help temporarily, but she has not undergone any new testing. In addition, her menstrual periods have not been regular. Her family history consists of peptic ulcer disease, diabetes, and hypertension. Her vital signs are significant for mildly elevated temperature, hypotensive, and tachycardia. On physical examination, she is pale and has epigastric tenderness. Her hemoglobin and hematocrit is low, and an endoscopy shows multiple ulcers in the duodenum. Her calcium and gastrin level is elevated.

What condition does this patient *most likely* have?

A. Duodenum ulcers
B. *Helicobacter pylori* infection
C. Atrophic gastritis
D. Pernicious anemia
E. Werner's syndrome

29. A 27-year-old man presents to the emergency department with an abrupt and severe headache, nausea, and vomiting. He has no

history of migraine headache and denies any trauma. Family history is significant for cystic kidney disease, hypertension, and rheumatoid arthritis. On physical examination, the patient's pupils are dilated with diminished light reflex. The rest of the neurological examination is grossly normal.

Where has the pathology *most likely* occurred?

A. Internal carotid artery
B. Anterior communicating artery
C. Posterior communicating artery
D. Superior cerebellar artery
E. Anterior inferior cerebellar artery

30. A 30-year-old male comes to your clinic because he has an ataxic gait, hyperreflexia with impaired position and vibration sense and elevated MCV.

Which of the following statements is correct?

A. This disease is caused by illegal drug use.
B. Ataxia is caused by a cerebral neoplasm.
C. Anti-intrinsic factor and antiparietal cell antibodies are present.
D. A normal Schilling test will occur.
E. A normal bone marrow will be present.

31. A 50-year-old woman has type 1 diabetes mellitus for 20 years. She complains of pain and numbness in her feet.
Following a physical examination, you note that she has the most common form of peripheral nerve damage in diabetes.

Her peripheral nerve damage will show

A. symmetrical involvement.
B. asymmetrical motor and/or sensory involvement.
C. motor function affected more than sensory.
D. reduced muscle tone.
E. inability to rise unaided from a squatting position.

32. A 53-year-old woman complains of left leg pain for the past 2 weeks. The pain is sharp and at the middle of the leg with no radiation. An OTC pain reliever gives only temporary relief. She notes weakness for the past month, and now has difficulty with ambulation due to the leg pain. She denies fever or chills. Her last menstrual period was at age 45. The patient denies smoking or drinking alcohol. Vital signs show mild elevation of temperature, tachycardia, and tachypnea. Physical examination shows normal skin tone and temperature with no tenderness on palpation of affected area. Muscular strength is decreased on the left leg with normal reflexes. An x-ray of her left leg shows deformity of the tibia and areas of lytic, mixed, and sclerotic changes.

Which of the following laboratory findings would be consistent with this patient's condition?

	Serum Vitamin D	Serum Calcium	Urinary Calcium	Alkaline Phosphatase
A.	N	N	N	N
B.	High	High	High	High
C.	Low	Low/N	Low	High/N
D.	N	N	Low	High
E.	N	High	High	High

33. A 20-year-old male comes to you complaining of swollen, black and blue joints, muscle hematomas, and hematuria.
    Which of the following do you expect to find?
    A. Bleeding time will be normal.
    B. This disease is autosomal dominant.
    C. Prothrombin time will be prolonged.
    D. Partial thromboplastin time will be normal.

34. An elderly couple is brought to the ER with complaints of headache, nausea, and dizziness. The husband states that they recently moved to a new home and, because of the cold weather, they have had to use the heater. On physical examination, vital signs show mildly elevated temperature, tachycardia, and tachypnea. The patients are ataxic and have generalized weakness; they are alert to person and place. The remainder of the physical examinations are normal.
    Which laboratory test would be helpful in diagnosing these two patients?
    A. Measurement for carboxyhemoglobin
    B. Oxygen saturation by pulse oximetry
    C. Oxygen saturation by arterial blood gas
    D. Chemistry panels for electrolytes level
    E. Complete blood count

35. A 40-year-old female visits your office complaining of a thyroid nodule. On physical exam the nodule feels firm to palpation and she has mild vocal cord paralysis. The nodule does take up iodine on a radioactive scan. A biopsy of the nodule shows ground glass Orphan Annie nucleus and psammoma bodies.
    Which of the following does this patient have?
    A. Medullary cancer
    B. Graves' disease

C. Follicular cancer
D. Papillary cancer
E. Beta thalassemia

36. A 35-year-old man complains about abdominal pain and frequent bowel movements. He has had chocolate-colored stool for the past 3 days, but now has bright-red bloody stool. His abdominal pain is generalized and is relieved with bowel movement. His appetite is decreased, but he has no nausea or vomiting. He reports mild fever and general weakness. He denies any past medical history and has not taken any NSAIDs recently. This patient's family history is significant for a sister with colon cancer at age 27. His vital signs are significant for mild elevation of temperature, hypotensive, and tachycardia. He is dehydrated. Abdominal exam shows hyperactive bowel sound, diffuse abdominal tenderness, and no rebound tenderness. Stool guaiac is positive. Laboratory tests show decreased hemoglobin/hematocrit, mild leukocytosis, and electrolytes abnormalities. Stool ovum and parasite culture is negative. A colonoscopy shows a continuous patch of friable mucosa; diffuse, uniform erythema replacing the usual mucosal vascular pattern and pseudopolyps in the sigmoid colon. A biopsy shows mucosa/submucosa lesions.

    What other findings would be associated with this man's condition?

    A. High risk for development of fistula
    B. High risk for development of fissure
    C. High risk for development of malignancy
    D. Biopsy would also show granuloma
    E. High risk for development of lesions in the small intestine

37. A 45-year-old female presents to you with a complaint that her rings and shoes no longer fit. On physical exam you note a coarsening of facial features, joint erosions, and bitemporal hemianopsia.

    Women with this syndrome are at a greater than expected risk of dying from

    A. carcinoma of the colon.
    B. AIDS.
    C. cardiovascular disorder.
    D. pulmonary insufficiency.
    E. carcinoma of the breast.

38. A 23-year-old female comes to your clinic complaining of obesity, infertility, and hirsutism. Laboratory studies indicate elevated LH, FSH, and testosterone. A course of oral contraceptive pills relieves many of her symptoms.

What is the main cause of her symptoms?

A. 21-alpha hydroxylase defect
B. Ovarian tumor secreting testosterone
C. Uterine leiomyosarcoma
D. 11-beta hydroxylase deficiency
E. Elevated LH

39. A 47-year-old man was diagnosed 3 weeks ago with a simple case of viral influenza. He now presents with a fever of 104° F, cough with mucopurulent sputum, HR 99, RR 24, BP 140/82. His lung exam is significant for dullness to percussion over the right middle lung, egophony, and increased tactile fremitus. A chest x-ray is ordered and in addition to the right middle lung consolidation identified on physical exam, it also shows a small right pleural effusion that layers when the patient is in the left lateral decubitus position. You admit this patient to the hospital and tap the effusions, which show the following.
pH: 7.1
glucose: 35
specific gravity: 1.025
protein: 5.0
LDH: 225

A common pathogen post viral pneumonia would reveal which of the following results during Gram stain?

A. Gram-negative rods
B. Gram-positive cocci in clusters
C. Gram-positive rods with tumbling motility
D. Gram's stain is negative; this is viral
E. Gram's stain is negative, the bacteria has no cell wall

40. A 58-year-old woman presents with episodes of blurry vision in her left eye. Besides a headache behind the eye, she notes some head pain that worsens on the left side when she puts on her glasses. In general, she is tired, has malaise, and has a decreased appetite that she attributes to a cold 10 days ago. On examination, she has a low-grade fever. The patient has a grossly normal eye examination with a mild papilledema and tenderness on palpation of the left temporal area. The remainder of the neurological examination is normal.

What is an appropriate next step to further evaluate this woman's condition?

A. CT scan of the head
B. Check a Westergren erythrocyte sedimentation rate (ESR)
C. Perform a lumbar puncture
D. Prescribe nonsteroidal anti-inflammatory agents (NSAIDs)

41. A 28-year-old pregnant woman presents to the ER complaining of uterine bleeding. She felt a sharp pain in the lower abdomen 1 hour ago, and uterine bleeding has not stopped since then. She still feels some movement of the baby. The gestation period is 29 weeks. The have been no pregnancy complications thus far, and no medications. While she is being evaluated in the ER, her blood pressure gradually decreases. She also experiences a strong contraction.

    What is the *most likely* diagnosis?

    A. Placenta previa
    B. Premature labor
    C. Ectopic pregnancy
    D. Abruptio placentae
    E. Vasa previa

42. A woman in the medical intensive care unit was diagnosed with encephalitis and has been ventilator dependent for the past 7 days. The course has been complicated by ARDS, which developed on day 2 but has since dramatically resolved. She has been steadily improving and each day the house officer has decreased her FiO_2 and minute ventilation all the while she has maintained adequate oxygenation. On the following graph, identify her functional residual capacity.

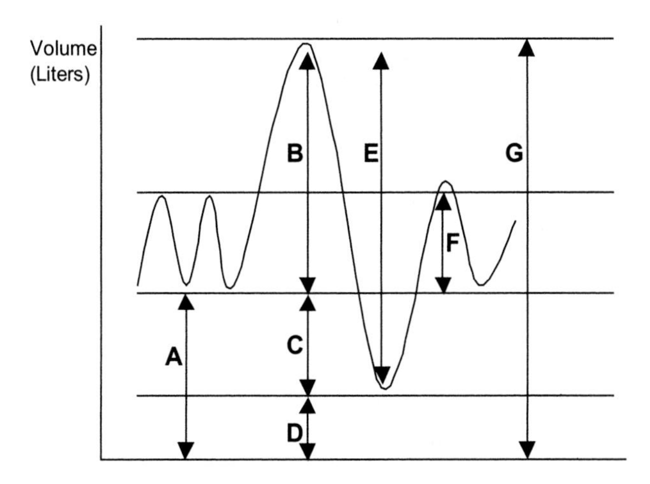

43. A 29-year-old man complains of a painless lesion on his penis. He denies any penile discharge and has no other lesions, no fever, chills, or dysuria. He has no significant medical history or family

medical history. He is single and drives a commercial truck. The patient had sexual intercourse 3 weeks ago with a new partner. Vital signs are normal. Genitourinary examination reveals no inguinal lymphadenopathy and normal genitalia. There is no discharge but there is a red and sharply demarcated 0.5 cm painless ulcer on the ventral side of the penis. A sample is taken from the papule, and laboratory tests are drawn.

Which of the following organisms would be found on microscopic examination of the sample?

A. Spirochete
B. Flagellated protozoa
C. Gram-negative coccobacilli
D. Gram-negative diplococci
E. Obligated intracellular, membrane-bound organisms

44. A 12-year-old boy visits his pediatrician for a checkup. He denies any illness or hospitalization within the past year and has no complaints. His medical history is significant for multiple hospitalizations for fractures. His father also sustained multiple fractures and died young after an automobile accident. The patient has short stature but his vital signs are within normal limits. Eye examination shows a blue sclera. His muscular strength is symmetrically equal with normal reflexes.

    What is the *most likely* cause of this boy's condition?

    A. Deficiencies of acid hydrolases
    B. Deficiencies of vitamin D
    C. Deficiencies of carbonic anhydrase II
    D. Deficiencies of collagen synthesis
    E. Deficiencies of hydroxylation of lysine/proline

45. A 25-year-old man who recently emigrated to the United States from Central America is in your office for a pre-employment physical. His physical examination is unremarkable. Blood tests are all within normal limits but examination of his chest x-ray reveals a calcified granuloma in the right mid-lung field with ipsilateral hilar adenopathy. Additionally, his PPD site is indurated with a diameter of 15 mm.

    The evolution of the characteristic Ghon complex seen on this patient's chest radiograph is due to

    A. defective macrophage phagocytosis.
    B. the patient's relative state of immune deficiency.
    C. cell-mediated immunity 2 to 6 weeks after primary infection.
    D. invasion of the organism into pulmonary lymphatics.
    E. invasion of the organism into blood vessel walls.

46. A 28-year-old man presents with a sinus infection. He is interested in learning more about sinus surgery because he has had these

infections his entire life and this is his fourth infection so far this year. On further history you find that he is moderately depressed because he has had no luck getting his wife pregnant after 2 years of trying. He is satisfied being a stepfather to her son from a previous marriage, however. He has a cough that he states has troubled him since childhood. He tells you an interesting story about how he almost didn't get out of a burning building in time because he never smelled the smoke.

Which of the following is the *most likely* cause of this man's chronic sinusitis?

A. Defective chloride channels
B. Lack of mucociliary escalator
C. Meatal obstruction
D. Osler-Weber-Rendu syndrome
E. Nasal polyp

47. A 27-year-old man comes to the emergency department in an agitated state because his eyes have become painful and he has associated hazy vision with dark black floaters. He has his hands over his eyes because he has become exquisitely sensitive to bright light. The patient denies any trauma, contact lens use, allergies, or new medications. There is no discharge coming from his eyes. Fluorescein stain is unremarkable. The only significant part of this man's history is that he has a history of Reiter's syndrome and is HLA-B27 ⊕.

The cause of this patient's eye symptoms is

A. conjunctivitis.
B. uveitis.
C. corneal abrasion.
D. keratitis.
E. scleritis.

48. A 39-year-old woman complains of progressive weakness in both legs that is now affecting her arms. She also reports increased sensation as well as persistent burning sensation in the legs. Her past medical history is significant for an appendectomy and a bout of gastroenteritis 3 months ago. Physical exam shows significant symmetrical weakness of the lower legs and forearms. She has depressed deep-tendon reflex of the Achilles, knee jerk, and biceps. No sensory loss is found. Her work-up includes laboratory tests, nerve conduction test, lumbar puncture, and imaging.

What would her cerebrospinal fluid show?

A. Mononuclear pleocytosis
B. Decreased protein level
C. Increased protein level

D. Elevated opening pressure
E. Decreased total cell count
F. Elevated glucose level

49. A 12-year-old boy with a history of chronic otitis media is found to have a left-sided conductive hearing loss on a routine well child examination prior to the start of school. He is in no acute distress, afebrile, HR 70, RR 12, BP 120/70. He states that his ears do not ring and do not hurt and he has suffered no recent trauma to the ear. You believe he may have a cholesteatoma.

    The *most likely* finding in this case would be

A. a dark blue tympanic membrane.
B. cholesterol crystals.
C. a lateral neck mass with an associated neuroendocrine tumor.
D. a retraction pocket in tympanic membrane containing keratin with mild inflammation.
E. a benign tumor at the cerebellopontine angle affecting cranial nerve VIII.
F. a normal tympanic membrane.

50. A 33-year-old woman complains of a 6-month history of difficulty with swallowing. She has not only been unable to swallow solid food but now also fluids. She also notes chest pain with eating and vomits undigested food during and sometimes after eating. Her weight has decreased significantly. She denies any other medical conditions or family history of similar illness. Her vital signs are within normal limits. On physical exam, she is cachectic with halitosis but otherwise normal. Laboratory tests show that electrolytes—including proteins—are on lower end of normal. Barium swallow shows "bird's beak" or "rat tail" appearances throughout the lower esophageal sphincter (LES).

    What would you expect to find on the manometry study of this patient?

	Peristalsis or Contraction	Intraesophageal Pressure	Basal LES Pressure	LES Relaxation
A.	Disorganized	Elevated	Elevated	Absent/incomplete
B.	Impaired	Normal	Decreased	Transient
C.	Nonperistaltic	Normal	Elevated	Incomplete
D.	Reduced	Normal	Decreased	Absent/incomplete
E.	Increased	Decreased	Normal	Normal

51. A 41-year-old man with a history of pheochromocytoma and parathyroid hyperplasia has a new neck mass. Physical examination shows a right-sided thyroid nodule that is rock hard. It has decreased uptake on radioiodine uptake scan (scintigraphy). Pathology revealed that it was malignant and did not form papillae or follicles. Of significance, the polygonal granular cells that composed the majority of the tumor were neurosecretory in origin.

This man's tumor is *most likely* derived from

A. thyroid hormone-secreting cells.
B. beta cells.
C. alpha cells.
D. parafollicular "C" cells.
E. chief cells of the parathyroid gland.

52. A 25-year-old man has numerous areas of denuded skin that are secondarily infected. He tells you that large flaccid "bubbles" have been appearing all over his body recently that easily "pop" leaving areas of raw skin behind. He is very ill-appearing; therefore, you admit him for intravenous steroids and antibiotics. A biopsy specimen of one of the skin lesions reveals a tombstone fluorescent pattern surrounding the epidermal cells.

Which of the following is *true* of this patient's disorder?

A. It is bullous pemphigoid.
B. It is pemphigus vulgaris.
C. It is rarely fatal even if left untreated.
D. IgG titers have no correlation with the course of this disease.
E. His urine probably also fluoresces a distinct orange-pink color.

53. A 51-year-old woman presents to the clinic concerned about a new erythematous and eczematous area on her left areola involving the nipple. She has not changed laundry detergents, soaps, or purchased any new brassieres. Two years ago she had a biopsy of the right breast that was diagnosed as ductal carcinoma in situ. This patient decided to go forward with biopsy of the new lesion. The pathology report describes large cells with clear cytoplasm that are irregularly shaped with hyperchromatic nuclei.

This lesion is which of the following?

A. Paget's disease; her alkaline phosphatase level is most likely elevated.
B. Paget's disease; an uncommon type of ductal carcinoma that can either be invasive or in situ.
C. An intraductal papilloma; because it was a solitary lesion, her cancer risk is not increased.

D. Acute mastitis; the patient needs to take antibiotics that cover *Staphylococcus* and *Streptococcus*, the most commonly isolated organisms.
E. An allergic contact dermatitis type IV, cell-mediated hypersensitivity reaction.

54. A 68-year-old woman comes to your office with the chief complaint of an increased cough. Her normal cough usually goes away before noon but this time the cough has been lasting all day, and now she is coughing up slight amounts of blood-tinged sputum. The patient has smoked 1.5 packs/day for 45 years, drinks no alcohol, and lives with her husband of 40 years. She has noted no change in her appetite although she states she has lost 15 pounds in the past 6 months. Physical examination reveals a barrel-chested, thin woman in no acute distress. Her skin is warm, pink, and dry. Lung examination reveals decreased breath sounds with a slight wheeze and prolonged expiratory phase. A chest x-ray shows a central, cavitated lesion. Biopsy of the lesion shows keratin pearls and desmosomes.

    A common chemistry abnormality associated with her lesion is

A. increased 5-HIAA levels in her urine.
B. increased levels of calcium due to parathyroid hormone related protein secreted by the lesion.
C. decreased levels of calcium due to parathyroid hormone related protein secreted by the lesion.
D. hyponatremia due to ADH secretion by the lesion.
E. high levels of carcinoembryonic antigen.
F. hyperglycemia due to ACTH secretion, resulting in a cushingoid picture.

55. A 42-year-old woman complains of nausea, fever, and a sharp right upper abdominal pain for the past 3 days. The pain is persistent and does not radiate. She also notes abnormal vaginal discharge. She denies any travel history or eating new food. An OTC pain reliever has not helped, and her appetite is not affected. She never had these symptoms before, and her medical history is significant for pelvic inflammatory disease. She is sexually active, and her last intercourse a week ago was with a new partner. Vital signs show elevated temperature, tachycardia, and tachypnea. Abdominal exam reveals normal active bowel sound and tenderness to right upper quadrant with no rebound tenderness. Genitourinary examination reveals some whitish discharge and normal external genitalia. Pelvic examination reveals discharge and inflammatory changes of vaginal mucosa. Bimanual examination elicits cervical and adnexal motion tenderness with no masses.

The patient's laboratories are significant for significant elevations of AST and ALT.

Which of the following is *most likely* a diagnosis of this woman's condition?

A. Toxic shock syndrome (TSS)
B. Ectopic pregnancy
C. Appendicitis
D. Fitz-Hugh-Curtis syndrome
E. Endometriosis

56. A 73-year-old man complains of difficulty with urination for the past 2 days. He states that he has the urge to urinate but has difficulty starting. The urine stream is weak, the bladder takes a long time to empty and feels full after urination. The patient denies any pain on urination and has no blood in the urine. There is no discharge. He also denies fever, chills, or weight loss. The man stopped smoking 20 years ago, and his medical history is significant for hypertension. Vital signs are within normal limits. Genitalia examination reveals normal genitalia with no lesions and no scrotal masses. A hard nodule is palpated in the man's prostate. A urine analysis is normal, and prostate-specific antigen (PSA) level is elevated.

Where is the *most likely* location of the malignancy?

A. Central zone
B. Transitional zone
C. Peripheral zone
D. Periurethral zone
E. Ejaculatory duct

57. A 19-year-old woman complains of vaginal itching and discharge. She states that the discharge is yellow, smells bad, but does not contain blood. She also notes pain upon urination but denies frequency or blood in her urine. She has never before experienced these symptoms. The young woman works as a clerk at a fast-food store and had sexual intercourse with a new partner about 10 days ago. Vital signs are within normal limits. Genitourinary examination reveals normal external genitalia with foul-smelling, frothy discharge. The vaginal vault is erythematous, and the cervix has multiple petechiae. A sample of the discharge was taken for analysis.

What is the *most likely* organism causing this condition?

A. Candida albicans
B. Gardinella vaginalis
C. Trichomonas vaginalis
D. Treponema pallidum
E. Calymmatobacterium granulomatis

58. A 53-year-old man complains of difficulty with urination for the past 3 months. He states that he has the urge to urinate but has difficulty starting. The urine stream is weak, and he has to press on the bladder to empty. He feels incomplete emptying his bladder and sometimes soils his underwear during the day. He frequently has to wake up at night to urinate. The patient denies any pain on urination and has no blood in the urine. There is no discharge. He also denies fever, chills, or weight loss. He does not drink or smoke, and his medical history is significant for hypertension. Vital signs are within normal limits. His genitalia are normal, and his prostate is diffusely enlarged but soft. Both a urine analysis and prostate-specific antigen (PSA) levels are normal. Postvoidal residual volume is elevated.

    Which of the following enzymes is responsible for this man's condition?

    A. 5 α-reductase
    B. 21-hydroxylase
    C. 17 β-hydroxylase
    D. Aromatase
    E. 3 β-hydroxysteroid dehydrogenase

59. A 6-year-old child whose family recently emigrated from Bolivia presents to your office with her parents. She has had a high fever for the past few days and now has a maculopapular rash that began on her head and neck and is now spreading down her torso. She is coughing, has a runny nose, and her eyelashes are crusted from a discharge coming from her eyes.

    This child's disease is caused by

    A. a togavirus.
    B. coxsackie A virus.
    C. human herpes virus 6.
    D. parvovirus B-19.
    E. a paramyxovirus.
    F. varicella-zoster virus.

60. A mother brought her 9-week-old baby boy to the pediatrician with complaints of vomiting. She states the vomitus is frothy and has similar consistency and color as the feeding. The infant's vomitus seems forceful and lands about 2 feet away. He acts as though he's hungry upon feeding. Further history is that he's the firstborn, was carried full term, and the pregnancy was uncomplicated. The vital signs are within normal limits. On physical exam, growth and head circumference are stable at 45th percentile and 60th percentile, respectively. He is mildly dehydrated, and the rest of the examination is normal.

What would an abdominal ultrasound show in this infant?

A. Normal ultrasound
B. Thickened and elongated pyloric muscle
C. A small gastral cardiac web
D. Pyloric atresia
E. Esophageal hiatal hernia

61. A 54-year-old man presents to the ER with abdominal pain. The pain is sudden, nonradiating, and localizes to left lower side. He has subjective fever but no chills. He is nauseated but does not vomit. There is no change in bowel habits. He denies recent antibiotic use. Vital signs are significant for elevated temperature, tachycardia, and tachypnea. The patient has hypoactive bowel sounds and tenderness on palpation of the left lower quadrant. Rebound tenderness is noted. The liver size is within normal limits, and there is no palpable mass. Stool guaiac is positive for heme.

    Which of the following is the *most likely* diagnosis for this patient?

    A. Diverticulitis
    B. Appendicitis
    C. Irritable bowel syndrome
    D. Lactose intolerance
    E. Pyelonephritis
    F. Pseudomembranous colitis

62. A 29-year-old homeless man comes to the ER with upper abdominal pain, nausea, and vomiting. The pain is sharp and radiates toward the back. He denies fever or chills. He has had these symptoms before but not as severe. The patient drinks alcohol almost daily if he can afford it. Vital signs are significant for mildly elevated temperature, tachycardia, and tachypnea. On abdominal exam, bowel sound is hypoactive, and he has tenderness over epigastric area with some guarding. An abdominal x-ray shows a loop of distended bowel adjacent to pancreas.

    Which of the following laboratory findings is *most likely* associated with this patient's condition?

    A. Decreased serum amylase
    B. Decreased serum lipase
    C. Hypoglycemia
    D. Hypocalcemia
    E. Decreased serum trypsin

63. An 18-year-old female presents to the emergency department with a 1-day history of decreased vision in her left eye. She states that double vision began yesterday and is still troubling her. She has no

significant medical history. Her only medication is birth control pills and occasionally acetaminophen for headaches. On funduscopic examination, you observe modest hyperemia. Examination of the cranial nerves reveals a left pupil that constricts when light is directed into the right eye but dilates when light is shown directly into the left. The right pupil is normal. There is also an inability to adduct either eye past the midline in a test of conjugate gaze.

The lesion that is causing this extraocular muscle abnormality is in which of the following locations?

A. CN II
B. CN III
C. CN VI
D. The median longitudinal fasciculus
E. The tectum in the midbrain
F. CN VI nucleus
G. CN III nucleus

64. A 19-year-old male complains of pain in his right lower thigh for the past month. The pain is dull with no radiation. He notes some swelling of the leg for the past 4 days, and simple walking has been difficult. He denies any history of trauma to the leg and has no fever, chills, or weight loss. The patient is otherwise healthy with no significant medical history. Vital signs show tachycardia and tachypnea. Musculoskeletal examination shows a mildly erythematous distal right femur with normal temperature. There is tenderness on palpation of affected area. Musculoskeletal strength and reflexes are symmetrical and grossly normal. Laboratory tests show normal complete blood count, negative blood culture, elevated alkaline phosphatase. An x-ray of the right femur was taken.

The *most likely* radiographic finding would be which of the following?

A. Sunburst pattern
B. Onion skinning
C. Salt and pepper appearance
D. Soap bubble
E. Lytic lesions

65. A firefighter is brought to the trauma bay for extensive burns and smoke inhalation. After the initial survey you note a large area of burned tissue. The situation looks grim as his extremities and part of his torso are totally black and look like pieces of leather. Surprisingly, the patient is not writhing in pain as you would have expected considering the extent of his burns. He responds in the negative when you ask if the area of burn is painful.

This type of burn

A. is a first-degree burn.
B. is a second-degree burn.
C. involves the full thickness of the dermis.
D. involves partial thickness of the dermis.
E. will heal on its own without consequence.

66. A 44-year-old man complains of a painful, red, and swollen right knee. The pain is persistent and is mildly alleviated with an OTC pain reliever. The pain does not radiate, and the patient ambulates with no difficulties. He denies any trauma and has no fever or chills. He has never had these symptoms before. He smokes and drinks a beer a day during dinner. His father had gout and died of lung cancer. The patient denies other problems and has no significant medical history. Vital signs show elevated temperature, tachycardia, and tachypnea. Musculoskeletal exam shows that the right knee is warm to touch, swollen with effusion, and tender to palpation. He has full range of motion of the joints. Muscular strength is grossly normal and symmetric. A complete blood count shows leukocytosis, elevated Westergren erythrocyte sedimentation rate, and hyperuricemia. The fluid is drained from the joints and sent for analysis.

Microscopic analysis of the synovial fluid would show which of the following?

A. Needlelike negatively birefringent crystals
B. Positive birefringent crystals
C. Envelope-shaped crystals
D. Diamond-shaped crystals
E. Coffinlid-shaped crystals
F. Hexagon-shaped crystals

67. An 8-year-old white female is brought to your office by her father. She has a long history of sinusitis growing pseudomonas, and is now presenting with a productive cough and difficulty in clearing secretions. She is in the 5% range for both height and weight. The girl embarrassingly tells you that she is frequently constipated and must flush the toilet four or five times after defecating. Physical examination reveals moderate respiratory distress. Lung examination reveals coarse rhonchi throughout both lung fields. The patient has clubbing of her upper extremities bilaterally. Her father tells you that he had a brother who was chronically ill since birth and died of pneumonia when he was 5 years old. You suggest a sweat chloride test to diagnose presumed cystic fibrosis.

Which of the following describes the lung pathology in this disease?

A. Noncaseating granulomas composed of epithelioid cells
B. Mucous plugging and inflammation of the bronchioles with irreversible cystic dilation
C. Mucous plugging and inflammation of the bronchioles with cystic dilation that can be reversed with prompt and proper treatment
D. Multiple alveoli filled with hyaline membranes
E. Mucus gland and smooth muscle hyperplasia, eosinophils, and thickening of the basement membrane

68. A mother brings her 3-year-old son into the clinic because, for the past 5 days, he has had a fever up to 103° F. He now has a bilateral conjunctivitis, a large palpable node in the anterior cervical triangle, and the tips of his fingers and toes are peeling. You diagnose this patient as having Kawasaki's syndrome.

Which of the following is *true* regarding Kawasaki's syndrome?

A. There is an associated thrombocytopenia
B. Steroids are a mainstay of treatment in this disease
C. It is a vasculitis of large-sized vessels
D. It is a vasculitis of medium-sized vessels
E. Patients may have a pulse-fever dissociation

69. A 27-year-old woman has been successfully treated with haloperidol for paranoid schizophrenia. She no longer has paranoid delusions, has few negative symptoms, and is in a stable and supportive relationship with her husband and two children. Recently she has noted a milky nipple discharge and wonders if she could be pregnant even though she had her tubes tied after the birth of her last child 5 years ago. The patient has had no change in her menses, which occur regularly every 28 days, and no breast tenderness. Her physical examination is otherwise unremarkable.

You tell the patient that this discharge is *most likely* due to

A. an anterior pituitary tumor that is secreting prolactin, and that an MRI of her brain is needed immediately.
B. an undiagnosed hypothyroidism, and that she should begin replacement thyroid hormone.
C. haloperidol, which has an antagonizing effect on dopamine and has resulted in an increase of prolactin because of decreased inhibition.
D. pregnancy; tubal ligations are highly unreliable for contraceptive purposes.

E. haloperidol, which has an antagonizing effect on dopamine and has resulted in an increase of prolactin because of increased inhibition.

70. A 53-year-old African American male with a history of Type II diabetes mellitus, multiple myeloma, and chronic renal failure presents to your office for routine follow-up. His serum chemistries are as follows.
sodium: 142
potassium: 5.4
chloride: 112
bicarbonate: 13
blood urea nitrogen: 89
creatinine: 5.6.
Which of the following acid-based disorder(s) is (are) present?
A. Anion gap metabolic acidosis
B. Nonanion gap metabolic acidosis
C. Both an anion gap metabolic acidosis and a nonanion gap metabolic acidosis
D. Both an anion gap metabolic acidosis and a metabolic alkalosis
E. Metabolic alkalosis

71. For the same patient in question 70, what is (are) the *likely* cause(s) of his acid-based disorder(s)?
A. Lactic acidosis
B. Uremia
C. Dehydration (contraction alkalosis)
D. Uremia and type IV renal tubular acidosis
E. Conn's syndrome and uremia

72. A 19-year-old female presents to your office complaining of body swelling. She had been fine until 3 weeks ago when she developed a sore throat and fever. She took OTC ibuprofen and her fever resolved after 4 days. Several days ago the patient began to develop swelling of her legs and face. Her urine then turned a dark color, like cola. On examination, her face has a puffy appearance, especially around the eyes. The woman's urine dipstick shows 4+ blood with trace protein and a few white cells. Her serum albumin is 3.7 and her cholesterol is 200. Being an astute clinician, you centrifuge the patient's urine and, on microscope analysis, find the presence of red blood cell casts.
This renal disorder is which of the following?
A. Minimal change nephrotic syndrome
B. Mesangial (type II) lupus glomerulonephritis

C. Primary membranous glomerulonephritis
D. Membranous (type V) lupus glomerulonephritis
E. Poststreptococcal glomerulonephritis

73. You are working in the emergency department when the paramedics bring in a 22-year-old male with altered mental status. No history is obtainable because the patient is delirious. He is agitated and in distress. His vital signs are as follows.

temperature: 98° F
pulse: 140
blood pressure: 90/40
respiratory rate: 26

His oral mucosa is dry and his jugular vein is flat. The patient is tachycardic with no murmurs and is taking rapid, deep respirations. He moans a little when you press on his belly. His laboratories are remarkable for the following serum chemistries.

sodium: 145
potassium: 5.3
chloride: 99
bicarbonate: 10
BUN: 26
creatinine: 1.3
glucose: 390

Which of the following is his active diagnosis?

A. Cushing's disease
B. Diabetic ketoacidosis
C. Addison's disease
D. Schmidt's syndrome
E. Conn's syndrome

74. A 34-year-old female with no medical history presents to your office with myriad complaints. She has developed rashes on her body, she aches everywhere—in the joints and in her muscles—she is constantly tired, and her feet and legs have begun to swell. She admits to depression and wants to talk to you extensively about this because her husband won't listen to her. He thinks she's exaggerating her problems. Although you have 20 patients scheduled that morning, you decide to perform a quick examination to rule out serious illnesses before you dismiss this patient with a prescription for sertraline for her depression. On examination, the woman is afebrile and has normal vital signs. She has a rash on her face on both cheeks that she says gets worse when she goes into the sun. She has swelling of her wrists, elbows, and knees. She has a couple of superficial oral ulcers. You then run a quick urinalysis that shows 3+ protein on dipstick.

Which two serum laboratory tests should you order immediately?

A. ANA and anti-SCL-70
B. Anti-Ro and anti-La
C. ANA and rheumatoid factor
D. ANA and anti–double-stranded DNA
E. ANA and ESR

75. A 36-year-old female with a history of type I diabetes mellitus is referred to you for evaluation of her anemia. The patient admits to a long-standing history of heavy menses. On examination she has marked pallor. Her hemoglobin is 10 mg/dL (normal 13.5–14.0), her MCV is 128 (normal 82–96), and she has hypersegmented neutrophils on her peripheral smear. Her smear and other laboratory tests show no evidence of hemolysis. Her iron and TIBC are both low. Her serum B_{12} level is at the lower limits of normal.

Which of the following tests should you order to confirm your diagnosis?

A. Methylmalonic acid
B. Serum ferritin
C. Coombs' test
D. Bone marrow biopsy
E. TSH

ANSWERS

1. **B.**

   Streptococcus viridans is the most common infecting agent causing subacute bacterial endocarditis.

   A, C, D, and E, are not a cause of subacute bacterial endocarditis.

2. **B.**

   An insulinoma is the most common islet cell tumor.

   A. C peptide would be increased in an insulinoma.
   C. The patient is not injecting herself with insulin as evidenced by high C-peptide levels.
   D. CNS abnormalities will reverse with glucose administration.
   E. Increased insulin would not be consistent with diabetes.

3. **D.**

   Auspitz sign is pinpoint bleeding with removal of an overlying psoriatic scale due to the thin epidermis above the dermal papillae.

   A. Köbner's phenomenon is also described in this question. It describes psoriatic lesions that appear at sites of cutaneous trauma.
   B. Microabscesses of Monro are also associated with psoriasis. They are neutrophil aggregates within the stratum corneum.
   C. Koplik spots are the pathognomonic white spots on an erythematous base found in the buccal mucosa before the rash of measles appears.
   E. Pastia's lines describe the rash of scarlet fever when it is more pronounced in the folds of the axilla and groin.

4. **C.**

   The elevated blood pressure, weak pulses, and notching on the lower borders of the ribs in a young patient is characteristic of coarctation of the aorta.

   A. Pulmonary stenosis is characterized by a systolic ejection murmur and canon "a" wave.
   B. The most common symptoms of atrial septal defect in adults is the development of palpitations related to atrial arrhythmias as a result of right atrial enlargement.
   D. Eisenmenger's syndrome develops after ventricular septal defects, is a right-to-left shunt characterized by systemic hypoxemia and cyanosis.
   E. Patients with VSDs complicated by pulmonary hypertension and reversed shunts may present with dyspnea and cyanosis.

5. **B.**

   With this patient's history of a recent MI he is most likely in congestive heart failure. His symptoms are due to pulmonary edema and his pleural tap confirms that the effusion is transudative.

   A. Pneumonia with empyema would cause an exudative effusion.
   C. Hypoalbuminemia secondary to liver failure is a cause of a transudative pleural effusion but this patient has no history of ascites or portal hypertension. Therefore, it is not the best answer in this scenario.
   D. A malignancy would have an exudative effusion.
   E. Esophageal rupture most commonly occurs in the scenario of a bulimic, an alcoholic, or in hyperemesis gravidarum due to violent vomiting. The effusion would be significant for increased amylase.
   F. Pulmonary embolus is associated with an exudative effusion.

6. **D.**

   The vast majority of acute Q-wave MIs occur as a result of occlusive thrombus within a coronary artery. Agents such as TPA can restore blood flow and limit myocardial damage.

   A. β-blockers are used acutely but restoration of blood flow is more important.
   B. ACE inhibitors are used for chronic management.
   C. Nitrates only provide symptomatic relief and have no proved impact on mortality.
   E. HMG CoA reductase inhibitors are used after the patient is discharged from the hospital.

7. **E.**

   Anticoagulation is recommended as the initial treatment to protect from stroke before attempting to restore sinus rhythm, whether through antiarrhythmic agents or cardioversion.

   A. β-blockers are not the first-line treatment for atrial fibrillation.
   B. If atrial fibrillation has persisted for at least 48 hours or for an unknown duration, patients should undergo anticoagulation for at least 3 weeks before cardioversion. Anticoagulation should be continued for 3 weeks following successful cardioversion.
   C. ACE inhibitors are not the first-line treatment for atrial fibrillation.
   D. Furosemide is not an option in atrial fibrillation.

8. **D.**

   This is the classic description of a thyroglossal duct cyst. This congenital disorder can present in childhood as a midline mass that is noncompressible and moves with swallowing or protrusion of the tongue. As the thyroid gland migrates during fetal development it courses from the base of the tongue to its final resting position in the base of the neck. The thyroglossal duct usually involutes but cysts can form anywhere along the tract.

A. Branchial cleft cysts are commonly found lateral in the neck, not midline.
B. Cystic hygromas are compressible and located in the lateral neck. They are derived from occluded lymphatics and usually present by age 2.
C. Dermoid cysts are located in the lateral neck and do not move with swallowing.
E. The thyroid gland is midline and moves with swallowing. However, there is no reason to believe that this is a goiter because of the child's otherwise healthy state.

9. **E.**

Multiple sclerosis is a recurrent, often progressive, inflammatory demyelinization of the white matter of the brain and spinal cord. The condition affects young adults with a predilection for females. Whereas the etiology is unknown, risk factors include Northern European descent, living in a temperate zone, and family history of the disease. Symptoms vary and are due to upper-motor neuron lesions. Besides imaging and lumbar puncture, work-up must include labs to rule out infectious causes. The classic finding in CSF is an increase in CSF immunoglobulins with mostly IgG, but often IgA and IgM, and results in oligoclonal bands on electrophoresis.

A. Mild mononuclear pleocytosis is seen in some patients, but this is not the best answer.
B. Other CSF abnormalities include increased total protein level and myelin debris.
C. Slight elevation of opening CSF pressure is possible but is not diagnostic for multiple sclerosis.
D. No significant changes in cell count is found in multiple sclerosis.

10. **A.**

Hypertrophic cardiomyopathy patients may have a sustained apical impulse.

B. Aortic stenosis has a narrow pulse pressure and ejection type murmur during systole.
C. Atrial septal defect has fixed splitting of the second heart sound on physical exam.
D. Tricuspid stenosis presents with a diastolic murmur heard best along the left sternal border.
E. Aortic regurgitation presents with a laterally displaced point of maximal impulse.

11. **A.**
ACE inhibitors slow the onset of nephropathy by decreasing angiotensin II, which normally vasoconstricts the efferent arteriole that releases pressure on the glomerulus.
B. β-blockers would not affect the efferent arteriole and prevent the onset of glomerulosclerosis.
C. Diuretics would also have no effect.
D. Digoxin would have no effect.
E. Aldosterone would have no effect.

12. **A.**
Primary biliary cirrhosis (PBC) is a chronic progressive disease affecting the small intrahepatic bile ducts. The majority of patients are women, frequently those between the ages of 40 to 60 years. PBC is more common in Northern Europeans but rare in those of African descent

Antimitochondrial antibodies is the best serologic test for diagnosis of PBC, with a sensitivity of 90% to 95%, and a specificity of 98%.
B. This answer is incorrect because antinuclear antibodies are found in many autoimmune diseases. It is only positive in 20% to 25% of patients with PBC.
C. An ESR is incorrect because it is a very nonspecific test.
D. An MRI of the liver is incorrect because imaging can only be used to rule out obstructive causes, but not to make the diagnosis.
E. A liver biopsy is invasive and would not be an appropriate next step.

13. **F.**
The number-one risk for all breast cancers is female gender (men account for 1% of all breast cancers). (F) Advanced age is the number-one risk factor for women. This is followed by (C) young (age <11) menarche; (H) old (age >30 years) first pregnancy; (D) late (age >50 years) menopause; and family history. (G) Family history is defined as a first-degree relative diagnosed with breast cancer at a young (<45 years old) age. However, 95% of all breast cancers are not familial. Inheritance of the BRCA1 gene places a woman at an 85% lifetime risk of developing breast cancer and is suspected to be the cause of half of all inherited breast cancers. There is no increased risk of breast cancer with (A) caffeine intake, (B) alcohol, or (E) fibrocystic disease (there is increased risk if there is fibrocystic change with atypia). A recent study suggests that long-term cigarette smoking may also increase risk. (I) No increased risk with breastfeeding.

14. **E.**

The classic triad of signs in Wernicke's encephalopathy includes confusion, ataxia, and ophthalmoplegia. Ataxia consists of predominantly stance and gait disturbances. Other ophthalmoplegia signs are strabismus and ptosis. Additionally, other signs such as indifference to the surroundings, confabulation, and retrograde amnesia would constitute the Wernicke-Korsakoff syndrome. Patients may also exhibit signs of alcoholism and nutritional deficiency including various forms of liver disease, angular stomatitis, and spider telangiectasia. While prompt thiamine replacement can reverse the symptoms, glucose replacement, if needed, must be secondary to thiamine replacement to reduce the risk of precipitously worsening the symptoms of Wernicke encephalopathy.

The central nervous lesion occurs in the mamillary bodies, the periventricular regions of the thalamus, the floor of the fourth ventricle, and the anterior region of the cerebellum.

A. Lesion of Wernicke's encephalopathy is not found in the pineal gland.
B. Lesion of Wernicke's encephalopathy is not found in the occipital lobe.
C. Lesion of Wernicke's encephalopathy is not found in the medulla.
D. Lesion of Wernicke's encephalopathy is not found in the frontal lobe.

15. **C.**

This case—with the BUN/Cr ratio of 10:1 and the low urine output—suggests acute tubular necrosis. This is often a result of hypovolemia that can occur during or after surgery. Acute tubular necrosis urinalysis shows Una >40 mEq/L, FENa >1, and Uosm 350.

A. Prerenal azotemia presents with FENa of <1, Una <40, and Uosm >500.
B. Acute glomerulonephritis presents with FENa of <1, Una <40, and Uosm >500.
D. Postrenal azotemia presents with FENa of <1, Una <40, and Uosm >500.
E. Focal segmental glomerulosclerosis presents with nephrotic syndrome and mild hypertension.

16. **D.**

Hypophosphatemia directly increases renal calcitriol production, which enhances intestinal calcium and phosphate absorption and bone reabsorption.

A. The consequent rise in plasma calcium concentration will suppress PTH release.

B. Choice B is incorrect because there would normally be a decreased urinary phosphate excretion, not increased as choice B states. Reduce urinary phosphate excretion by removing the normal inhibitory effect of PTH.
C. The intestinal, bone, and renal changes will all raise the plasma phosphate concentration toward normal. An undesired elevation in the plasma calcium concentration is prevented by the fall in PTH secretion.

17. **A.**

Systemic lupus erythematosus (SLE) is a multisystem, autoimmune inflammatory condition with fluctuating, chronic course. This disease has a higher occurrence in women compared to men (9:1). Most cases are idiopathic but drugs such as procainamide, hydralazine, and D-penicillamine can induce similar symptoms.

Antihistone antibodies must be used to differentiate drug-induced SLE from idiopathic SLE.

B. Antimitochandrial antibodies are diagnostic of primary biliary cirrhosis.
C. ESR can be elevated in this patient but would not be helpful in differentiating the causes of SLE.
D. C reactive protein is a non-specific marker of inflammation and is not diagnostic of lupus or drug-induced lupus.
E. PTT prolongation is consistent with a diagnosis of lupus (due to antiphospholipid antibodies), but can also be seen in a variety of other conditions (i.e., not a specific finding).

18. **D.**

Inhaled steroids are a mainstay in treatment for this patient's asthma symptoms. They are potent agents reducing both acute and chronic inflammation.

A. This is the perceived mechanism of the bronchodilating action of theophylline.
B. This is the mechanism of action of beta agonists that are selective to the pulmonary system (metaproterenol).
C. This is the mechanism of action of beta-antagonists that are cardioselective (atenolol).
E. This is the mechanism of action of the leukotriene inhibiting drugs (zileuton).
F. This is the mechanism of action of cromolyn sodium.

19. **B.**

A contraction metabolic alkalosis would occur. The loop of Henle reabsorbs sodium chloride. This is the major mechanism of the countercurrent gradient that allows concentrated urine to be excreted. Therefore, the major manifestations of injury to the loop of Henle include sodium wasting, hypokalemia, and metabolic alkalosis due to excess sodium leaving the loop and reabsorbed in the cortical collecting duct in exchange for potassium and hydrogen. The polyuria would be due to decreased concentrating ability.

A. Metabolic acidosis would not occur.
C. Respiratory alkalosis would not occur.
D. Respiratory acidosis would not occur.
E. Normal acid base balance would not occur.

20. **B.**

DCIS is a true premalignancy that can lead to invasive ductal carcinoma in either breast. Lumpectomy with wide excisions and radiation therapy is usually recommended. Mammography and self-breast exam are important parts of continuing detection.

A. She is at risk for cancer in either breast, regardless of where the DCIS lesion was found initially.
C. DCIS is a premalignant lesion. She is at risk for cancer in either breast.
D. DCIS is in situ and by definition has not metastasized.

21. **C.**

Basal cell carcinoma (BCC) is the most common malignant skin tumor. If left untreated this can progress to disfiguring "Rodent Ulcers." However, these are local tumors and rarely ever metastasize.

A. BCCs are not usually found on the extremities.
B. Actinic keratosis are a frequent precursor to squamous cell carcinomas (SCC). SCC may also be found on the lips and metastasize more frequently than BCC but are not as common as melanoma.
D. BCCs and SCCs are commonly due to sun exposure and found in sun-exposed areas of the skin (e.g., the face and neck of farmers). Choice D says that they are not related to sun exposure.
E. SCCs have histologically characteristic keratin pearls.
F. Seborrheic keratosis is common in the elderly and have a characteristic "stuck on" appearance. They are not related to BCC.

22. **C.**

Wilms' tumor is common in this age group and presents as described.

A. Adenoma is often small and asymptomatic.
B. Renal cell carcinoma usually presents in age group 50–70. It is characterized by polygonal clear cells.

D. Transitional cell carcinoma often presents clinically with hematuria. It is associated with toxic exposures.
E. Squamous cell carcinoma comprises a small minority of urinary tract malignancies. It is associated with chronic bacterial infection.

23. **B.**
There is an increased risk for the development of pigment stones in the gallbladder because of the increased bilirubin, due to increased spleen recycling of Hb, which will precipitate out.
A. There will be no hemoglobinuria because the RBC destruction is extravascular in the spleen that will recycle the Hb. Hb will be present in the urine during intravascular hemolysis where the Hb will then be filtered in the kidney.
C. MCHC is the most significant index because there is loss of surface area with normal Hb the Hb concentration essentially goes up. This indicates spherocytosis.
D. Splenomegaly occurs because of the destruction of all the spherocytes.
E. Increased RBC osmotic fragility occurs in spherocytosis, not decreased.

24. **D.**
There is no increased risk of male breast cancer with gynecomastia. However, 1% of all breast cancers are diagnosed in males so, although his risk is small, it is not zero. Gynecomastia is common in pubertal males and conditions, such as alcohol use, where there is an imbalance of testosterone and estrogen. If the conditions resulting in gynecomastia are addressed within 1 year the breast tissue may regress.
A. Although his breasts have increased in size, he has no increased risk of male breast cancer.
B. Gynecomastia in liver disease is a result of increased peripheral conversion of androstenedione into estrogens; however, there is no increased risk of breast cancer.
C. It is true that gynecomastia has no increased risk of breast cancer, but just because he is a man does not mean that his risk is zero.

25. **E.**
Dermatomyositis is an uncommon inflammatory myopathy with involvement of the skin and the skeletal muscles. This disease has a predilection for females than males with a ratio of 2:1. Skeletal muscle involvement occurs in proximal muscle symmetrically including dysphagia, dysphonia, and proximal limbs muscle weak-

ness. Work-up must be extensive to rule out neurological and musculoskeletal causes.

A muscle biopsy is necessary for confirmation, and findings include inflammation predominantly around small blood vessels and in the perimysial connective tissue.

A. Inflammation of endomysium connective tissue is found in polymyositis.
B. Rimmed vacuoles are found in inclusion-body myositis.
C. Amyloid deposits within myocytes are found in inclusion-body myositis.
D. This choice is incorrect because the pathology is not normal.

26. **A.**

This case is most likely chronic myelogenous leukemia (CML) because of slow onset and the fact that the marrow is not completely abnormal. Bone marrow cellularity, primarily of the myeloid and megakaryocytic lineages, with a greatly altered myeloid to erythroid ratio, is increased in almost all patients with CML.

B. Acute myelogenous leukemia would present with fever, splenomegaly, Auer rods, thrombocytopenia, and myeloblasts in the blood and bone marrow.
C. Hodgkin's lymphoma would present with Pel-Ebstein fevers, leukocytosis, and Reed-Sternberg cells.
D. Non-Hodgkin's lymphoma would present with nontender lymphadenopathy and proliferation of neoplastic cells with a low rate of mitosis.
E. Acute lymphoblastic leukemia would present with fever, fatigue, infections, leukocytosis, decreased platelets, and increased blasts in bone marrow.

27. **A.**

Polycythemia vera is characterized by an elevated hematocrit (>52%). It is caused by a clonal expansion of the trilineage myeloid stem cell associated with a primary increase in RBC mass, plasma volume, granulocytes, and platelets to a lesser extent.

B. Chronic myelogenous leukemia would present with elevated white blood cell count; varying degrees of immaturity of the granulocytic series are present at diagnosis. Usually <5% circulating blasts and <10% blasts and promyelocytes are noted.
C. Acute lymphoblastic leukemia would present with leukocytosis, anemia, and decreased platelets. Bone marrow biopsy would show increased blasts.

D. Iron-deficiency anemia would present with decreased serum iron and ferritin, increased total iron-binding capacity, and peripheral smear would show target cells.
E. Essential thrombocythemia would present with platelet count $> 5 \times 10^5$ cells/μL, splenomegaly, and ecchymosis.

28. **E.**

It is essential to find the etiology of peptic ulcer disease in order to provide the appropriate treatment. As this patient's symptoms are consistent with duodenal ulcers, causes such as medication-induced (NSAID, glucocorticoids), *H. pylori* infection, alcohol-induced gastritis seems less likely because of the additional symptoms of amenorrhea and elevated calcium and gastrin level. The triad of tumors or hyperplasia of the pituitary, parathyroid, and pancreatoma describes Werner's syndrome or multiple endocrine neoplasia syndrome type I and can describe the symptoms and signs in this patient. Gastrinoma is the most common tumor of the pancreas. This tumor produces high levels of gastrin and stimulates the secretion of gastric acid to cause ulcers. The condition is called Zollinger-Ellison syndrome when there is only gastrinoma. Parathyroid tumor produces a high level of parathyroid hormone that acts to conserve and maintain a high level calcium. The most common pituitary tumor is prolactinoma. Besides amenorrhea, other symptoms include galactorrhea, osteopenia, or osteomalacia due to decreased estrogen level. Symptoms in men include impotence, gynecomastia, and galactorrhea.

A. Duodenum ulcers only describe part of the diagnosis and do not explain the rest of the problems.
B. *H. pylori* can cause ulcers but is not linked to Werner's syndrome.
C. Atrophic gastritis is unlikely in this patient based on the signs, symptoms, and work-up.
D. Pernicious anemia is unlikely in this patient based on the signs, symptoms, and work-up.

29. **C.**

This patient most likely has an impending subarachnoid hemorrhage. Causes include trauma, aneurysm, arteriovenous malformation, hypertension, tumor, and blood dyscrasias. Based on the history, he probably has a congenital or berry aneurysm that has developed later in life due to a defect in the media of the arterial wall. The hallmark symptoms of subarachnoid hemorrhage are headache ("the worst headache of my life"), syncope, nausea, and vomiting. Aneurysm usually develops at the junction of vessels in the circle of Willis.

Findings of pupillary defects should raise suspicion of oculomotor nerve defect (CN III) caused by an aneurysm of the posterior communicating artery.

A. Aneurysm at the internal carotid artery is possible but not likely in this patient.
B. Berry aneurysms at other vessels are possible; that is, 40% at the junction of anterior communicating artery and anterior cerebral artery, 34% at the first bifurcation of the middle cerebral artery, and 20% at middle cerebral artery and posterior communicating artery.
D. Aneurysm at the superior cerebellar artery would be unlikely in this patient.
E. Aneurysm at the anterior inferior cerebellar artery is unlikely in this patient.

30. **C.**

Anti-intrinsic factor and antiparietal cell antibodies will be present in B_{12} deficiency due to pernicious anemia.

A. Drug abuse is unlikely to present as jaundice unless the patient has hepatitis.
B. Ataxia is caused by subacute combined degeneration of the cord, not by a cerebral neoplasm.
D. The Schilling test would be abnormal.
E. Bone marrow will show pancytopenia and hypersegmented neutrophils.

31. **A.**

This is a case of peripheral nerve damage due to diabetes, which is a symmetrical involvement.

B. The sensory involvement would be symmetrical, not asymmetrical.
C. Sensory would be affected more than motor.
D. Muscle tone is usually not affected.
E. The ability to rise from a squatting position would not be affected.

32. **D.**

Paget's bone disease (osteitis deformans) is a nonmetabolic bone disease characterized by repeated episodes of osteolysis and excessive attempts to repair that result in a weakened bone of increased mass. The disease occurs more often in males than females in a 2:1 ratio. This condition can involve one bone or many and is usually in the spine, pelvis, skull, femur, and tibia. Symptoms develop mainly from the effects of complications such as skeletal pain and bowing of long bones due to fracture, increased heat of extremity due to increased vascularity, skull enlargement due to bone enlargement, and high cardiac failure due to chest and spine deformity and blood shunting. These laboratory changes reflect the osteoclastic and osteoblastic process.

A. These changes occur in patients with ascorbic acid (vitamin C) deficiency.
B. These changes occur in patients with von Recklinghausen's disease of the bone (osteitis fibrosa cystica), an osteolytic bone disease caused by hyperparathyroidism.
C. These changes occur in patients with osteomalacia/rickets due to vitamin D deficiency.
E. These changes occur in patients with a malignancy of bones such as multiple myeloma.

33. **A.**

Patient has hemophilia A, so patient is deficient in Factor 8 (VIII). Bleeding time will be normal.

B. Hemophilia A is sex-linked recessive, not autosomal dominant.
C. Prothrombin time will be normal.
D. Partial thromboplastin time would be prolonged.

34. **A.**

Carbon monoxide (CO) is a colorless, odorless, tasteless, and nonirritating gas. Since CO has about 250 times the affinity for hemoglobin than oxygen, it displaces oxygen from hemoglobin and results in decreasing the oxygen-carrying capacity of the blood. It also shifts the oxyhemoglobin curve to the left, thus decreasing oxygen release to tissue. Binding of CO to myoglobin affects muscle activity. CO also binds to cytochrome oxidase impairing mitochondrial function. This gas is most toxic to organs with the highest oxygen consumption—especially the heart and the brain. CO poisoning is mostly seen during winter months as people start using gas heaters. Severity of symptoms usually, but not always, correlates with measured carboxyhemoglobin levels. The cherry-red skin color and bright red venous blood are infrequent and late finding of CO poisoning. With a good history and physical exam, one can suspect CO poisoning and administer hyperbaric oxygen treatment quickly. However, poisoning with other agents such as cyanide, hydrogen sulfide, methemoglobinemia, PCP, phenothiazines, and theophylline can produce similar symptoms.

Measurement of carboxyhemoglobin is vital for diagnosis and treatment.

B. Similar measurement using pulse oximetry is inaccurate because of the similar absorption characteristics of oxyhemoglobin and carboxyhemoglobin.
C. Oxygen saturation measurement by arterial blood gas may be inaccurate because it measures oxygen dissolved in plasma, which is not affected by CO.
D. Electrolyte levels are important if one suspects lactic acidosis.
E. A complete blood count is not useful for diagnosing CO poisoning.

35. **D.**

Papillary cancer is the most common cancer of the thyroid. It is pathologically distinguished by a ground glass Orphan Annie nucleus and psammoma bodies.

A. Medullary cancer is a cancer of the parafollicular "C" cells that secretes calcitonin.
B. Patients with Graves' disease have infiltrative ophthalmology and pretibial myxedema. It is caused by an autoimmune response to the TSH receptor.
C. Follicular cancer usually has a poor prognosis. It commonly has bloodborne metastases to bone and lungs.
E. Beta thalassemia has marked anemia due to folate deficiency and decreased hemoglobin synthesis.

36. **C.**

This patient has symptoms of ulcerative colitis (UC), a chronic idiopathic inflammatory disease affecting the large intestine. Similar to UC, Crohn's disease (CD) is a chronic idiopathic inflammatory disease that affects the GI system from oral to anus. Both are more common in Jewish-descent populations, and most cases are in the 15–35 age range or during ages 50–70. UC usually starts in the rectum and spreads proximally, whereas CD is commonly found in the terminal ileum. UC affects the mucosa and submucosa layers and causes continuous lesions, and biopsy can show pseudopolyps, abscesses with numerous neutrophils in the crypt of Lieberkühn. CD causes transmural inflammation and skip lesions, and biopsy can show noncaseating granulomas. Because of the transmural inflammation in CD, there is also a risk of inflammation to adjacent loops of bowels or organs that results in development of fistula and fissure.

Because of the predominant nature of UC in the large intestine, these patients have a higher rate of development of colon cancer. Various medical regimens are available for treatment, and total colectomy is a valuable surgical option not only to remove the affected colon segment but also to cure the patient.

A, B, D, and E findings are seen in Crohn's patients.

37. **C.**

Patients with acromegaly are known to have significant cardiovascular complications that include increased risk of hypertension and stroke. Visual symptoms in this patient are most likely due to pituitary adenoma.

A. Patients with acromegaly are not at increased risk for carcinoma of the colon.
B. Patients with AIDS are not at increased risk for carcinoma of the colon.
D. Patients with pulmonary insufficiency are not at increased risk for carcinoma of the colon.
E. Patients with carcinoma of the breast are not at increased risk for carcinoma of the colon.

38. **E.**

Elevated LH is responsible for polycystic ovarian syndrome.

A. 21-alpha hydroxylase defect causes virilization in females but oral contraceptives will not alleviate this patient's symptoms.
B. Ovarian tumor secreting testosterone will cause virilization but oral contraceptives will not alleviate this patient's symptoms.
C. Uterine leiomyosarcoma will cause pelvic pain and vaginal discharge.
D. 11-beta hydroxylase deficiency will cause virilization in females. Hypertension occurs due to salt and water retention. Oral contraceptives will not alleviate this patient's symptoms.

39. **B.**

This is a staphylococcal pneumonia that classically presents after a viral influenza infection. It is associated with an exudative pleural effusion.

A. If it were encapsulated, this could be *E. coli* or *H. influenzae*.
C. This is characteristic of *Listeria monocytogenes*.
D. This could be true, but is not the best choice in the presence of the patient's clinical appearance.
E. This is the picture of mycoplasma pneumonia.

40. **B.**

This patient most likely has temporal arteritis, a vasculitis commonly affecting the temporal artery. This disease frequently affects white women of Northern European descent who are usually older than 50. Patients report headaches, cephalagia, amaurosis fugax, jaw claudication, anorexia and weight loss, fever and sweats, and malaise, fatigue, and depression. The 1990 American College of Rheumatology criteria for classification of giant cell arteritis states that three of the following five items must be present: symptoms in patients older than 50 years, new onset of headache or localized head pain, temporal artery tenderness to palpation, decreased pulsations not related to arteriosclerosis of cervical arteries, and ESR greater than 50.

A definitive diagnosis of temporal arteritis requires temporal artery biopsy, however an ESR rate is highly suggestive and can be obtained much more quickly. Patients with an elevated ESR need to be on corticosteroid to prevent damage to the visual system that would result in blindness while awaiting confirmation biopsy.

A. CT scan may be beneficial to rule out malignancy, but would not be beneficial in this case.
C. Lumbar puncture would not be beneficial.
D. Supportive care including NSAIDs can relieve symptoms but cannot reduce the inflammation.

41. **D.**

Abruptio placentae is the separation of the placenta from the uterine wall before delivery of the fetus. The patients usually present with a triad of hypertonic uterine contractions or signs of preterm labor, uterine bleeding, and evidence of fetal compromise. The condition can be graded based on maternal and fetal status. It is imperative to recognize and to diagnose the condition because of the possible catastrophic nature to the mother and the fetus.

A. Placenta previa is a condition of abnormal placental implantation in the lower uterine segment in advance of the presenting fetal part. This condition causes painless vaginal bleeding.
B. Bleeding can be associated with premature labor, but most patients present with regular uterine contraction before 36 weeks of gestation.
C. Ectopic pregnancy is unlikely in this patient based on her history.
E. Vasa previa, the presentation of the blood vessels of the umbilical cord in front of the fetal head during labor, is unlikely in this patient based on her history.

42. **A.**
Functional residual capacity equals the expiratory reserve volume plus the residual volume.
B. Inspiratory capacity
C. Expiratory reserve volume
D. Residual volume
E. Vital capacity
F. Resting tidal volume
G. Total lung capacity

43. **A.**
Syphilis is a sexually transmitted infection of the spirochete, *Treponema pallidum*. The initial symptom of a red, painless, sharply demarcated ulcer (condyloma lata) can be overlooked, and patients may present with symptoms of secondary stage such as malaise, headaches, sore throat, fever, weight loss, musculoskeletal pain, red and papular rash in palms and soles, and lymphadenopathy. This disease occurs commonly among those with risk factors of unsafe sexual practices, multiple partners, and drug abuse. Various blood tests (e.g., RPR, VDRL, FTA-ABS) are currently used for diagnosis, but the spirochete can be seen on a sample taken from the condyloma lata under a dark-field microscopy.
B. These organisms are seen in microscopic examination of patients infected with *Trichomonas vaginalis*.
C. These organisms can be found in patients infected with *Calymmatobacterium granulomatis* (granuloma inguinale).
D. These organisms are seen in patients infected with *Neisseria gonorrhea*.
E. These organisms are seen in patients infected with *Chlamydia trachomatis*.

44. **D.**
Osteogenesis imperfecta (OI) is a group of genetically heterogeneous connective tissue disorders affecting bone and soft tissue. Symptoms include short to normal stature, skeletal fragility with multiple fractures, dentinogenesis imperfecta, hearing impairment, joint laxity, and blue sclera. OI is caused by the failure of maturation of procollagen to type 1 collagen and the failure of normal collagen cross-linking.
A. A deficiency of acid hydrolases occurs in patients with mucopolysaccharidoses. The deficiencies result in accumulation of dermatan sulfate, heparan sulfate, and keratin sulfate.
B. Patients with rickets/osteomalacia are vitamin D deficient.

C. Patients with a variant form of osteopetrosis are carbonic anhydrase II deficient.
E. Patients with scurvy disease (Barlow disease) are deficient in hydroxylation of lysine/proline. Vitamin C is needed in the hydroxylation of lysine/proline. This patient doesn't have this.

45. **C.**

The characteristic Ghon complex of primary TB is defined as the tubercle and the node into which it drains. The granuloma is formed 2–6 weeks after primary infection by the cell-mediated immune system. The infected macrophages (aka, Langerhans cells multinucleated giant cells from the fusion of many macrophages) are walled off by monocytes recruited by activated T cells. Histologically, the granuloma is surrounded by a ring of lymphocytes with central caseous necrosis.

A. The TB bacillus reproduces inside of the macrophage after phagocytosis. It is spared intracellular killing by inhibiting the fusion of the phagosome with lysosomes.
B. There is no information to conclude that the patient is immunosuppressed. Immunosuppression can, however, result in reactivation TB.
D. Invasion of the bacillus into pulmonary lymphatics results in miliary TB.
E. Invasion of the bacillus into the blood vessels results in systemic dissemination and disease.

46. **B.**

This patient has Kartagener's syndrome, a congenital disorder of immotile cilia due to the absence of dynein arms. It is associated with infertility, decreased olfaction, bronchiectasis, situs inversus, and sinusitis. Lack of cilian motility disables normal mucociliary escalator.

A. Defective chloride channels is associated with cystic fibrosis and can cause a pansinusitis and bronchiectasis in childhood. It is not associated with anosmia.
C. Meatal obstruction can cause chronic sinusitis, but is not the best answer in this case.
D. Osler-Weber-Rendu is an autosomal-dominant disorder of telangiectasias on the lips, skin, mucous membranes, and internal organs. It presents with severe epistaxis, hemoptysis, and unexplained GI bleeds.
E. Nasal polyps could cause meatal obstruction, but is not the best answer in this case.

47. **B.**
Reiter's syndrome is nongonococcal urethritis, arthritis, uveitis, and conjunctivitis. This patient's signs and symptoms would point you toward an uveitis instead of a conjunctivitis.
A. Conjunctivitis is associated with Reiter's syndrome; however, there would be no change in vision or photophobia if this was the cause of his current symptoms.
C. A corneal abrasion is associated with an acutely painful, red, watering, and photophobic eye, but this patient denies trauma. There would have been a defect noted with fluorescein staining.
D. Keratitis is caused by viral (HSV or adeno) or bacterial (due to poor contact lens hygiene) infection. You would have observed an inflamed cornea and dendritic branching on fluorescein stain (if it were HSV).
E. Scleritis is an extremely painful condition that can be associated with collagen vascular disease.

48. **C.**
In contrast to multiple sclerosis, Guillain-Barré syndrome is an acute inflammatory demyelinating polyradiculopathy predominantly affecting motor function. Motor weakness is symmetric, initially involving proximal muscles but subsequently involves both proximal and distal muscles and results in difficulty in ambulating, rising from a chair, or climbing stairs. Reflexes are depressed or absent bilaterally. Some patients report glove and stocking anesthesia. Other manifestations are autonomic abnormalities such as bradycardia or tachycardia, hypotension, or hypertension. Late symptom of respiratory insufficiency caused by weakness of intercostal muscles can be fatal. The etiology of Guillian-Barre syndrome is unknown, but it is clearly associated with infections such as upper respiratory or diarrheal illness, vaccinations, malignancies, surgery, drugs. The work-up must rule out other causes of neuropathy.

The pathognomonic CSF findings are elevated protein level especially IgG without an increase in cells (albumin-cytologic dissociation).
A. Mononuclear pleocytosis is not the pathognomic CSF finding.
B. Increased protein rather than decreased protein level is the pathognomic CSF finding.
D. Elevated opening pressure is not the pathognomic CSF finding.
E. No significant change in cell count is found in Guillain-Barré syndrome.
F. Elevated glucose level is not the pathognomic CSF finding.

49. **D.**

Cholesteatomas are the most common growths in the middle ear and usually present after a chronic episode of otitis media. Treatment is surgical as it can destroy bone causing deafness and facial nerve palsy if left untreated.

A. Idiopathic hemotympanicum is the idiopathic bluish color of the TM common to a cholesterol granuloma. The blue color is a foreign-body reaction to cholesterol crystals.
B. The blue color is a foreign-body reaction to cholesterol crystals.
C. A lateral neck mass with an associated neuroendocrine tumor is characteristic of a glomus tympanicum tumor.
E. A benign tumor at the cerebellopontine angle describes an acoustic neuroma.
F. Patients with chronic otitis media commonly have a perforated eardrum.

50. **A.**

Achalasia is an uncommon disorder of esophageal transport due to the failure of esophageal smooth muscle function to move food from the oral cavity to the stomach. Classic symptoms include long-standing, slowly progressive dysphagia for both solids and liquids; however, it is more frequent with solids. Regurgitation is common and unprovoked, occurring during or shortly after a meal. Chest pain similar in nature to cardiac angina is frequent, but heartburn is rare. Achalasia has no predilection for gender, and its etiology is still unknown. Patients affected with Chagas' disease due to protozoan parasite *Trypanosoma cruzi* may end up with a form of esophageal motility disorder that is indistinguishable from achalasia. Barium swallow with fluoroscopy can help diagnosis before manometry.

Manometry study usually shows low-amplitude disorganized contraction, high intraesophageal resting pressure, high LES pressure, and inadequate LES relaxation after swallow.

B. These findings describe a patient with gastroesophageal reflux disease.
C. These findings describe a patient suffering diffuse esophageal spasm.
D. A patient with progressive systemic sclerosis (scleroderma) may have these findings.
E. May be seen with irritability of esophagus, but not in achalasia.

51. **D.**

This man has MEN IIa, also known as Sipple syndrome. His thyroid nodule is derived from parafollicular "C" cells that secrete calcitonin.

A. Medullary carcinoma does not involve the thyroid hormone-secreting cells.

B. Beta cells are the insulin-secreting cells of the pancreas.
C. Alpha cells are the glucagon-secreting cells of the pancreas.
E. Chief cells secrete PTH. This patient has a history of parathyroid hyperplasia, but this is not the source of this neoplasm.

52. **B.**
This is pemphigus vulgaris. It is a rare autoimmune disorder that primarily affects persons age 20–40 years. IgG autoantibodies are directed against desmoglein III, a cadherin.
A. Bullous pemphigoid is a milder form of pemphigus vulgaris in which the bullae are firm and do not break easily. It commonly affects the elderly and immunofluorescence demonstrates a linear band along the basement membrane.
C. Pemphigus vulgaris is commonly fatal if left untreated.
D. IgG titers correlate with the courses of disease.
E. Urine that fluoresces a distinct orange-pink color is characteristic of cutaneous porphyria tarda, an autosomal dominant defect in heme synthesis. The urine fluoresces due to increased levels of uroporphyrins.

53. **B.**
Paget's disease of the nipple is histologically described with an accurate clinical picture. The patient's history of DCIS in the contralateral breast gives her an increased risk of subsequent cancers in both breasts.
A. Paget's disease of the breast is not related to Paget's disease of the bone where one would expect to find increased levels of alkaline phosphatase.
C. An intraductal papilloma would have the additional history of a serous or bloody discharge from the nipple. A solitary intraductal papilloma does not increase cancer risk; however, multiple intraductal papillomas do.
D. Acute mastitis is more frequently seen in the postpartum period. It is caused by blocked ducts that become infected most commonly by *Staphylococcus* and *Streptococcus* species. It is usually treated with warm compresses and expression of breast milk but can progress to abscess in which case antibiotics would be required.
E. There is no history of allergen exposure in this patient.

54. **B.**
The patient has squamous cell carcinoma, most commonly found centrally in smokers and may cavitate. This lesion may cause hypercalcemia due to release of a parathyroid hormone related protein.
A. Bronchial carcinoid tumors secrete serotonin (5-HT) causing symptoms of intermittent diarrhea, skin flushing, wheezing, and

heart disease; 5-HIAA is a serotonin metabolite that is secreted in the urine.

C. See B. PTH causes hypercalcemia, not hypocalcemia.
D. A syndrome of inappropriate antidiuretic hormone (SIADH) picture is more characteristic of small cell carcinoma. The histological picture of which is small, dark-blue cells like lymphocytes. It is a neoplasm of neuroendocrine (Kulchitsky) cells.
E. Carcinoembryonic antigen is a marker that can be a followed (but not screened for) adenocarcinoma. Adenocarcinoma presents in the subpleura and periphery and is the most frequent cancer in nonsmokers.
F. ACTH is secreted by small cell tumors. Seen mostly in small cell tumors not squamous cell carcinoma. See D.

55. **D.**

This patient most likely has Fitz-Hugh-Curtis syndrome, *Chlamydia* or gonorrhea perihepatitis as a complication of pelvic inflammatory disease (PID). As the infection spreads outside the reproductive system, it causes inflammation of the abdominal organs such as the liver in Fitz-Hugh-Curtis syndrome. Long-term complications include chronic pelvic pain, ectopic pregnancy, and recurrent PID.

A. TSS is a systemic reaction to enterotoxin produced by *Staphylococcus aureus*, found in certain tampons. This patient does not have any history or physical examination results consistent with such a diagnosis.
B. Ectopic pregnancy is unlikely in this patient based on her symptoms and signs, but complications from her PID may cause an ectopic pregnancy in the future.
C. Appendicitis is unlikely in this patient because the pain associated with appendicitis is usually localized to right lower quadrant.
E. Endometriosis is due to ectopic growth of endometrial tissue; symptoms occur cyclically with the menstrual cycle.

56. **C.**

Prostate cancer is the most common cancer in males and is the second most common cause of cancer death. This disease usually affects people in the age range of 60–70 years. African Americans have the highest incidence of prostate cancer, whereas the incidence is low in Asians. Because the disease is usually silent and becomes known only in the advanced stage, it is imperative to perform regular screening (digital rectal examination and PSA level) for prostate cancer. Early symptoms relate to urine outflow obstruction, and bone pain and pathologic fracture can indicate metastasis. The prostate is divided into four anatomic zones: the central, transitional, peripheral, and periurethral zones; 70% to 85% of prostate cancer arises in the peripheral zone.

A. Only a small number of prostate cancer cases arise from the central zone.
B. Benign prostatic hyperplasia usually arises from the transitional zone.
D. Only a small number of prostate cancer cases arise from the periurethral zone.
E. The ejaculatory duct has nothing to do with prostate cancer and is therefore (1) not a perfect prostate and (2) zones refer to areas of prostate tissue.

57. **C.**

Trichomonas vaginalis is a flagellated protozoan that is highly motile in vaginal secretions. The organism is transmitted sexually, and most are asymptomatic. Typical symptoms in women are copious, frothy, yellow, or gray discharge; vaginal itching; dysuria; and vaginal odor. Pelvic exam shows "strawberry cervix" (petechiae). Symptoms in men are urethral discharge, dysuria, and rarely epididymitis. An analysis of the discharge can help to quickly differentiate which sexually transmitted disease is under inspection.

A. A yeast infection caused by *Candida* usually creates cheesy white material in the vagina and vaginal itching; these appear as pseudohyphae on a 10% KOH prep.
B. Bacterial vaginosis is caused by proliferation of different bacteria in the vaginal vault; *Gardinella* is the predominant organism. The discharge has a "fishy" smell on KOH prep. Microscopic examination shows large vaginal epithelial cells covered with lots of bacteria (clue cells).
D. Syphilis is caused by *Treponema*, a spirochete that can be seen on dark-field microscopy.
E. *Calymmatobacterium granulomatis* causes granuloma inguinale (Donovanosis), a condition of genital ulceration and soft tissue/bone destruction; a gram stain of the ulcer shows Donovan bodies (stained organisms within macrophages).

58. **A.**

Benign prostatic hyperplasia (BPH) is the growth of the prostate usually in the periureteral and transitional zones. The resulting enlargement causes obstruction of urine outflow and obstructive incontinence. Common symptoms include difficulty with initiating urination (hesitancy), decrease in caliber and force of stream, incomplete emptying of bladder, postvoid "dribbling," and nocturia. The prostatic hyperplasia is due to androgen action. As circulating testosterone is taken into prostatic stromal cells, it is converted by 5 α-reductase type 2 to dihydrotestosterone (DHT), a metabolite of testosterone and a mediator of prostatic growth. DHT acts in an autocrine fashion on the stromal cells and in paracrine fashion by diffusing into nearby epithelial cells. DHT, similar to androgen, is able to bind to nuclear receptor and promote growth factors necessary for mitotic activity of both epithelial and stromal cells. Because DHT is 10 times more potent than testosterone in promoting prostatic growth, treatment for BPH relies on agents blocking 5 α-reductase activity.

B. Deficiency of 21-hydroxylase, an enzyme converting 17 α-hydroxyprogesterone to deoxycortisol, is found in patients with congenital adrenal hyperplasia.
C. 17 β-hydroxylase is a necessary enzyme for testosterone synthesis, converting androstenedione to testosterone.
D. Aromatase converts androstenedione to estrone.
E. 3 β-hydroxysteroid dehydrogenase converts dehydroepiandrosterone to androstenedione.

59. **E.**

This is a case of measles with the diagnostic signs of the 3Cs: cough, coryza, and conjunctivitis. Measles is caused by a paramyxovirus and should be considered when immunization status is unknown.

A. A togavirus is the etiological agent in rubella, or German measles.
B. Coxsackie A causes hand-foot-and-mouth disease.
C. Human herpes virus 6 is the cause of roseola infantum also known as exanthem subitum.
D. Parvovirus B-19 causes erythema infectiosum, also known as fifth disease. The classic finding is "slapped cheek" appearance.
F. Varicella-zoster causes chickenpox.

60. **B.**

This infant most likely has congenital pyloric stenosis, an idiopathic disorder of the pylorus. Hypertrophy of the muscular layers of the pylorus causes obstruction of the pylorus, preventing food from entering the duodenum. Because this infant presents with common symptoms, other signs and symptoms—such as weight loss, visible peristalsis, and palpable "olive" nodule in mid-epigastrium—are also observed. Diagnosis can be made by ultrasound; however, prompt fluid resuscitation and correction of electrolytes are also important in severely dehydrated infants.

A. Imaging even with ultrasound would show abnormality of pyloric stenosis. A normal ultrasound would not be seen in this patient.
C. An antral web is more likely in this patient than a cardiac web.
D. Pyloric atresia is unlikely in this patient as this would present at birth.
E. Esophageal hiatal hernia is unlikely in this patient because it is more common in adults.

61. **A.**

Colonic diverticula are herniations of mucosa and submucosa through the muscularis, and are usually found along the anatomic weak point: the colon's mesenteric border where the vasa recta penetrates the muscle wall. Diverticula are common in older people, and an association has been made of diverticula with diets low in fiber. When inflammation occurs, abdominal pain is usually located in left lower quadrant but can be anywhere in the lower abdomen because of the redundancy of the sigmoid colon. As the inflammation progresses, other symptoms such as muscle spasm, guarding, and rebound tenderness can develop. CT scan is helpful in diagnosis, and typical findings are thickening of the bowel wall, fistulas, or abscess formation. Treatments are aimed to reduce inflammation and prevent infection. Complications include bleeding, perforation, peritonitis, and fistula.

B. Appendicitis is unlikely due to this patient's location of the abdominal pain; a CT scan can help rule out appendicitis.
C. Irritable bowel syndrome is unlikely due to history of presentation. IBS usually presents with alternation between constipation and diarrhea.
D. Lactose intolerance is commonly associated with postdairy diarrhea and flatulence.
E. Pyelonephritis is unlikely based on this patient's symptoms.
F. Pseudomembranous colitis is unlikely based on this patient's symptoms and because the patient denies any history of taking antibiotics.

62. **D.**

Acute pancreatitis is an inflammatory process of the pancreas with intrapancreatic activation of enzymes that may also involve peripancreatic tissue and/or remote organic systems. Biliary tract disease or alcohol abuse cause most cases; other causes include drugs, abdominal trauma, surgery, ERCP infections, penetrating peptic ulcers, and scorpion bites. As pancreatic enzymes autodigest the pancreas, both endocrine and exocrine tissues are affected with leakage of enzymes into the vascular system to cause elevation of serum amylase and lipase. Fat necrosis of the pancreas also occurs as a saponification reaction with the severe alkaline pH of the enzymes acting on the fat tissue in the omentum. The deposition of calcium salts in this tissue results in the white coloration seen grossly.

When serum calcium is depleted in the saponification process, hypocalcemia results.

A. Damage of the exocrine system would cause leakage of amylase into the vascular system and result in an increase of serum amylase rather than decrease of serum amylase.
B. Damage of the exocrine system would cause leakage of lipase into the vascular system and result in an increase of serum lipase rather than decrease of serum lipase.
C. As pancreatic endocrine tissues are destroyed, serum glucose level is not regulated resulting in hyperglycemia but not hypoglycemia.
E. While serum trypsin, an uncommon test for diagnosis of pancreatis, would be elevated, serum trypsin level, measured by radioimmunoassay, is the most accurate laboratory indicator for pancreatitis.

63. **D.**

This is internuclear ophthalmoplegia. It is caused by a lesion in the median longitudinal fasciculus, which results in a lack of communication between the ipsilateral CN III nucleus and the contralateral CN VI nucleus. It is classically found in multiple sclerosis (MS). Of note, this question also describes optic neuritis and a Marcus Gunn pupil, which are also found in MS.

A. CN II is the optic nerve. Inflammation of CN II within the eye is the cause of her optic neuritis and hyperemia.
B. CN III is the occulomotor nerve.
C. CN VI is the abducens nerve.
E. A lesion in the tectum in the midbrain would cause Parinaud's syndrome and bilateral paralysis of upward gaze.
F. and G. See D.

64. **A.**

Primary malignant bone tumors are rare, and osteosarcoma (osteogenic sarcoma) is the most common primary malignant bone tumor among the four types. This disease often affects the metaphysis of long bone such as distal femur and proximal tibia in males between the ages 10–20 years. Osteosarcomas show loss of retinoblastoma and p53 suppressor genes; these are, grossly, bulky tumors with gritty texture and gray-white coloration. The mesenchymal tumor cells can differentiate to produce osteoid. As the tumors grow, they destroy the overlying cortex and produce a soft tissue mass.

On x-ray, findings of osteosarcoma include Codman's triangle (periosteal elevation by the tumor) and "sunburst pattern."

B. Onion skinning occurs in patients with Ewing's sarcoma, an extremely anaplastic small cell tumor.
C. Salt and pepper appearance is found in patients with primary hyperparathyroidism.
D. The soap bubble pattern is found in patients with chondromas.
E. Lytic lesions are found in conditions such as Pott's disease and multiple myeloma.

65. **C.**

This is a third-degree burn that involves the full thickness of the dermis. The cutaneous nerves are damaged so they are characteristically not painful.

A. A first-degree burn is limited to epidermal damage.
B and D. A second-degree burn causes damage extending partially into the dermis.
E. First- and second-degree burns heal on their own. Third-degree burns require debridement, thorough cleansing, and fluid replacement. Pseudomonas is the most common infection.

66. **A.**

Gout is an inflammatory condition in which crystals of monosodium urate deposit in tissue as a result of hyperuricemia. Primary gout develops from an inborn error of metabolism and results in excessive uric acid production, a decrease in the renal excretion of uric acid, or both. Secondary gout develops from other conditions predisposing the patient to hyperuricemia. This disease often affects the first metatarsophalangeal joint (podagra) causing pain and skin erythema. Attacks can be recurrent, and maintenance treatment requires differentiating the causes of gout. Confirmation of gout can be done with microscopic analysis of synovial fluid aspirate.

Gout crystals are needlelike negatively birefringent crystals.

B. Pseudogout, caused by calcium pyrophosphate dihydrate crystal deposition, produces positively birefringent crystals. Pseudogout occurs more often in large joints like the knee.
C. Envelope-shaped crystals are seen in microscopic urine analyses of patients with kidney stones composed of calcium oxalate.

D. Diamond-shaped crystals are seen in microscopic urine analyses of patients with kidney stones composed of uric acid.
E. Coffinlid-shaped crystals are seen on microscopic urine analyses of patients with kidney stones composed of struvite.
F. Hexagon-shaped crystals are seen in microscopic urine analyses of patients with kidney stones composed of cystine.

67. **B.**
Cystic fibrosis is the most common autosomal recessive disorder in Caucasians. It causes bronchiectasis, which is irreversible.
A. Noncaseating granulomas composed of epithelioid cells are characteristic of sarcoid.
C. This choice is incorrect because this condition is irreversible.
D. Multiple alveoli filled with hyaline membranes is characteristic of adult respiratory distress syndrome (ARDS).
E. Mucus gland and smooth muscle hyperplasia, eosinophils, and thickening of the basement membrane is the histological picture of untreated asthma.

68. **D.**
Kawasaki's syndrome is a vasculitis of the medium-sized vessels. Its most deadly complication is coronary artery aneurysm.
A. Thrombocytosis not thrombocytopenia is characteristic of Kawasaki's.
B. Steroids are contraindicated in Kawasaki's. Aspirin is the mainstay of treatment; IVIG may also help prevent cardiac disease.
C. Takayasu arteritis is a vasculitis of the large arteries arising from the aorta also known as the "pulseless" disease.
E. Pulse-fever dissociation is associated with typhoid fever and also brucellosis. It is a high fever with relative bradycardia.

69. **C.**
Haloperidol's antagonism of dopamine—the origin of its antipsychotic properties—can also disrupt the regulation of prolactin. Dopamine is a prolactin inhibitor and, by antagonizing dopamine and releasing the inhibitory effects on prolactin, galactorrhea may result. Because of the positive result on this patient's schizophrenia with current medical management, it should only be changed if the side effects become unbearable.
A. While an anterior pituitary tumor is a cause of hyperprolactinemia and galactorrhea, it is less likely with this patient's history of haloperidol use. There might also be associated oligomenorrhea and visual changes (bitemporal hemianopsia due to mass effect), which is not so in this case.
B. While hypothyroidism is also a possible cause of hyperprolactinemia associated with galactorrhea due to the increase in thyrotropin-releasing hormone (TRH), it is not likely in this case.

D. Lactation usually begins after delivery due to increased prolactin levels.
E. Dopamine inhibits prolactin release from the anterior pituitary. Decreased amounts of dopamine will have a decreased inhibitory effect on prolactin release resulting in an increased amount of circulating prolactin.

70. **C.**
The key to answering this question, and the key to most acid-base questions, is to begin by first calculating the anion gap. Anion gap = the sodium − (the chloride + the bicarbonate) = 142 − (112 + 13) = 142 − 125 = 17. A normal anion gap is ≤ 12 (other things can affect the gap, such as decreased albumin, changes in calcium levels, or metabolic alkalosis, but this may never be asked on USMLE Step 1!). Hence, the gap of 17 is elevated, and this patient does in fact have a primary anion gap metabolic acidosis. However, you must now calculate the so-called delta gap (Δgap or ΔΔ). The delta gap attempts to determine what the bicarbonate *would* be if there were no anion gap acidosis, thereby establishing whether or not a second acid-based problem is being masked by the gap acidosis. The way to do this is to subtract the normal anion gap (12) from the actual anion gap (17): 17 − 12 = 5. This number, 5, represents the number of bicarbonate units being used up by the anion gap acidosis. By adding this number to the current bicarbonate, you get the corrected bicarbonate, which represents what the bicarbonate *would* be if no anion gap acidosis was present. Remember, a low bicarbonate (<21) would represent an acidosis, and a high bicarbonate (>29) would represent an alkalosis. Hence, if the corrected bicarbonate is <21, there is *also* a primary nongap metabolic acidosis. If the corrected bicarbonate is >29, there is *also* a primary metabolic alkalosis. In this case, the ΔΔ is 5, the corrected bicarbonate is 5 + 13 = 18; hence, there is also a primary nonanion gap metabolic acidosis.

71. **D.**
The patient has no reason to have a lactic acidosis, but he is likely to be uremic with a high serum BUN and creatinine. Uremia is a common cause of anion gap metabolic acidosis in patients with renal failure. But you know from question 70 that the patient also has a nongap metabolic acidosis. The most common causes of a nongap metabolic acidosis is either iatrogenic hyperchloremic acidosis (from you giving too much saline to patients) or renal tubular acidosis. Diabetes and multiple myeloma both cause type IV renal tubular acidosis.

72. **E.**

This patient has nephritic syndrome, not nephrotic syndrome. She has classic "cola-colored" urine, with red cells, minimal protein, and virtually pathognomonic red cell casts. Her edema is most impressive in the facial area, giving her a puffy-faced appearance. This is a classic presentation of nephritic syndrome. Nephrotic syndrome presents with general anasarca, massive proteinuria with few red cells, a low serum albumin, and high serum cholesterol. Further, the patient had an antecedent illness consistent with Group A strep throat. Thus the diagnosis is likely poststreptococcal glomerulonephritis.

A. Minimal change is a nephrotic syndrome, not a nephritic syndrome.
B. Mesangial (type II) lupus glomerulonephritis is a nephrotic syndrome, not a nephritic syndrome.
C. Primary membranous glomerulonephritis is a nephrotic syndrome, not a nephritic syndrome.
D. Membranous (type V) lupus glomerulonephritis is a nephrotic syndrome, not a nephritic syndrome.

73. **B.**

Everything about this gentleman is classic for diabetic ketoacidosis. The patient is clearly dehydrated (dry oropharynx, flat jugular veins, ↑ creatinine, BUN/creatinine ratio = 20), caused by prolonged osmotic diuresis from his hyperglycemia. On examination, this patient reveals classic Kussmaul hyperpnea, with rapid, very deep breaths. He has abdominal pain, which is common in diabetic ketoacidosis. He has a large anion gap (36) acidosis caused by the ketoacids, and his corrected bicarbonate is 34 (36 − 12 + 10), meaning he also has a primary metabolic alkalosis. This metabolic alkalosis is a contraction alkalosis caused by his severe dehydration.

A. Cushing's disease presents with hypertension, truncal obesity, abdominal striae, ecchymoses, and a buffalo hump.
C. Addison's disease presents with hyponatremia, hyperkalemia, darkening of the skin, a nongap metabolic acidosis, and often eosinophilia.
D. Schmidt's syndrome is autoimmune polyendocrinopathy, and can present with any mixture of Hashimoto's disease, pernicious anemia, vitiligo, diabetes, or Addison's disease.

74. **D.**

You had better not dismiss this woman's depression. She has cause to be depressed, since she very likely has systemic lupus erythematosus. Patients with diffuse complaints and fatigue are often depressed on presentation. This patient exhibits three of the diagnostic components on exam: malar rash, symmetric arthritis, and oral ulcers. Her proteinuria is highly suspicious for lupus nephritis, but you can't use this as a criterion until a kidney biopsy confirms the pathology. Blood tests for ANA and double-stranded DNA should be sent. The ANA is >98% sensitive, meaning if the ANA is negative the diagnosis is almost ruled out. However, the ANA is not specific; therefore, even if it is positive, it does not by itself make the diagnosis. Anti–double-stranded DNA is not sensitive (about 50%), so a negative test does not rule out the diagnosis; however, it is highly specific >98%, so a positive test virtually clinches the diagnosis. Ro and La antibodies are sent for Sjögren's disease, and SCL-70 is specific for CREST syndrome. The ESR is often elevated in lupus, but is not part of the diagnostic criteria.

75. **A.**

Remember, elevation of methylmalonic acid is more sensitive than low B_{12} level to diagnose B_{12} deficiency (this is because of the huge range of "normal" B_{12} levels in the population). This patient clearly has a megaloblastic anemia, with a very high MCV and pathognomonic hypersegmented neutrophils on her peripheral smear. She has low iron and a history of "heavy menses"; however, her low TIBC argues against iron deficiency anemia, as does her high MCV. This patient most likely has anemia of chronic disease, in which both iron and TIBC are low. The coexistence of B_{12} deficiency with type I diabetes should raise the specter of Schmidt's syndrome, or autoimmune polyendocrinopathy. The patient most likely has autoimmune pernicious anemia, which may explain her chronic disease.

B. Use in the work-up of iron deficiency anemia.
C. The Coombs' test is for autoimmune hemolytic anemia.
D. A bone marrow biopsy would be checked only if all other non-invasive diagnostic modalities failed to determine a diagnosis.
E. A TSH should probably be checked to rule out thyroid involvement in the Schmidt's syndrome, but will not help diagnose the anemia because thyroid-induced anemias are usually normocytic, and rarely microcytic. Additionally, iron-deficiency anemia, hemolytic anemia, and thyroid disease would not explain hypersegmented neutrophils on a peripheral smear.

INDEX

A

C

D

E

F

G

H

I

J

K

O

P

Q

R

S

T

U

V

W

X

Y

Z